T0253914

Changing the Global Approach to Medicine

Volume 2

Medical Vector Therapy

Also Introducing the Quantum Gene and the Quadsistor

Lane B. Scheiber II, MD

Lane B. Scheiber, ScD

iUniverse, Inc.

Bloomington

Changing the Global Approach to Medicine, Volume 2
Medical Vector Therapy
Also introducing the Quantum Gene and the Quadsistor

VIReSOFT Developers of Medically Therapeutic RNA Vector Technologies, Medical Vector Therapy, Quantum Gene, and Quadsistor.

Copyright © 2011 by Lane B. Scheiber II, MD and Lane B. Scheiber, ScD

All rights reserved. No part of this book may be used or reproduce by any means, graphic, electronic, or mechanical including photocopying, recording, taping or by any other information storage retrieval system without the explicit written consent of the authors. All figures represent schematic concept representations of proposed objects.

This text is intended for educational and entertainment purposes. This text is not intended to take the place of a physician's evaluation or a physician's advice regarding any medical condition. It is recommended the reader consult their physician before starting any medication for any medical condition. All medications have potential side effects. Healthcare providers should review current prescribing information before prescribing medications; patients should review the latest prescribing information and side effects before taking any medication.

At the time of copyright the authors believed the concepts to be unique and different from prior art. All figures are meant to be illustrative concepts of otherwise sometimes very complex structures.

iUniverse books may be ordered through booksellers or by contacting:

iUniverse
1663 Liberty Drive
Bloomington, IN 47403
www.iuniverse.com
1-800-Authors (1-800-288-4677)

Because of the dynamic nature of the Internet, any Web addresses or links contained in this book may have changed since publication and may no longer be valid. The views expressed in this work are solely those of the authors and do not necessarily reflect the views of the publisher, and the publisher hereby disclaims any responsibility for them.

ISBN: 978-1-4502-8219-2 (pbk)

ISBN: 978-1-4502-8220-8 (ebk)

Printed in the United States of America

iUniverse rev. date: 3/8/11

Suggested Additional Reading:

CHANGING THE GLOBAL APPROACH TO MEDICINE, Volume 1

New Perspectives on Treating AIDS, Diabetes, Obesity, Aging, Heart Attacks, Stroke, and Cancer

by Lane B. Scheiber II, MD and Lane B. Scheiber, ScD

IMMORTALITY: QUATERNARY MEDICINE CODE

by Anthony Scheiber

THE HUMAN COMPUTER

by Anthony Scheiber

EARTH PRO: The Rings of Sol

By Anthony Scheiber

Dedication

Thanks to our wives, Karin and Mary Jane, for
all of their love and support without which this
effort could never have been done;

and Pat for use of Oceana, with its
spectacular view of the Atlantic.

Forward

Today's medical approach to treating a disease is to flood the body with a medication in an effort to deliver a drug or protein to the cells that would either benefit from treatment or be terminated by the action of the treatment. Medications are introduced through an oral route, by infusion, injection, sniffed up the nose, absorption through a dermal patch or deposited rectally. Essentially this might be referred to as the Whole Body Approach to medical care. Unfortunately, all too often, this Whole Body Approach generates undesirable side effects. While the Whole Body Approach generally delivers a medication to all of the cells comprising the body, usually only a single cell type is actually the target of the medical therapy.

A Cell Specific Approach, which delivers a medical therapy only to the cells in need of treatment, would be expected to increase the medical therapy's effectiveness and lower the incidence of side effects.

In nature viruses utilize a Cell Specific Approach to deliver genetic material and support proteins to specific cells that act as the host for a particular virus for the purpose of replicating the virus. Understanding the construction, behavior and life-cycle of viruses offers a platform upon which a Cell Specific Approach medical treatment strategy can be devised.

Volume 1 of this series discussed the Human Immunodeficiency Virus in detail. The initial objective of the first book was to explore means to defeat HIV by understanding how the virus was constructed and deriving treatment strategies to neutralize the HIV virion based on this knowledge. Studying HIV led to the recognition that viruses carry more than DNA as their payload. Some viruses, such as HIV and Hepatitis C, carry RNA as well as support proteins as their payload. The study of Hepatitis C led to realizing that viral genomes do not have to utilize the biologic machinery of the nucleus of a host cell in order to generate copies of the virus.

Understanding that the nucleus of a cell could be bypassed and that a virus's payload could act independent of the nucleus of a cell led to exploring RNA therapy as its own entity. Recognizing that some viruses carry support proteins to assist their genome in being utilized, led to the concept that viruses could carry medically beneficial proteins to specific cells to produce therapeutic effects. Further, if viruses can carry proteins, they should be able to carry reasonably sized chemical molecules and nutrients. Modifying viruses and incorporating them to carry chemical molecules and proteins to specific cell types draws the medical profession closer to achieving a very versatile and effective, broad spectrum Cell Specific Approach to medical care.

Medical Vector Therapy, introduced here in Volume 2 of the series, describes a Cell Specific Approach to medical care that not only takes advantage of the fact that the payload of a virus can be changed, but that the surface probes can be altered. Such a device is referred to as a vector, which leads to the concept Medical Vector Therapy. By modifying the surface probes, a virus-like transport device can be configured to deliver its payload to any cell-type in the body. Medical Vector Therapy offers a practical means of achieving a Cell Specific Approach to delivering medical therapy. Such a Cell Specific Approach provides the means to treat a body with smaller, more exact doses of a particular medical therapy delivered to specific target cells and to improve the effect of the treatment, while at the same time reducing the occurrence of side effects.

Table of Contents

Introduction

Hippocrates, considered the father of medicine, introduced to the world the concept that disease states were the result of a treatable dysfunction of the body's state of health, rather than the result of evil spirits punishing man or playing pranks on mankind. Prior to the teachings of Hippocrates, the world existed in a dark merciless era of early healers conjuring potions and mystical chants in an effort to relieve the ill of their state of dysfunction by attempting to appease what was thought to be a form of cruel deity. Hippocrates took a bold step forward; introducing uncommon concepts of healing that were often counter to the presiding culture of his time and linger in some cultures since Hippocrates's time.

For the last 3,000 years, the foundation of treating disease has been based on the use of natural herbs and other plant and animal extracts. Most treatments were derived from observations that a certain herb or extract interdicted in a positive manner to counter the ill effects of a disease process. Early natural herbs such as salicylic acid, derived from various plant species of *Spiraea*, and derivatives of Belladonna, accessed from the tall bushy herb *Atropa belladonna*, including hyoscyamine (sedative), hyoscine (stimulant), atropine (antispasmodic) were available prior to modern pharmacology. Dating back to at least 200 A.D., with some believing as far back as 500 B.C., individuals afflicted with gout sucked on the underground stem of the autumn crocus (*colchicum autumnale*) to access the plant's drug colchicine, in an effort to ease the bitter pain of an inflamed joint from a crystal arthritis.

In the last two hundred years formulated chemicals taken orally, infused, injected, administered through a transdermal means or administered rectally, have been developed in ever growing numbers and utilized to treat or manage a wide variety of disease states.

In contrast to chemical agents, protein products were introduced starting in 1921, when Banting, Best, and Macleod isolated insulin. Prior to insulin becoming available as a treatment modality, individuals diagnosed with diabetes mellitus faced a virtual death sentence. Even today, those residents of third world countries face a grim one year survival following a diagnosis of diabetes mellitus. Other protein substances such as calcitonin and tumor necrosis factor alpha blockers have been successfully developed to treat osteoporosis and inflammatory arthritis, respectfully.

Medical treatment has evolved from being rooted in superstition administered as prayers and chants, to being administered as oral drugs, injectable products, transdermal products, rectal suppository products, to inhaled medications. At this point in time, Medicine has now reached a critical crossroad.

The body is comprised of approximately 240 different cell types. Each functional element of the body has its own cell type or types. Many disease states arise from a particular cell type and/or afflict a particular type of cell.

Often side effects caused by medications are the result of the medical therapy coming in contact with cells that suffer a negative reaction to the action of the therapy and often see no benefit from the drug. The current Whole Body Approach to treatment, which exposes most cells of the body to a particular treatment, places bystander cells at risk of suffering unwanted side effects due to chemical or biologic actions from a medical therapy.

In an effort to improve the actions of medications and reduce unwanted side effects, the development of a means of delivering medication to specific cell types rather than to the whole body is imperative. The only means of delivering any agent directly to a specific cell type occurs in nature as the actions of a virus. For decades, viruses have been the fall-guy for many disease states. Generally when a physician has assessed an acute medical problem that was short-lived, and there was no adequate explanation for the phenomenon, the term 'virus' has been commonly used in an attempt to explain the phenomenon. Certainly the mere mention of a stomach virus or stomach flu conjures up distressful thoughts or memories for most people.

Viruses have been portrayed as evil and at times the root of human misery. Some viruses are known to be deadly, such as the Human Immunodeficiency Virus (HIV). Yet, studying viruses in detail suggests that viruses are an indispensable teaching tool. Knowledge of how viruses are constructed, how they function, how they infect cells and how they replicate can be used to develop means to achieve a Cell Specific Approach to medical treatment.

A vector is often thought of as an insect or animal that transmits a microorganism from one animal to another. The term vector may also refer to a virus or plasmid that contains modified genetic material that can be utilized to introduce exogenous genes into the genome of an organism. Expanding this definition, a vector can be used to deliver many different types of therapeutic material to specific cell types that would benefit from such materials, which gives rise to the concept of Medical Vector Therapy as illustrated in Figure 1.

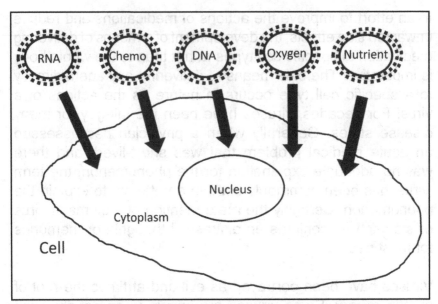

**Figure 1: Medical Vector Therapy utilizing virus-
like vectors to insert RNA, Chemotherapy,
DNA, Oxygen or Nutrients into cells**

This document opens with a discussion of the evolution of Medical Vector Therapy. This is followed by a discussion of how Medical Vector Therapy can facilitate the delivery of RNA, DNA, medications, oxygen, and nutrients to specific cells in the body.

I. Evolution of Medical Vector Therapy

Today's approach to medical treatment generally involves blindly placing a chemical or protein entity into the body in an attempt to treat an illness or disease state. Chemical entities are generally swallowed or administered rectally. Proteins are broken down by the acid and digestive enzymes secreted by the stomach and GI tract. In order to successfully utilize protein entities as medical therapies such treatments are generally injected, infused or sniffed up the nose as a means of introducing the entity into the body.

Once inside the body, the chemical or protein entity has the opportunity of making contact with any or all tissues comprising the body. The objective of the current approach is that by introducing a chemical or protein entity into the body that the beneficial effects of the entity will outweigh the potential harmful effects this entity might cause to tissues other than the target tissues the chemical or protein is intended to interact with as it transits the body. Such potential harmful effects are alternatively referred to as adverse side effects.

Second, it is hoped that a sufficient amount of the chemical or protein substance will reach the intended tissues to provide an expected benefit, rather than be absorbed by other tissues or eliminated by the natural excretion mechanisms before a sufficient concentration can occur in the target tissues. Since there exits variability amongst individuals regarding the prowess of the body's immune system, renal and liver excretion rates, blood flow through tissues, and body chemistries, responses to chemical and protein medical treatment entities vary. Some of the responses are what is expected, some results are better than expected, some results are less than expected, some treatments result in unacceptable, unwanted side effects.

An improved approach to the generalized administration of a medical treatment is to package a chemical or protein entity into a delivery device. Such a delivery device could transport the treatment entity directly to the tissues that would benefit from the presence of the medical treatment. By delivering a medication directly to target tissues, rather than dispersed throughout the body, smaller total concentrations of the medication are required to achieve the expected effect. Smaller concentrations of a drug result in minimizing or avoiding unwanted side effects. Packaging drugs in a delivery device shields non-target cells from the adverse side effects of the drugs.

Nature provides numerous examples of means to transport materials to target cells. Viruses represent a versatile transport mechanism to carry genetic material and enzymes to specific cells. See Figure 2. Viruses locate their host cell by the probes mounted on their exterior shell or envelope. A virus's exterior probes seek out and engage surface receptors on cell membranes. Viruses utilize their exterior probes to make contact with their host. Once contact is made, some viruses are absorbed into the host, while other viruses open an access portal in a cell's outer membrane, through which the virus injects its payload into its host cell.

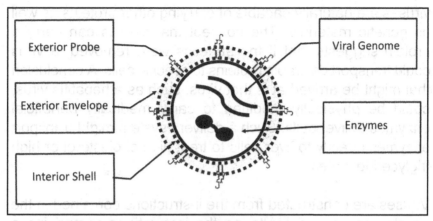

Figure 2: Model of a virus

In Nature, the objective of a virus is to locate a cell that will act as a host. A host is defined as a cell that has available the proper resources to provide the environment to manufacture complete copies of the virus. Viruses tend to be very selective, and usually target only one type of cell to act as a suitable host cell. The Human Immunodeficiency Virus virion searches the human body it has infected seeking a T-Helper cell. Since viruses conduct no internal biologic process, they therefore have no energy requirements and can exist as a predator for as long as it takes before either locating an appropriate host cell or being destroyed by environmental factors or being detected by a sensitized immune system.

The genetic code a virus inserts into its host cell is either in the format of deoxyribonucleic acid (DNA) or ribonucleic acid (RNA). Whether DNA or RNA, the genetic code is comprised of a set of instructions that command the host cell to manufacture viral proteins which are used to generate copies of the virus. A virus's genetic code represents a biologic program, the endpoint of the program being the assembly and release of numerous copies of the virus into the environment.

The fact that viruses are capable of carrying enzymes to assist in the utilization of the genetic code the virus carries, suggests viruses are naturally capable of carrying other proteins as well as genetic materials. The concept that a virus can carry a protein suggests that if the genetics were removed, a virus could transport desirable proteins to specific cells. A conclusion that might be arrived at is that virus, such as a hepatitis virus, could be physically modified to carry medically beneficial enzymes to liver cells. Such a delivery system might transport enzymes directly to liver cells to treat high cholesterol or high triglyceride states.

Viruses are constructed from the instructions contained in the virus's genetic code. Altering the instructions comprising a virus's genetic code would alter the form the virus virion would take once produced and released by a host cell. A virus's instructions could be modified so as to create the shell and exterior probes of a virus, but replace the genetic instructions and viral enzymes with a medically beneficial payload comprised of exogenous genetic material, enzymes or other molecules or some combination thereof. See Figure 3. Inserting modified genetic code into a host cell would produce a modified therapeutic virus that would be comprised of naturally occurring outer envelope, inner shell, and exterior probes, but carry medically beneficial enzymes. Such modified viruses would then be capable of seeking out the virus's natural host cells and deliver to such host cells medically beneficial enzymes.

As an example, the RNA genetic instruction code for Hepatitis C virus could be modified to produce a Hepatitis C virion that carried enzymes intended to take lipids and convert them to high density lipoproteins (HDL). Hepatitis C virions carrying such enzymes as a payload could be used to deliver such enzymes to liver cells in individuals with high cholesterol levels. Hepatitis C viruses naturally infect liver cells. Upon injecting a load of modified virus into an individual, the modified Hepatitis C virions would deliver their payload of medically beneficial cholesterol enzymes directly to the individual's liver cells. Such a direct approach to administering a medical therapy would concentrate the treatment in target cells and avoid side effects of the medical treatment by isolating the cells that would be exposed to the effects of the medical treatment.

The advantage of utilizing modified viruses to deliver medical treatments is limited by the probes that are mounted on the surface of naturally occurring viruses. The probes that are mounted on the surface of a naturally occurring virus represent the means the virus utilizes to seek out and engage the specific cell type that is appropriate for the virus to insert its payload into in order for the virus to replicate itself. For a virus to properly carry out its mission of replication, the exterior probes must single out and engage specific cell surface receptors on the type of cell that will act as the host cell for the virus. Thus, a naturally occurring virus, whose payload is altered to carry medically beneficial enzymes, is only capable of delivering its payload to the cell type that the exterior probes are designed to engage. See Figure 3.

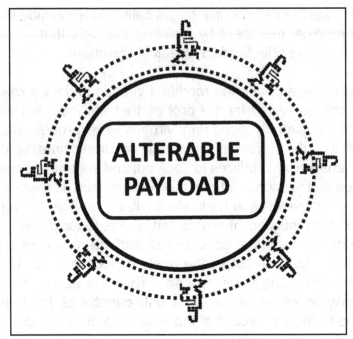

**Figure 3: Modifying a virus, altering the original
payload to a medically therapeutic material**

Cells possess numerous cell-surface markers. Most cell-types
have a unique combination of cell-surface markers embedded
in their exterior membrane, which acts as a means of cell
recognition. Cell recognition is important for the body for
architectural purposes to produce a body that is constructed
in the proper manner such that cells are positioned around the
body in their proper place for purposes of the body functioning
in an appropriate manner. Cell recognition is also important to
facilitate cells receiving hormonal signals and nutrients they
require to maintain a healthy life-cycle and participate in body
functions. Cell surface markers also assist in the immune
system being able to distinguish between cells that comprise
the body and pathogens that have breached the body's outer
defenses.

Cell-surface markers act as probes or receptors. Cell-surface
markers can be proteins or glycoproteins. Protein cell-surface

markers are anchored in a protein shell and project outward from the protein shell. In some cases, protein cell-surface markers are anchored into a protein shell and extend through an exterior lipid layer to project outward from the lipid layer. Glycoprotein cell-surface markers are comprised of a protein molecule coupled to a lipid molecule. See Figure 4. In the case of a glycoprotein cell-surface marker, the lipid segment is embedded in a lipid layer which acts as an anchor, while the protein portion of the marker projects outward and away from the lipid layer.

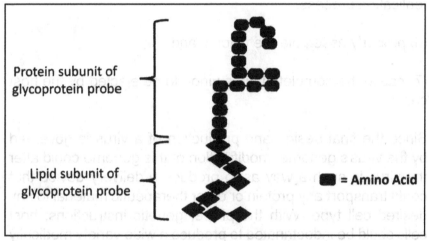

Figure 4: Glycoprotein probe

The exterior probes can be changed to facilitate a modified virus to target any specific cell. The payload of the virus can be changed so that the modified virus can be fashioned to carry a medically therapeutic messenger RNA. Altering the exterior probes of a virus and altering the payload of a virus produces a means whereby any therapeutic payload can be delivered to any specific cell in the body.

Exterior probes mounted on the surface of a virus are either protein structures or glycoproteins. Like all other components of a virus, the exterior probes are manufactured in a host cell as dictated by the instructions carried in the virus's genome.

A virus's genome must possess the proper instructions to:

(1) generate the virus's exterior envelope,

(2) generate any inner shells that might be necessary,

(3) manufacture the exterior probes,

(4) manufacture the viral genome,

(5) manufacture any enzymes needed to assist with the replication process,

(6) properly assemble the virions, and

(7) cause the completed virus virion to be ejected by the host cell.

Since the final design and production of a virus is governed by the virus's genome, modification of this genome could alter the virus in such a way as to produce a delivery device that could transport any protein or other therapeutic material to any desired cell type. With the proper genetic instructions, host cells could be indoctrinated to produce a wide variety medically therapeutic configurable delivery devices.

Modified viruses are considered to be delivery devices where the naturally occurring genetic payload of a particular type of virus has been replaced by a therapeutic payload. Modified viruses offer a means of administering a medically therapeutic payload to a specific cell type, but such a transport mechanism is limited to only the cell type the virus utilizes as its host cell. Modifying an existing virus to act as a delivery system is also limited by the naturally occurring size of the virus, which limits the type of payload the transport device is able to carry. Further, a naturally occurring virus can generate an immunologic response to the presence of the modified virus once inserted into a body. The immunologic response generated by the body to eliminate modified viruses significantly limits the utility of this type of delivery system.

Constructing virus-like transport devices, built similar to naturally occurring viruses, but variable in design and function, offers a modifiable approach to the delivery of medical treatment. Virus like transport devices that can be constructed to deliver a specific medically beneficial payload to any cell type provide a radically new approach to medical care. Any set of exterior probes can be mounted on a configurable delivery device to offer the advantage of targeting any of the approximately 240 cell types in the body. The size of a configurable delivery device is adjustable in order to accommodate differing payload sizes. Configurable delivery devices generated from stem cells possess the least number of naturally occurring surface markers so as to reduce the possibility of stimulating the immune system to its presence. A low rate of antigenicity leads to repeated uses of the configurable delivery device in the same individual while invoking minimal to no immune response.

II. Configurable Delivery Devices

Lessons Learned From Viruses

Despite all that is thought that a virus is capable of in a negative sense, viruses are simply a segment of genetic code carried inside a transport medium. The genetic code carried inside a virus's core is comprised of the set of the instructions and the data necessary to recreate copies of the virus. A virus is incapable of carrying out any biologic processes on its own and thus not able to reproduce itself. A virus requires the biologic machinery found inside a living cell to replicate copies of its virion.

The primary function of a virus is to generate copies of itself. Ill effects of viruses are generally related to the presence of the virus and the type of host cell the virus virion interacts with, not necessarily the result of any action taken by the virus.

With respect to at least one virus, this concept is a bit more complicated. The HIV genome, in addition to coding for viral replication, codes for an FASL receptor. The FASL receptor, when mounted on the surface of an infected T-Helper cell acts as a trigger to kill other T-Helper cells. The FASL receptor, when it comes in contact with a FAS receptor on a neighboring T-Helper cell, transfers a signal to the neighboring T-Helper cell to engage in apoptosis, which results in the death of the T-Helper cell. Clearly, HIV is an example of a virus of which the effects go beyond simply infecting T-Helper cells and replicating. The actions of the HIV virion are not what one might expect, such as generating a toxin to damage or slow down immune cell operation. Instead, the HIV virion actions are more of a cloak and dagger function, which actively assassinates noninfected T-Helper cells, resulting in a global dysfunction of the immune system.

A virus generally targets a particular type of cell to act as a host in order to carry out the replication process. Probes jutting forth from the exterior surface of the virus are used to seek out a target host cell. Once the virus locates the appropriate target cell, the virus breaches the exterior membrane of the cell and inserts its genetic material into the target cell. The viral genome then takes command of the host cell's internal biologic machinery and dictates to the host cell the instructions necessary to generate copies of the virus. In essence, most viruses simply seek out, engage and infect a host cell for the sole purpose of replication and this is the extent of their life-cycle. Some viruses, like HIV, cause alterations to their host, which results in the host cell acting in a noxious manner to do harm to the body which the virus has infected.

Viruses carry one of three forms of genetic material, which include double-stranded deoxyribonucleic acid (dsDNA), single stranded deoxyribonucleic acid (ssDNA), or ribonucleic acid (RNA). Nuclear DNA is comprised of double-stranded DNA.

Viruses which carry dsDNA as their payload have the potential of inserting their genetic material directly into the nuclear DNA of the host cell. Viruses that carry ssDNA or RNA must have their genetic material modified before their viral genetic code can be inserted into the host cell's nuclear DNA. A virus carrying ssDNA or RNA generally must convert these forms of genetic material into dsDNA prior to inserting the genetic material into the host cell's double-stranded nuclear DNA. Enzymes termed proteases, transcriptases and reverse transcriptases are used to modify ssDNA and RNA into dsDNA.

Once a virus's genetic material is in the proper dsDNA form, enzymes termed integrases transport the viral genome to the nucleus of the host cell and insert the viral genetic code into the host cell's nuclear DNA. Nuclear DNA in a cell is transcribed by transcription complexes. Transcription complexes decode the genetic information stored in the nuclear DNA and generate RNA molecules.

Viral RNA genomes occur in at least two general forms, which can be represented by HIV and Hepatitis C. HIV carries a form of RNA genome that exists as two strands of RNA, which once the genome gains access to a T-Helper cell's cytoplasm the RNA strands are converted to DNA by the action of the enzyme reverse transcriptase. HIV's viral DNA migrates to the cell's nucleus where it becomes integrated into the T-Helper cell's nuclear DNA. The genome of the Hepatitis C Virus, like HIV, is positive stranded RNA. Unlike HIV, Hepatitis C's viral RNA is not converted to DNA. Once Hepatitis C's viral genome gains access to a hepatic cell's cytoplasm, each RNA strand is enzymatically degraded into segments. Segments of the Hepatitis C viral RNA function as messenger RNA. The segments of Hepatitis C viral genome act as templates to produce the proteins needed to make copies of the virus.

HUMAN IMMUNODEFICIENCY VIRUS

The Human Immunodeficiency Virus (HIV is comprised of an outer coat made of a shell wrapped with an outer envelope. Mounted on the outer envelope are glycoprotein 120 (gp120) probes and glycoprotein 41 (gp41) probes. See Figure 5. The HIV virion uses the gp120 probes to seek out its host, a T-Helper cell. The gp120 attaches to a CD4+ cell-surface receptor on a T-Helper cell. Once the gp120 probe has made contact with a CD4+, a conformational channel change occurs in the gp120 probe, which allows the gp41 probe to become exposed and intercept the surface of the T-Helper cell. The gp41 probe interacts with either a CCR5 or CXCR4 cell-surface receptor on the exterior of the T-Helper cell. Once the gp41 probe successfully makes contact with the surface of the T-Helper cell, the gp41 probe's action aids in the opening of an access port in the wall of the T-Helper cell. With an access port open, the HIV virion injects the RNA genome and proteins that it carries into the T-Helper cell. The proteins are used to modify the RNA genome once the virus's genetic code is physically inside the T-Helper cell.

The HIV virion carries in its core two RNA strands and three different modifier enzymes. See Figure 5. Each RNA strand is a positive strand RNA approximately 9500 nucleotides in length. The three different proteins include an integrase enzyme, a reverse transcriptase enzyme and a protease enzyme. Once the HIV virion's genetic material has been inserted into the cytoplasm in a T-Helper cell, the reverse transcriptase and protease enzymes convert the HIV RNA to dsDNA. The integrase enzyme helps to transport the HIV dsDNA into the nucleus of the T-Helper cell and to insert the HIV's dsDNA into the T-Helper cell's nuclear DNA. Once HIV's genetic material is integrated into the T-Helper cell's nuclear DNA it lays dormant until activated. HIV's genome may sit dormant for years, thus the virus is classified as a latent virus.

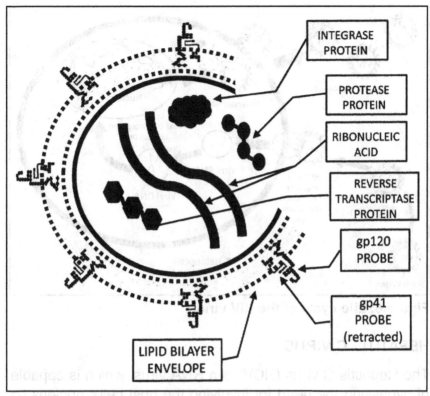

Figure 5: Illustration of an HIV virion

HIV's DNA, when triggered by the replication process, takes command of the T-Helper cell's biologic machinery to produce numerous copies of the HIV virion. Upon release, the HIV virion becomes enveloped with a portion of the exterior membrane of the T-Helper cell. Figure 6 provides a diagram of the life cycle of the Human Immunodeficiency Virus.

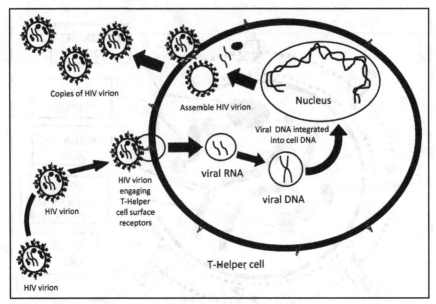

Figure 6: Life cycle of the HIV virion

HEPATITIS C VIRUS

The Hepatitis C virus (HCV) is a RNA virus, which is capable of bypassing the need for involving the host cell's nucleus by having its RNA genome function as messenger RNA. Hepatitis C infects liver cells. The Hepatitis C viral genome becomes divided once it gains access to the interior of a liver host cell. Portions of the subdivisions of the Hepatitis C genome directly interact with liver cell ribosomes to produce proteins necessary to construct copies of the virus.

HCV belongs to the Flaviviridae family and is the only member of the Hepacivirus genus. There are considered to be at least 100 different strains of Hepatitis C virus based on genome sequencing variability.

HCV is comprised of an outer lipoprotein envelope and an internal nucleocapsid. The genetic payload is carried within the nucleocapsid. In its natural state, present on the surface of the outer envelope of the Hepatitis C virus are probes that detect receptors present on the surface of liver cells. The glycoprotein E1 probe and the glycoprotein E2 probe have been identified as being affixed to the surface of HCV. The E2 probe binds with high affinity to the large external loop of a CD81 cell-surface receptor. CD81 is found on the surface of many cell types including liver cells. Once the E2 probe has engaged the CD81 cell-surface receptor, cofactors on the surface of HCV's exterior envelope engage either or both the low density lipoprotein receptor (LDLR) or the scavenger receptor class B type I (SR-BI) present on the liver cell in order to effect the mechanism to facilitate HCV breaching the cell membrane and creating a pathway through the plasma cell membrane of the liver cell. Upon successful engagement of the HCV surface probes with a liver cell's cell-surface receptors, HCV inserts the single strand of RNA and other payload elements it carries into the liver cell which will act as its host cell. The HCV RNA genome then interacts with enzymes and ribosomes inside the liver cell in a translational process to produce the proteins required to construct copies of the protein components of HCV. The HCV genome undergoes a method of transcription to replicate copies of the virus's RNA genome. Inside the host, pieces of the HCV virus are assembled together and ultimately loaded with a copy of the HCV genome. Replicas of the original HCV then escape the host cell and migrate the environment in search of additional host liver cells to infect and continue the replication process.

The HCV's naturally occurring genetic payload consists of a single molecule of linear positive sense, single stranded RNA approximately 9600 nucleotides in length. By means of a translational process a polyprotein of approximately 3000 amino acids is generated. This polyprotein is cleaved post translation by host and viral proteases into individual viral proteins which include: the structural proteins of C, E1, and E2; the nonstructural proteins NS1, NS2, NS3, NS4A, NS4B, NS5A, NS5B, and p7; and the ARFP/F protein. Hepatitis C virus's proteins direct the host liver cell to construction copies of the Hepatitis C virus. A membrane associated replicase complex consisting of the virus's nonstructural proteins NS3 and NS5B facilitate the replication of the viral genome. The membrane of the endoplasmic reticulum appears to be the site of protein maturation and Hepatitis C viral virion assembly.

The Hepatitis C virus life-cycle demonstrates that copies of a virus virion can be generated by inserting RNA into a host cell that functions as messenger RNA in the host cell. See Figure 7. The Hepatitis C viral RNA genome functions as messenger RNA, acting as the template in conjunction with the biologic machinery of a host cell to produce the components that comprise copies of the Hepatitis C virion and the Hepatitis C viral RNA provides the biologic instructions to assemble the components into complete copies of the Hepatitis C virions. The Hepatitis C virus life-cycle clearly demonstrates that viral virions can be manufactured by a host cell without involving the nucleus of the cell. Certainly simpler, but possibly more intriguing, is the concept that a virus's genome is capable of producing proteins and genetic material without utilizing the nucleus of a cell.

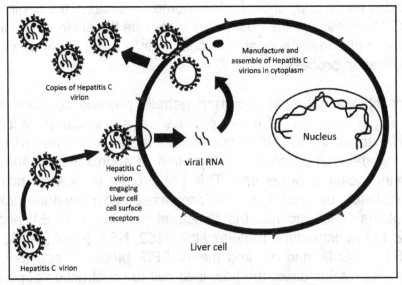

Figure 7: Hepatitis C virus Life cycle.

Lessons learned from studying naturally occurring viruses are (1) these submicroscopic pathogens are very effective at seeking out the cells they require to effect replication of their virion, (2) viruses locate and engage their host cell due to the probes mounted on the exterior of the pathogen, (3) they carry genetic materials as well as a variety of proteins as their payload, and (4) there are a variety of mechanisms viruses use to infect cells and effect replication of their virion, which medical science can utilize as effective treatment strategies.

Design of Configurable Delivery Devices

Configurable Delivery Devices (CDD) are to be constructed similar to naturally occurring viruses. See Addendum No.1. The CDD has a bilipid outer envelope. Glycoprotein probes are embedded in the outer envelope with the protein segment extending outward and away from the exterior envelope. Inside the CDD there are one or more protein shells that act to both support the spherical structure of the device as well as create an inner cavity where the payload is carried.

Advantages of a CDD include a versatile universal design that allows the transport device to carry a wide variety of payloads and the configurable exterior probes allow the CDD to be constructed in a manner that enable the CDD to deliver its payload to any specific target cell type.

The Configurable Delivery Device in Figure 8 demonstrates two differing sets of exterior probes mounted on the surface of the CDD. This illustration demonstrates that unlike naturally occurring viruses where the probes are limited to one set, the exterior probes on a CDD can be constructed at the time of manufacture to any form that can be utilized to seek out and engage a specific cell type.

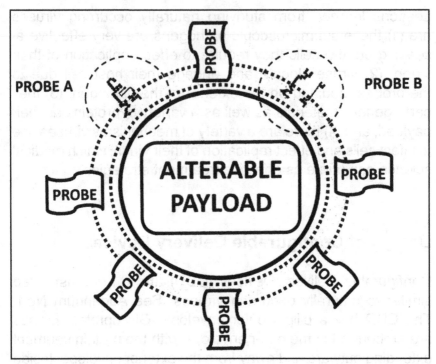

Figure 8: Configurable Delivery Device demonstrating two possible sets of exterior probes

A configurable delivery device would be comprised of an exterior envelope and inner shells similar to a naturally occurring virus, but have mounted on its surface a set of probes that would target a desired cell type. The viral genome would be replaced by a payload that would produce a desired medical effect. The exterior probes mounted on the surface of a configurable delivery device could be configured to target any cell type in the body. The payload such a device would carry could include proteins, genetic material, chemicals and nutrients.

Table 1. provides a comparison of the features of a naturally occurring virus versus a modified virus versus a configurable delivery device. As Table 1 demonstrates, naturally occurring viruses are pathogens, they are limited to seeking out and engaging one type of cell that acts at their host cell, they have a fixed size and therefore a fixed payload capacity, and they are generally antigenic. The presence of a naturally occurring virus often stimulates a response by a body's immune system, this immunologic response aimed at ridding the body of the virus. An immune response to a foreign entity can cause a vigorous reaction to the foreign entity, which can result in clinically visible distress to the body.

Naturally Occurring Virus	Modified Virus	Configurable Delivery Device
Pathogenic	Therapeutic	Therapeutic
One type of cell as host cell	One type of cell as target cell	Mount any set of probes to target any cell type
Fixed size, therefore fixed size of payload.	Fixed size, therefore fixed size of payload.	Alter size to accommodate differing payload sizes and types
Antigenic: Stimulates immune system	Antigenic: Stimulates immune system	Eliminate unnecessary cell-surface markers which reduces or eliminates the antigenicity

Table 1
Table comparing natural and artificially generated genome transport mechanisms.

III. RNA Vector Therapy

Introducing RNA Vector Therapy

Ribonucleic acid (RNA) Vector Therapy refers to a medical treatment strategy comprised of utilizing a vector to carry messenger RNA to accomplish a medically therapeutic task. A vector may be an existing virus modified to carry medically therapeutic RNA or a lipid or protein shell that acts as a medium to transport medically therapeutic RNA or a configurable delivery device to act as a medium to transport medically therapeutic RNA. A vector would be equipped with probes mounted on its surface intended to seek out cells that would benefit from the therapeutic RNA the vector carries as a payload in its core.

As an example, consider messenger RNA. Messenger RNA molecules are divided into three regions. The three regions include (1) the 5' untranslatable region, (2) the coding region, and (3) the 3' untranslatable region. An 'untranslatable region' represents a segment of a messenger RNA molecule that does not code for a protein and is not used to yield a protein and therefore 'translation' does not occur in such a region. The 'coding region' is the portion of the mRNA that is decoded by the ribosomes by the process known as translation to produce a particular protein molecule. A sequence of three nucleotides present in the coding region of a mRNA molecule represents a unit of information referred to as a codon. Codons code for all of the 20 amino acids used to construct protein molecules and also for START and STOP commands. The configuration of the 3' untranslatable region, in part, determines the half-life survival of the messenger RNA molecule.

In the process known as translation, a ribosome decodes the codons present in the coding region in the mRNA, initiating the protein manufacturing process at a START codon, then interfacing with charged transport RNAs (tRNA) carrying the amino acids that match the sequence of codons in the mRNA as the ribosome traverses the length of the coding region of the mRNA molecule. The ribosome functions as a protein factory by taking amino acids delivered by charged tRNAs and binding the amino acids together in the order dictated by the sequence of codon instructions coded into the mRNA template as directed by the manner of the nucleic acid arrangement in the mRNA molecule. Protein synthesis ceases when a ribosome encounters a STOP code. The protein molecule is then released by the ribosome. Ribosomes do not decode the nucleotide sequences to produce proteins in a mRNA's 5' untranslatable region or a mRNA's 3' untranslatable region.

In the case of medical diseases which are the result of a protein deficiency, the management of such medical diseases would be greatly enhanced if cells responsible for the protein deficiency could be stimulated to generate the necessary proteins to correct the deficiency. Proteins are constructed inside cells as a result of ribosome molecules decoding the instructions present in mRNA templates and assembling amino acid chains sequenced from the mRNA instructions. A protein deficient state could be corrected by utilizing Configurable Delivery Devices to insert mRNA, coded for the deficient protein, into cells having the deficient state. See Addendum No. 2 and Addendum No.3.

To correct a protein deficient state, a Configurable Delivery Device could be produced that carried the specific mRNA that could be used by the cell as a template to generate the needed protein. Once inserted into the body, the Configurable Delivery Device would utilize its surface probes to seek out those target cells that would benefit from the mRNA that it was carrying. Once the surface probes of the Configurable Delivery Device located and engaged a target cell's cell-surface receptors the Configurable Delivery Device would insert its payload of mRNA into the target cell. See Figure 9. Following insertion into the target cell's cytoplasm the therapeutic mRNA would undergo the process of translation, like any cellular messenger RNA. Cellular ribosomes would decode the biologic information in the translatable region of the therapeutic mRNA and the necessary proteins would be generated.

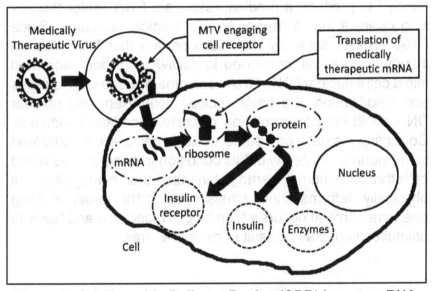

Figure 9: Configurable Delivery Device (CDD) inserts mRNA, capable of producing a needed protein, into a targeted cell

Diabetes mellitus is generally regarded as a medical condition where an individual is lacking in the protein 'insulin'. Sickle cell anemia is a devastating medical condition where a genetic mutation creates abnormal hemoglobin, the protein red blood cells rely on to carry oxygen. Osteoarthritis is a very common condition, generally associated with aging, where cartilage is worn off the surface of the bone over time which leads to joints of the body wearing out, causing pain and disability in individuals. Recent treatments of inflammatory arthritis and inflammatory bowel disease have enlisted the use of tumor necrosis factor alpha blocker proteins to manage the destructive inflammation associated with these diseases. A number of medical conditions would significantly benefit from being treated with RNA vector therapy.

RNA vector therapy offers two distinct approaches to medical disease. RNA vector therapy offers the capacity to treat medical conditions to see a relatively immediate response by providing mRNA that cells could act on very quickly to generate proteins needed to produce a medical response. RNA vector therapy also offers a long-term solution to medical problems. Since RNA viruses, such as HIV, demonstrate that RNA can be inserted into a cell, converted to dsDNA and then integrated into a cell's nuclear DNA, RNA vector therapy can lead to repair and modification of a cell's nuclear DNA. Repairing nuclear DNA could lead to resolution of certain medical conditions. Correcting the base pair defect in sickle cell anemia could lead to individuals afflicted with this condition to generate red blood cells that carry normal hemoglobin rather than hemoglobin that physically deforms under stress causing the telltale sickling phenomenon that occurs which blocks blood flow and leads to painful episodes as a result of oxidative stress.

Modifiable Messenger RNA Vector Therapy

An argument against the use of RNA Vector therapy is that the service-life of certain messenger RNA molecules can be relatively short, in the order of minutes, which would make the strategy of delivering mRNAs to cells impractical for clinical medicine. Nature provides a solution to this paralyzing limitation. Analyzing the components of the messenger RNA molecule of several types of mRNAs offers a clue to how to adjust the service life as well as to adjust other features of the mRNA molecule in order to make this treatment strategy more proficient at improving protein deficient states.

Messenger RNA molecules are comprised of three regions (or segments). These three regions include: (1) a 5' untranslatable region, (2) a coding region and (3) a 3' untranslatable region. The 5' untranslatable region acts as the initiation point for a ribosome to attach to the mRNA. The 'coding region' acts as the template from which a protein is constructed. An 'untranslatable region' represents a segment of a messenger RNA molecule that does not code for a protein and is not used to yield a protein and therefore 'translation' does not occur in such a region. RNA enzymes, termed RNAases, are proteins that exist in the cytoplasm and act to degrade messenger RNA molecules. The composition of the 3' untranslatable region is associated with the rate of degradation of messenger RNA molecules.

Different mRNAs have different service-life expectancies. The half-life of the naturally occurring mRNA that acts as the template responsible for the production of the protein 'glucokinase' is two hours. The half-life of the naturally occurring mRNA that acts as the template to produce the protein 'alcohol dehydrogenase' is ten hours. The half-life of the naturally occurring mRNA that acts as the template to produce the protein 'glucuronidase' is thirty hours.

Thus, modifying the nucleotides that comprise the 3' untranslatable unit of an mRNA, the service-life of the mRNA can be altered. By adjusting the 3' untranslatable unit of the mRNA, the service-life of the mRNA molecule can be lengthened or shortened depending upon the need for the quantity of protein and the timeframe over which the mRNA is required to produce the protein coded in the protein template of the mRNA's coding region. It is reasonable to expect that the half-life of an mRNA utilized to produce insulin could be at least thirty hours by altering the 3' untranslatable region of a naturally occurring insulin producing mRNA to the configuration of the 3' untranslatable region of the mRNA responsible for generating glucuronidase. Longer half-lives are certainly possible with a better understanding of the interactions of the 3' untranslatable region with RNAase molecules that act to degrade RNAs.

Research has demonstrated that natural proteins can be altered to produce medically beneficial effects. The parathyroid hormone (PTH) is one example. Intact PTH is produced by cells in the parathyroid glands. There are four parathyroid glands present in the neck, generally in the vicinity of the thyroid gland. The term 'para-' means 'next to', so early anatomists identified the four glands as 'parathyroid glands' because they were generally found 'next to' the thyroid gland in the neck. Parathyroid hormone is released in response to the cells of the parathyroid gland sensing a decline in the level of serum calcium. Parathyroid hormone, in its natural state, acts to stimulate osteoclast cells present in bone to release calcium from bone, thereby acting as a mechanism to return the serum calcium level to the normal range whenever the serum calcium drops below the normal range. On the other hand, it has been quite well demonstrated that if (1) the amino acid chain of the parathyroid hormone is shortened and (2) the shorter parathyroid hormone molecule is pulsed, by injecting it into the body once a day, the action of this modified parathyroid hormone molecule is opposite of the intact parathyroid hormone. One such form of a shorter length parathyroid hormone molecule is termed 'teriparatide'. Teriparatide (1-34) has the identical sequence from 1 to the 34th N-terminal amino acid of the 84-amino acid endogenous human parathyroid hormone. The skeletal effects of the modified protein molecule act on bone cells to preferentially cause osteoblastic activity over osteoclastic activity, which results in storage of calcium into bone, rather than a release of calcium from bone if the teriparatide is administered once a day. Teriparatide has been a recognized and widely used treatment of osteoporosis since at least as far back as the year 2000.

Modifying the 'coding region' of a messenger RNA will modify the protein the messenger RNA will produce when the ribosomes decode such a modified messenger RNA. As demonstrated by the case of modifying the naturally occurring parathyroid hormone by administering a molecule that is comprised of fewer amino acids than the original PTH molecule, modifying proteins the messenger RNAs produce may provide health care providers with an entirely new and widely expanding armamentarium of medically beneficial therapies.

The 5' untranslatable region of a messenger RNA molecule is used to identify the messenger RNA and utilized as a point of attachment by ribosomes to the messenger RNA molecule. Modifying the 5' untranslatable region by altering the nucleotide sequence in the 5' untranslatable region may make it easier to identify a modified messenger ribonucleic acid molecules in a fashion that the modified ribonucleic acid molecules can be engaged by ribosomes. Altering the nucleotide sequence of the 5' untranslatable region of a modified messenger ribonucleic acid molecule to create a unique identifier would facilitate ribosomes to preferentially engage the modified messenger ribonucleic acid molecule to preferentially produce the protein for which the modified messenger ribonucleic acid molecule is acting as a template.

Having configurable delivery devices insert modified RNA molecules into specific target cells enhances medical therapy by providing mRNA molecules that can have a longer service life than naturally occurring mRNAs, are easily recognizable by rRNAs and will produce improved effects by having the coding region altered to a superior state of function. See Addendum No. 4.

Ribosomal RNA Vector Therapy

Ribosomal RNAs (rRNA) are generated by polymerase molecule deciphering the instruction code present in the DNA. The rRNAs generally migrate to locations where mRNAs are to be utilized as templates. The rRNA molecules connect to their respective ribosome proteins and this macromolecule complex, referred to as a ribosome or ribosome complex, surrounds the beginning segment of a mRNA molecule. Utilizing inherent coding, the rRNA molecules direct the ribosome pieces to build the ribosome complex around a particular strand of mRNA or particular type of mRNA. The inherent coding the rRNA molecules harbor is a sequence of nucleotides which represent a unique name, unique base-four number or unique combination of a name and base-four number that corresponds to a particular mRNA or particular type of mRNA. In this manner, rRNA acts to control which mRNA molecule will undergo translation to produce proteins, rather than a ribosome complex randomly engaging any mRNA template that happens to be available. With the DNA producing rRNA molecules that cause a ribosome to attach to a particular mRNA molecule or particular type of mRNA molecule, the DNA is able to exert control over the manufacturing capacity of the cell and produce proteins as needed, rather than producing proteins in a random fashion. Producing proteins as needed by the cell, rather than in a random fashion, conserves valuable resources and conserves energy inside the cell.

Having configurable delivery devices transport mRNA molecules and rRNA molecules to specific cells improves cell function by providing a deficient cell type templates to produce a desired protein and the means to recognize the mRNAs to assemble ribosomes to generate the desired proteins. See Addendum No. 5 and No. 6.

RNA Vector Therapy to Treat Diabetes

Diabetes is generally considered a state where there is a lack of sufficient amount of the protein 'insulin' to limit the amount of glucose circulating in the blood stream. Insulin is generated in the pancreas. The pancreas is located in the mid portion of the abdomen.

Glucose generally enters the body and then the blood stream as a result of the digestion of food. For purposes of this description, 'blood' and 'blood stream' refer to the same substance, which is generally considered to be blood as a whole including plasma and blood cells.

Specifically Beta cells located in the Islets of Langerhans in the pancreas produce insulin. As the insulin is generated the protein is stored in vacuoles in the Beta cells. In a person who does not have diabetes, the Beta cells utilize surface probes to monitor the level of glucose present in the blood. If the level of glucose present in the blood rises above acceptable limits, Beta cells release insulin stored in the vacuoles and introduce the insulin into the blood stream. Generally, it is accepted that the normal range for a fasting blood sugar level is between 60 mg/dl to 110 mg/dl.

Glucose is a six carbon sugar molecule that is utilized in the respiration process to produce the energy a cell requires to perform the metabolic functions necessary to maintain health. Glucose circulating in the blood stream enters into cells by means of insulin receptors that exist on the surface of cells. When glucose is available in the blood stream, and sufficient insulin is present in the blood stream, the insulin interacts with the insulin receptor on the surface of cells in order to cause glucose to be transported from the blood through the outer membrane of the cell and into the cytoplasm inside the cell.

Diabetes is considered to occur in those individuals that persistently demonstrate blood glucose levels that exceed the normal limits. Blood sugar levels higher than the normal limits is usually the result of an inadequate supply of insulin to meet the demands of transporting the circulating glucose molecules into cells. In the case of failure of the Beta cells to produce insulin this is generally considered insulin dependent diabetes mellitus (IDDM) and requires the individual to administer insulin into their body by an injection. Since insulin is a protein it would be broken down by the hydrochloric acid the stomach produces, therefore administration of insulin must involve a root that bypasses the stomach. Though administering insulin by a nasal spray has been investigated, this has not yet evolved to become a practical method. Injection into the subcutaneous tissues remains the preferred method.

Noninsulin dependent diabetes mellitus (NIDDM) refers to the state where Beta cells produce a quantity of insulin, but the supply of insulin produced by the Beta cells is inadequate to fully manage the level of glucose circulating in the blood stream. To treat NIDDM, often individuals take oral medications that stimulate Beta cells to generate additional amounts of insulin. When the dosing of oral medications fail to control the disease, injectable insulin is required to control blood glucose levels.

The use of oral medications and injectable insulin, in adjunct with a calorie restricted diet and exercise represents the current approach to the management of diabetes. The level of glucose circulating in the blood is a twenty-four hour management problem. An individual generally checks their blood sugar level one to four times a day, depending upon the level of blood sugar control that is required. Injectable insulin is generally administered two to four times a day depending upon the individual's need for control of their blood sugar. Despite strict control of blood sugar utilizing current medical management, many individuals suffer from microvascular damage to internal organs. Individuals may develop kidney failure, heart disease, poor wound healing, and nerve damage to name a few of these conditions.

In numerous individuals with IDDM, despite strict regular insulin dosing and restricted caloric intake, serum glucose levels remain elevated. In cases where treatment with injectable insulin is inadequate to maintain the blood glucose level in the normal range, the management of circulating blood glucose requires a more elaborate approach.

Transport of a glucose molecule from the blood stream into a cell is facilitated by insulin interacting with an insulin receptor mounted on the surface of the cell. Once insulin protein has activated the insulin receptor the glucose molecule is transported through the cell membrane into the cytoplasm inside the cell. In the cytoplasm inside the cell, the glucose molecule is acted upon by an enzyme glucokinase. Glucokinase begins the metabolic process of respiration in which the glucose molecule is broken down through glycolysis, the Krebs's cycle and oxidative phosphorylation. The Krebs's cycle and oxidative phosphorylation are accomplished by a series enzyme reactions that utilize oxygen, with the result being one glucose molecule will result in 38 adenosine triphosphate (ATP) molecules. ATP molecules represent the currency of energy used to drive chemical reactions throughout the cell.

The lack of insulin therapy to fully control serum glucose levels in some individuals may be related to failure of glucose to be adequately metabolized in these individuals. Utilization of glucose may be hampered by inadequate or dysfunctional insulin receptors or inadequate or dysfunctional enzymes comprising the respiration process.

RNA vector therapy could be used to insert into cells the messenger RNA that would be used by Beta cells to produce insulin and, if necessary, the surface probes that monitor blood sugar levels. RNA vector therapy may also be used to produce additional insulin receptors in cells and, if necessary, additional enzymes to carry out the processes of respiration.

Diabetes mellitus is generally classified as Type One and Type Two. Type One diabetes mellitus is insulin dependent, and refers to the condition where there is an insufficient quantity of insulin molecules circulating in the blood stream compared to the quantity required to maintain the blood glucose level within the recognized normal range. In Type One diabetes mellitus insulin must be provided to the body in order to properly regulate the blood plasma glucose level. When insulin is required to regulate the blood glucose level in the body, this condition is often referred to as insulin dependent diabetes mellitus (IDDM). Type Two diabetes mellitus is not dependent upon insulin and is often referred to as noninsulin dependent diabetes mellitus (NIDDM), meaning the blood glucose level can be managed without treatment with exogenous insulin, and is generally managed by means of diet, exercise or intervention with oral medications. Type Two diabetes mellitus is considered a progressive disease, with the underlying pathogenic mechanisms including pancreatic beta cell (often designated as β-Cell) dysfunction and insulin resistance.

The pancreas serves as an endocrine gland and an exocrine gland. Functioning as an endocrine gland, the pancreas produces and secretes hormones including the hormones insulin and glucagon. Insulin acts to reduce levels of glucose circulating in the blood. Beta cells secrete insulin into the blood when a higher than normal level of glucose is detected in the serum. Glucagon is an antagonistic hormone to insulin, which acts to stimulate an increase in glucose circulating in the blood. Alpha cells in the pancreas secrete glucagon into the blood when a low level of glucose is detected in the blood.

Insulin is a protein. An insulin molecule consists of two chains of amino acids, an alpha chain and a beta chain, linked by two disulfide (S-S) bridges. The alpha chain consists of 21 amino acids. The beta chain consists of 30 amino acids.

Insulin interacts with the cells of the body by means of a cell-surface receptor termed the 'insulin receptor' located on the exterior of a cell's 'outer membrane', otherwise known as the 'plasma membrane'. Insulin interacts with muscle and liver cells by means of the insulin receptor to rapidly remove excess blood sugar when the glucose level in the blood is higher than the upper limit of the normal physiologic range. Recognized functions of insulin include stimulating cells to take up glucose from the blood, convert glucose to glycogen (an extensively branched glucose storage polysaccharide molecule), to facilitate the cells in the body to utilize glucose to generate biochemically usable energy, and to stimulate fat cells to take up glucose and synthesize fat.

Diabetes Mellitus may develop in an individual as the result of one or more factors. Causes of diabetes mellitus may include: (1) mutation of the insulin gene itself causing miscoding, which results in the production of ineffective insulin molecules; (2) mutations to genes that code for the 'transcription factors' needed for transcription of the insulin gene in the DNA to create messenger RNAs which facilitates the manufacture of the insulin molecule; (3) mutations of the gene encoding for the insulin receptor, which produces inactive or an insufficient number of insulin receptors; (4) mutation to the gene encoding for glucokinase, the enzyme that phosphorylates glucose in the first step of glycolysis; (5) mutations to the genes encoding portions of the potassium channels in the plasma membrane of the beta cells, preventing proper closure of the channel, thus blocking insulin release; (6) mutations to mitochondrial genes that as a result, decreases the energy available to be used to facilitate the release of insulin, therefore reducing insulin secretion; and (7) failure of glucose transporters to properly permit the facilitated diffusion of glucose from plasma into the cells of the body.

The use of a configurable delivery device to carry the messenger RNA to beta cells in the Islets of Langerhans, would improve insulin production in the beta cells. See Figure 10. Supplying beta cells with messenger RNA that function as the template to produce insulin molecules, the beta cells will be made capable of regulating blood sugars. With beta cells monitoring serum glucose levels and being able to respond in a timely fashion to elevated blood sugar levels by the adequate release of insulin, allows for the body's natural regulatory mechanisms to control serum glucose. Controlling blood sugar levels by means of the beta cells leads to a significant reduction in the unwanted, devastating side effects of chronic diabetes mellitus.

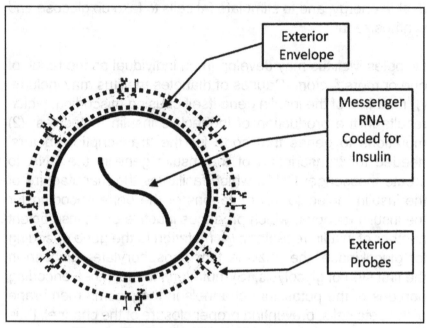

Figure 10: Configurable Delivery Device to carry messenger RNA to produce insulin

Other messenger RNAs that act as templates for the insulin receptor and the various enzymes that participate in glycolysis would be helpful in managing individuals who have diabetes mellitus based not on a lack of sufficient insulin production, but on a deficiency in removing glucose from the blood stream or a deficiency in sufficiently processing the glucose once the sugar is in the cell. Today, often some individuals with diabetes are still not able to adequately control their blood sugars though large amounts of exogenous insulin may be being administered, in split doses, throughout a day. Utilizing configurable delivery devices would be useful in supplying those diabetic individuals whom adequate insulin production is available but who still experience difficulty in controlling their blood sugars. Some of the brittle diabetic individuals or individuals demonstrating an insulin resistance, may indeed benefit from being supplied with messenger RNA that would construct additional insulin receptors or generate the enzymes utilized in glycolysis.

RNA Vector Therapy to Treat Obesity

Obesity has become an epidemic both in the United States and many of the industrialized nations around the globe. The term obesity is generally considered to refer to an individual whom has reached a body mass that is much larger than expected based on the age and height of the person. To be considered obese, the larger than expected body mass is generally comprised of excess adipose (fat) tissue.

As a person consumes energy sources in their diet such as fats and carbohydrates, the energy source is either metabolized by the cells to produce energy or the dietary energy source is stored for later use. When fats and carbohydrates are sent for storage, they are generally converted by processes in the liver to a form that can be stored in adipose tissues. Adipose tissues are generally found in the abdomen, pelvis and thighs, though adipose tissues can also appear in the arms, back, and legs.

When an individual is in a young stage of life, generally the cellular metabolic rate is high due to the need to convert dietary fats and carbohydrates into energy. The energy generated by cells is used to produce the proteins required to facilitate growth. Once the body's structures have fully matured, there is no longer a need for production of a high output of energy and the cellular metabolic rate declines as an individual ages.

In part, 'obesity' is the result of established dietary habits as the individual grows and matures that in the younger years leads to growth and maturation, but is no longer required once the state of adulthood has been reached. High input of dietary fats and carbohydrates combined with a decreased utilization of the fats and carbohydrates leads to an increase in the formation of adipose tissues.

The pancreas produces the protein insulin. Insulin directs glucose into cells so that the glucose can be converted to energy by means of the respiratory process. Though the pancreas in a healthy individual generally excretes into the blood the necessary amount of insulin required to control the blood glucose level, insulin circulating in the blood can be absorbed by adipose tissues before the insulin has the opportunity to effectively regulate blood sugar.

As an individual expands their body mass by adding adipose tissue, the problem of obesity becomes increasingly problematic due to the insulin being produced by the pancreas not available in adequate amounts in the circulation in order to direct the serum glucose into the cells to be utilized for energy metabolism rather than being converted into fat tissue. Therefore, as many obese individuals expand their body mass by generating more adipose tissue, they find themselves in a position that facilitates the generation of additional adipose tissue, while they sense they have less energy with which to function with on a day to day basis. Reduction in caloric intake, reduction in sodium intake and the utilization of a tolerable aerobic exercise are all important fundamentals in achieving success at weight loss.

Significant weight loss in patients left to their own devices is rare, and is generally considered an impossible task for the average individual. Even with medical management, significant weight loss is a very difficult task for anyone to achieve, except in the most motivated of patients. Often unexplained weight loss is a sign of a disease, or cancer or dramatic change in the body's metabolism and should be brought to the attention of the individual's physician.

At times of dieting, where fat and carbohydrate intake may be voluntarily restricted, generally it takes nine days before any of the energy stores present in the adipose tissues begins to be consumed. In the first eight days of a calorie restricted diet the body preferentially converts muscle tissue to energy, rather than converting adipose tissue to energy. Generally, if an individual wishes to reduce their weight by reducing the fat stores that comprise their excess body mass, the individual needs to adhere to their diet for more than nine days before there is any substantial reduction on their fat stores. During the period of weight loss aerobic exercise, in some reasonable fashion, should be performed in order to maintain muscle mass during the dieting process.

Paradoxically, as individuals gain excess weight, the body becomes less efficient in utilizing glucose, therefore individuals may increase their glucose, carbohydrate and fat intake in order to compensate for the sense of not having enough energy at their disposal. The increase in sugar and fat intake further contributes to the accumulation of fat stores resulting in even less insulin available to process glucose.

Dieting is extremely difficult to accomplish, even under the supervision of trained healthcare providers. Many obese individuals participate in various bariatric surgery methods in order to reduce the size of their stomach. Reducing the volume of food that can be consumed at any given time forces the individual to reduce the quantity of fat and carbohydrate intake. In motivated patients bariatric surgery can result in a decline in adipose tissue stores, which can result in weight loss.

RNA vector therapy could be utilized to increase an individual's metabolic rate in order to convert glucose and fats into energy. Enzymes utilized in the metabolism of glucose could be delivered to cells to increase the function of the mitochondria, which would result in a rise in the metabolic rate. As people age, their mitochondrial function declines. Increasing the metabolic rate in an obese individual would reverse the tendency to convert dietary fat and carbohydrates into additional adipose tissues and would lead to increased energy production, which could then facilitate exercise. Stepping up the exercise in obese individuals would lead to converting existing adipose tissues into sugar, which could be further metabolized within the cells. Reduction in adipose stores around the body would lead to weight loss, and with reasonable dietary restrictions would eventually eliminate the obesity in an individual.

RNA Vector Therapy to Treat Chronic Fatigue

Chronic fatigue is a relatively common complaint expressed by some patients, as they pass through their early adult and middle age years. The feeling of fatigue or as some report 'a loss of youthful energy' has been described by numerous terms in the medical literature. In the past chronic fatigue was termed 'Chronic Mononucleosis Syndrome'. In the eighties, 'Chronic Fatigue Syndrome' was a popular term. In the nineties, 'Fibrositis' and later the term 'Fibromylagia Syndrome' were used to identify individuals who complained of a chronic form of fatigue.

The medical world is somewhat lacking in their ability to arrive at a convincing diagnosis for individual's that report 'fatigue' as a chief complaint. When an individual complains about fatigue, clinicians are able to check for only a limited number of correctable medical conditions that may cause an individual to feel tired. Often a work-up for a chief complaint of fatigue involves measuring an individual's blood sugar to investigate for diabetes, checking for a thyroid disorder, checking for anemia, making sure there is no electrolyte imbalance or renal disease, and checking calcium and magnesium levels. Given the age and history of an individual, a series of screening tests may be performed to investigate for an occult cancer that could lead to fatigue.

It has been conjectured in the past that the pathogen Ebstein Barr Virus (EBV) may cause fatigue in adults. It is recognized in teenagers and young adults that EBV exposure may lead to the development of mononucleosis that may be manifested by symptoms of a debilitating fatigue that can in some individuals last for weeks. It remains unclear whether EBV causes fatigue in adults.

In the late eighties, the medical diagnosis of Chronic Fatigue Syndrome was applied to individuals, in their adult years, that complained to their doctor about chronic fatigue and tested positive for exposure to EBV. The numbers of individuals diagnosed with Chronic Fatigue Syndrome swelled at an alarming rate as the nineties came to a close. Review of the clinical symptoms correlated with EBV test results demonstrated that half the individuals reporting symptoms associated with Chronic Fatigue Syndrome tested positive for EBV, while half the individuals tested negative for EBV; such a study result effectively made the diagnosis of Chronic Fatigue Syndrome based on an EBV titer a none entity.

Fibrositis or fibromyalgia, both terms referring to the same medical condition, has required no lab test in order for a physician to make such a diagnosis. In fact, generally all of the normal screening tests used to investigate individuals for a complaint of chronic fatigue are suppose to be normal for a diagnosis of fibrositis to be made. Fibrositis is generally considered a form of fatigue caused by a lack of effective sleep.

Adequate sleep generally consists of several stages, the deepest stage being referred to as Rapid Eye Movement (REM) sleep. During REM sleep a person's eyes are thought to be fluttering under the eyelids, which is how this stage of sleep acquired its name. REM sleep is meant to represent the phase of sleep where the muscles have fully relaxed and are in a state where increased blood flow due to reduced resistance helps repair the muscles. If an individual is not able to achieve an adequate amount of REM sleep during the night, and this occurs chronically, this is felt to lead to a state of fatigue. There are currently no lab tests that reflect a state of lack of adequate sleep, so individuals with fibrositis as their primary diagnosis, will generally have a normal serum profile.

Some individuals experience poor sleep due to sleep apnea. Not to be confused with fibromyalgia, sleep apnea refers to the condition where an individual develops intermittent breathing difficulty while they sleep. Often the individual with sleep apnea is not aware they have this condition. Sleep apnea is often accompanied by violent snoring fits, which at times may cause a spouse to seek alternate bedroom arrangements due to the snoring being too loud for the spouse to sleep restfully. Sleep apnea is manifested by the individual discontinuing breathing, which eventually causes snoring and loud erratic breath sounds. Often the spouse will witness the individual exhibiting episodes of a lack of breathing and will alert the individual to the problem. Sleep apnea is a treatable condition, and the fatigue that can accompany such a condition may improve dramatically with proper management.

Fibrositis patients often become depressed due to a chronic insufficiency of a proper type of sleep that eventually leads to fatigue. The sense of a lack of adequate daytime energy fuels their depression. Antidepressants and sleep aides help improve sleep and a sense of well-being, but often do not improve an individual's exercise capacity or their desire to exercise. Regular daytime exercise can be helpful in relieving myalgias and possibly improve the quality of sleep.

Utilizing configurable delivery devices to insert into cells the messenger RNA to produce the enzymes to enhance glycolysis in middle-aged individuals may improve the desire for exercise by making available additional energy molecules to facilitate oxidative cell metabolism. Stimulating the muscles by supplying the muscles with additional energy molecules, may create a greater desire to utilize such muscles.

RNA Vector Therapy to Forestall Aging

The exact cause of aging has been an elusive subject. Some theories regarding aging include such concepts as a cell can only divide so many times before it reaches a point where it triggers the terminal program 'apoptosis' and kills itself. Recently, it has been discussed that the caps on the ends of the chromosomes, called telomeres, fray with each cell division and once the fraying reaches a critical point, the DNA comprising the genome becomes unreadable and this leads to cell death. Other theories have suggested that there is a generation of toxins, at one time referred to as ubiquitins, which accumulate inside cells over time, and when the toxins reach a certain concentration the cell's inner mechanisms are unable to function adequately enough to meet the needs of the cell and the cell dies. In recent years, ubiquitins are thought to tag proteins for degradation and usher such proteins to proteasomes, which chop proteins up into amino acids; the ubiquitins themselves are preserved in the process.

Mitochondrion (a single mitochondria) is a cellular organelle that is considered the energy producing organelle of the cell. Mitochondria assist in generating energy for cell metabolism by producing ATP molecules from glucose. Energy is most efficiently produced when a mitochondria degrades glucose in the presence of oxygen. See Figure 11.

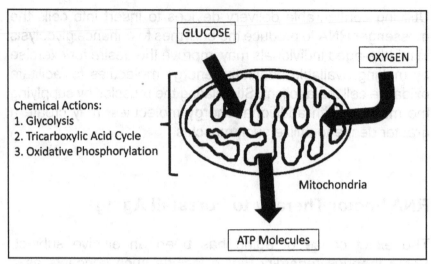

Figure 11: Mitochondria produce ATP by breaking down glucose in the presence of oxygen.

Within the cytoplasm and outer wall of the mitochondria glucose molecules undergo the process of glycolysis, and then inside the mitochondria byproducts of glucose are further broken down in the tricarboxylic acid (TCA) cycle and by oxidative phosphorylation to produce useable forms of energy molecules.

The exterior of a mitochondrion is referred to as an external membrane. Inside the outer membrane is an inner membrane. Folds in the inner membrane create crista, which expands the surface of the inner membrane and enhances the mitochondrion's ability to create ATP molecules. Inside the inner membrane is the mitochondrion matrix. The mitochondrion matrix contains a highly concentrated mixture of enzymes, ribosomes, tRNA and mitochondrial DNA. Glycolysis occurs in the cytosol of the cell and the membrane of the mitochondrion. The tricarboxylic acid cycle functions within the inner chambers and matrix of the mitochondrion. Oxidative phosphorylation occurs within the boundaries of the outer and inner membranes of the mitochondrion.

Many of the intermediates of the processes of glycolysis and the tricarboxylic acid cycle exist as anions at the pH found in cells, and readily associate with H^+ to form acids. The intermediates of glycolysis and the tricarboxylic acid cycle are therefore often written as either an anion or an acid. For the purposes of this description, the intermediates of the processes of glycolysis and the tricarboxylic acid cycle are generally written as anions (as an example pyruvate versus pyruvic acid).

As a result of the biochemical process of glycolysis during aerobic (a state where adequate oxygen is available) respiration conditions glucose is converted to pyruvate. The abbreviated processes of glycolysis include: (1) Glucose is converted to glucose-6-phosphate by the enzyme 'hexokinase', (2) Glucose-6-phosphate is converted to fructose-6-phosphate by the enzyme 'glucose-6-phosphate isomerase', (3) Fructose-6-phosphate is converted to fructose 1,6-diphosphate by the enzyme 'phosphofructo kinase', (4) Fructose 1,6-diphosphate is converted to two different entities including dihydroxyacetone-3-phosphate and glyceraldehydes-3-phosphate by the enzyme 'fructose bisphosphate aldolase', (5) Dihydroacetone-3-phosphate converts to D-glyceraladehyde-3-phosphate by the enzyme 'triose-phosphate isomerase', (6) Glyceraldehyde-3-phosphate is converted to 1,3-diphosphoglycerate by the enzyme 'glyceraldehyde-3-phosphate dehydrogenase', (7) 1,3-diphosphoglycerate is converted to 3-phosphoglycerate by the enzyme 'phosphoglycerate kinase', (8) 3-phosphoglycerate is converted to 2-phosphoglycerate by the enzyme 'phosphoglycerate mutase', (9) 2-phosphoglycerate is converted to phosphoenolpyruvate by the enzyme 'enolase', and (10) Phosphoenolpyruvate is converted to pyruvate by the enzyme complex referred to as 'pyruvate kinase'.

Pyruvate is then oxidized to an acetyl group, which is combined with Coenzyme A and produces acetyl Coenzyme A (acetyl-CoA). Pyruvate dehydrogenase which metabolizes pyruvate to acetyl-CoA is comprised of a multi-enzyme complex. The three protein complexes of pyruvate dehydrogenase are designated E1 (pyruvate dehydrogenase), E2 (dihydrolipoamide S-acetyltransferase), and E3 (dihydrolipoamide dehydrogenase). Acetyl-CoA enters the tricarboxylic acid cycle. Under aerobic respiration conditions from one glucose molecule the process of glycolysis generates 8 ATP molecules, conversion of pyruvate to acetyl CoA generates an additional 6 ATP molecules.

The tricarboxylic acid cycle otherwise known as the citric acid cycle or the Krebs cycle, was discovered in 1937 by Sir Hans Krebs, and is a biochemical process that provides complete oxidation of acetyl-CoA, which may be derived from sources such as fats, carbohydrates and lipids. For purposes of this discussion, acetyl-CoA is a byproduct of glucose metabolism during glycolysis, and enters the tricarboxylic acid cycle and (1) combines with oxaloacetate (also known as oxaloacetic acid) by the action of the enzyme 'citrate synthetase' which produces citrate (also known as citric acid), (2) Citrate is converted to cis-aconitate per the enzyme 'aconitase', (3) Cis-aconitate is converted to iso-citrate (also known as isocitur acid) again by the enzyme aconitase, (4) Iso-citrate is converted to alpha-ketoglutarate by the enzyme 'isocitrate dehydrogenase', (5) Alpha-ketoglutaric acid is converted to succinyl CoA by the enzyme '2-oxoglutarate dehydrogenase', (6) Succinyl CoA is converted to succinate (also known as succinic acid) by the enzyme 'succinyl-CoA synthetase', (7) Succinate is converted to fumarate (also known as fumaric acid) by the enzyme 'succinate dehydrogenase', (8) Fumarate is converted to malate (also known as malic acid) by the enzyme 'fumarate hydratase', and (9) Malate is converted to oxaloacetate by the enzyme 'malate dehydrogenase'. The result of metabolism of glucose by glycolysis and the tricarboxylic acid cycle yields ATP molecules and electron donor molecules such as the reduced form of the coenzyme nicotinamide adenine dinucleotide written NADH $+H^+$. The tricarboxylic acid cycle also produces electron donor molecules in the form of the reduced co-enzyme flavin adenine dinucleotide written $FADH_2$.

Oxidative phosphorylation is a metabolic pathway that uses energy released by oxidation to produce adenosine triphosphate (ATP). During oxidative phosphorylation electrons are transferred from electron donors to electron acceptors such as oxygen in redox reactions. In eukaryotes the redox reactions are carried out by a series of protein complexes located within mitochondria. These protein complexes represent a linked set of enzymes referred to as electron transport chains. The protein complexes utilized in oxidative phosphorylation include the nicotinamide adenine dinucleotide dehydrogenase enzyme molecule, the succinate dehydrogenase enzyme molecule, the cytochrome-c reductase enzyme molecule, the cytochrome-c oxidase enzyme molecule, and the ATP synthase enzyme molecule. Under aerobic respiration conditions one glucose molecule metabolized by the combination of glycolysis, the tricarboxylic acid cycle and oxidative phosphorylation yields as many as 38 ATP molecules.

An enzyme is a protein generated by cells that acts as a catalyst to induce chemical changes in other substances, itself remaining apparently unchanged in the process. There are several main groups of enzymes including oxidoreductase, transferase, hydrolase, lyase, isomerase, and ligase, sometimes referred to as synthetase. EC is an abbreviation for Enzyme Commission of the International Union of Biochemistry and it is used in conjunction with a unique number to define a specific enzyme identified in the Enzyme Commission's list of enzymes. Oxidoreductases generally have as their first EC identifying number, the number 1. Transferases generally have as their first EC identifying number, the number 2. Hydrolases generally have as their first EC identifying number, the number 3. Lyases generally have as their first EC identifying number, the number 4. Isomerase generally have as their first EC identifying number, the number 5. Ligases generally have as their first EC identifying number, the number 6. Several scientific names often exist to identify the same enzyme.

Enzymes utilized in the metabolism of glucose in the processes of glycolysis, tricarboxylic acid cycle, and oxidative phosphorylation include the named enzymes in the following paragraphs as described.

[1] Hexokinase (EC 2.7.1.1), is also referred to as hexokinase type IV glucokinase or in some cases simply glucokinase. Hexokinase converts glucose to glucose-6-phosphate in glycolysis.

[2] Glucose-6-phosphate isomerase (EC 5.3.1.9), is also known as phosphoglucoisomerase. Glucose-6-phosphate isomerase is an enzyme that converts glucose-6-phosphate to fructose-6-phosphate in glycolysis.

[3] 6-phosphofructokinase (EC 2.7.1.11), is also known as phosphofructokinase. 6-phosphofructokinase is an enzyme that converts fructose-6-phosphate to fructose 1,6-diphosphate in glycolysis.

[4] Fructose bisphosphate aldolase (EC 4.1.2.13), is also known as aldolase. Fructose bisphosphate aldolase is an enzyme that converts fructose 1,6-diphosphate to two different entities including dihydroxyacetone 3-phosphate and glyceraldehydes 3-phosphate in glycolysis.

[5] Triose-phosphate isomerase (EC 5.3.1.1). Triose-phosphate isomerase is an enzyme that converts dihydroacetone-3-phosphate converts to D-glyceraladehyde-3-phosphate.

[6] Glyceraldehyde-3-phosphate dehydrogenase (EC 1.2.1.12), may be abbreviated GAPDH or G3PDH. Glyceraldehyde-3-phosphate dehydrogenase is an enzyme that converts glyceraldehydes-3-phosphatate to 1,3-diphosphoglycerate in glycolysis.

[7] Phosphoglycerate kinase (EC 2.7.2.3). Phosphoglycerate kinase is an enzyme that converts 1,3-diphosphoglycerate to 3-phosphoglycerate in glycolysis.

[8] Phosphoglycerate mutase (EC 5.4.2.1). Phosphoglycerate mutase is an enzyme that converts 3-phosphoglycerate to 2-phosphoglycerate in glycolysis.

[9] Enolase (EC 4.2.1.11). Enolase is an enzyme that converts 2-phosphoglycerate to phosphoenolpyruvate in glycolysis.

[10] Pyruvate kinase (EC 2.7.1.40). Pyruvate kinase is an enzyme that converts phosphoenolpyruvate to pyruvate in glycolysis.

[11] Pyruvate dehydrogenase is comprised of three units. The three units include E1 (EC 1.2.4.1), (EC 1.2.1.51), E2 dihydrolipoamide S-acetyltransferase (EC 2.3.1.12), and E3 dihydrolipoamide dehydrogenase (EC 1.8.1.4). Pyruvate dehydrogenase molecular complex catalyzes the conversion of pyruvate to acetyl-CoA.

[12] Citrate synthetase (EC 4.1.3.7). Citrate synthetase is an enzyme that converts acetyl-CoA combines with oxaloacetate to produce citrate in the tricarboxylic acid cycle.

[13] Aconitase (EC 4.2.1.3). Aconitase exists in two isoenzyme forms in eukaryotes: mitochondrial and cytosolic. Aconitase is an enzyme that converts citrate to cis-aconitate in the Tricarboxylic acid cycle and converts cis-aconitate to iso-citrate in the tricarboxylic acid cycle.

[14] Isocitrate dehydrogenase (EC 1.1.1.41). Isocitrate dehydrogenase is an enzyme that converts isocitrate to alpha-ketoglutaric acid in the tricarboxylic acid cycle.

[15] 2-oxoglutarate dehydrogenase is a protein complex comprised of three units. The three units include E1 (EC 1.2.4.2), E2 (EC 2.3.1.61), and E3 (EC 1.8.1.4). 2-oxoglutarate dehydrogenase is an enzyme complex that converts alpha-ketoglutaric to succinyl CoA in the tricarboxylic acid cycle.

[16] Succinyl-CoA synthetase (EC 6.2.1.5). Succinyl-CoA synthetase is an enzyme that converts succinyl CoA to succinate in the tricarboxylic acid cycle.

[17] Succinate dehydrogenase (EC 1.3.5.1). Succinate dehydrogenase is an enzyme that converts succinate to fumarate in the tricarboxylic acid cycle.

[18] Fumarate hydratase (EC 4.2.1.2). Fumarate hydratase is an enzyme that converts fumarate to malate in the tricarboxylic acid cycle.

[19] Malate dehydrogenase (EC 1.1.1.37). Malate dehydrogenase is an enzyme that converts malate to oxaloacetate in the tricarboxylic acid cycle.

The proteins manufactured by the ribosomes from mRNA templates participate in the chemical reactions of glycolysis, the tricarboxylic acid cycle, oxidative phosphorylation and anaerobic respiration by acting as enzymes to catalyze these reactions or as other support proteins.

The mitochondria's internal biochemistry is fairly complex. If the mitochondria's energy producing mechanisms fail to operate at an optimal level, overall cell function suffers due to a decline in the supply of available energy. Glucose may indeed be available for utilization by the mitochondria, but actual utilization rate of the glucose will be reduced if the cell's mitochondria are not functioning properly, with the result that the necessary supply of ATP molecules may not be adequate to supply the needs of the cell, thus limiting the function and survivability of the cell.

If the mitochondria fail to produce energy at adequate levels the cell fails to perform its primary internal functions as wells as any secondary external functions. As in the case of an endocrine cell, if the mitochondria fail to produce adequate amounts of ATP, the secondary functions of hormone production and release may cease to occur. It has been thought that from the mid thirties to fifty, approximately half of the mitochondria in a cell have their output of ATP reduced to inadequate levels. From the mid sixties to ninety years of age an additional thirty to forty percent of the mitochondria shut down. According to these estimates, an 87 year old individual may be functioning with only ten to twenty percent of the energy output at the cellular level compared to what they had available in their youth, which certainly could account of a sense of lack of adequate energy individuals report in their later years. As the number of cells comprising an organ lose their internal source of energy, organ function degrades. Once the number of cells that are unable to function, due to lack of adequate energy supply, reaches a critical mass, organ failure ensues. At some point single organ failure, such as the heart or brain, or accumulated organ insufficiency reaches to point where the body is not able to sustain itself and death occurs.

Developing a method of correcting the cause of the decline in mitochondrial function would lead to increasing the body's utilization of glucose, which would result in a more optimal management of the sense of fatigue some individuals experience and would halt and possibly reverse some of the deleterious results of the aging process.

Essential function of the mitochondrion relies on mRNA being decoded by the ribosomes in order to produce proteins that act as enzymes and catalyze the biologic reactions of aerobic respiration. It does not appear that the mitochondrial DNA creates the majority of the required mRNAs to generate the enzymes required for aerobic respiration. The mRNAs are then either produced by the cell's nucleus and sent to the mitochondria or the required mRNAs are created at the time a new mitochondrion is constructed. Loss of proper regulation of the chemical pathways inside a mitochondrion may be related to degradation of the necessary mRNAs.

Energy facilitates function. A decline in energy production by the cell directly impacts the cell's health by limiting the number of ATP molecules available to participate in chemical reactions, thus reducing the cell's capacity to carry out biologic functions. Energy is essential for life.

A treatment and prevention of aging may be approached by utilizing configurable delivery devices as vehicles to transport biologically active mRNAs to mitochondria to bolster function of the mitochondria in critical cell types in the body. See Figure 12. There are numerous enzymes that participate in the processes of glycolysis, the tricarboxylic acid cycle, and oxidative phosphorylation. To restoke the fires of energy production in the mitochondria it may take inserting more than one type of mRNA to produce more than one type of enzyme that can be used in the energy producing processes of the mitochondria.

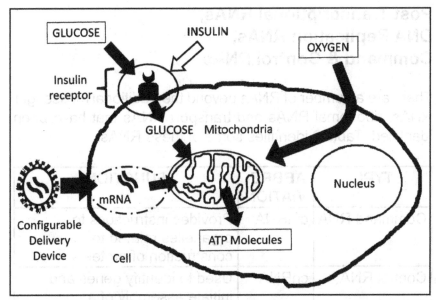

Figure 12: Configurable Delivery Device to insert into cells messenger RNA coded to generate mitochondrial enzymes

Alternatives include utilizing configurable delivery devices to transport to cells the oxygen and glucose needed to effect respiration, and even the transporting of ATP molecules themselves to cells endanger of respiratory collapse.

RNA Vector Therapy to Treat Most Protein Deficient States

There are an estimated 33,000 proteins the body is capable of generating. For each individual protein there exists at least one mRNA that is used as the design template to produce the protein. Therefore, there are at least 33,000 potential applications for RNA Vector Therapy, with each of these treatment therapies carrying a payload comprised of at least one type of mRNA molecule. For the construction of some proteins, it may require more than one type of mRNA to be delivered to a particular cell type to create the desired protein structure.

Post Transcriptional RNAs,
DNA Replication RNAs,
Command & Control RNAs

There are a number of RNAs beyond the traditional messenger RNAs, ribosomal RNAs and transport RNAs that have been identified. Table 2 identifies some of these RNAs.

TYPE	ABBRE-VIATION	FUNCTION
Command RNA	cmRNA	Provides instructions to organelles related to construction of proteins
Control RNA	cnRNA	Used to identify genes and initiate assembly of a transcription complex
Guide RNA	gRNA	mRNA nucleotide modification
Ribonuclease MRP	RNase MRP	tRNA maturation, DNA maturation
Ribonuclease P	RNase P	tRNA maturation
Small nuclear RNA	snRNA	Splicing and other functions
Small nucleolar RNA	snoRNA	Nucleotide modification of RNAs
Sm Y RNA	Sm Y	mRNA trans-splicing
Telomerase RNA	teloRNA	Telomere synthesis
Y RNA	yRNA	RNA processing, DNA replication

Table 2
Different types of RNAs.

The RNAs listed in Table 2 are candidates RNAs for RNA Vector Therapy. As research progresses the list of RNAs is expanding. Where a deficiency can be identified, RNAs involved in post-transcriptional modification of RNA, DNA replication or Command and Control functions of the cell can be transported to specific cells by the use of configurable delivery devices to effect a medical therapy.

IV. DNA Vector Therapy

Gene Therapy

Gene therapy has been a novel approach to treating medical diseases that has been explored over at least the last twenty years. The origins of gene therapy arose out of seeking a means to repair genetic defects that were responsible for a number of medical diseases.

Deoxyribonucleic acid (DNA) represents the genetic code present in a cell's nucleus. Human DNA, present in every cell of the body except red blood corpuscles, is generally segmented into 46 chromosomes. The 46 chromosomes are matched into 23 pairs. Most nucleated cells of the body carry all 23 pairs of chromosomes, except for the sex cells which carry only one of each of the 23 chromosomes.

DNA is present in the nucleus of the nucleated cells, termed nuclear DNA, and in a limited amount in the mitochondria of cells, termed mitochondrial DNA. Nuclear DNA in humans is comprised of two strands of nucleotides linked together. There exist four nucleotides: adenine, cytosine, guanine, and thymine. In the double stranded DNA of the nucleus of the cell, the nucleotide adenine present on one strand is always paired with the nucleotide cytosine present in the parallel strand. The nucleotide guanine is always paired with the nucleotide thymine. It is the sequencing of adenine, cytosine, guanine, thymine nucleotides that produces the genetic code used by the body to construct the cellular structures it needs and perform the functions required by the body to maintain an optimal state of health. The DNA, represented in the nucleus of each cell by 46 chromosomes is comprised of 3 billion base pairs. Each base pair comprising the 46 chromosomes could be thought of as one of 3 billion bits of genetic information.

Genes represent subsets of the DNA. A gene is a segment of the 3 billion base pairs that is considered to represent the genetic code that dictates a physical feature of the body or instructions to conduct a function in the cell. Each of the 46 chromosomes contains numerous segments that have been identified as individual genes. Of the 3 billion base pairs comprising the entire DNA genetic code, only 3% has been defined as being associated with a recognizable gene.

Genes are generally represented in pairs amongst paired chromosomes. Given there are 46 total chromosomes in a human cell nucleus, there are 26 pairs of chromosomes. Genes are generally mapped out similarly in the DNA sequences of paired chromosomes. Genes can be dominant or repressive. Dominant genes will be expressed in the presence of a repressive gene. In the case of the gene for eye color, the gene that codes for brown eyes is generally considered dominant, where the gene for blue eye color is considered repressive. If an individual has two genes for brown color present in their chromosomes, their eye color will be brown. If an individual carries one gene for brown eyes and one gene for blue eyes, the person will have brown eyes since the gene for brown eyes is dominant and the gene for blue eyes is recessive. A person with blue eyes carries in their chromosomes two genes that code for blue eyes.

A number of medical conditions are related to harmful mutations occurring in the genetic code of the genes present in the nuclear DNA. Sickle cell anemia is a condition where one set of base pairs in the gene that codes for hemoglobin has undergone a detrimental mutation. Hemoglobin is the protein that exists inside red blood corpuscles that acts as the transport mechanism to carry oxygen around the body. If an individual carries one gene that has the mutation for sickle cell anemia, generally such an individual is protected from being infected by malaria. If an individual carries two genes that have the sickle cell anemia mutation, then at times of stress, the red blood corpuscles can transform from round cells into a sickle shaped cell. Sickle shaped cells block the normal flow of blood and cause the individual pain in the joints, muscles and some organs inside their body.

Gene therapy was originated as an effort to try to discover a means to make corrections to gene mutations in order to treat people suffering from the ill effects of dysfunctional genes.

Currently DNA therapy is generally directed at utilizing existing viruses to transport genes. Existing viruses target only their natural host cells and therefore are limited in their role as a transport device.

DNA Vector Therapy

Utilizing configurable delivery devices to transport medically therapeutic segments of DNA to specific cells is meant to enhance the current state of gene therapy. By utilizing configurable delivery devices, gene therapy is no longer confined to being inserted into the host cells of common viruses, but gene therapy can be transported to any targeted cell type that would demonstrate a benefit from being modulated by the gene therapy.

In addition, DNA vector therapy involves loading a transport vector's core with a payload comprised of not only a medically beneficial DNA, but also various proteins that could assist the DNA in accomplishing the desired medically beneficial outcome. A simple example of an assisting enzyme would be the integrase enzyme that accompanies the exogenous DNA from the vector into the nucleus of the target cell and functions to insert the exogenous DNA into the proper position in the nuclear DNA of the target cell. Other assisting enzymes might modify the DNA once the therapeutic DNA is inserted into the cytoplasm of the target cell. Another category of assisting enzyme that may be required in some instances is the enzyme to convert single stranded DNA into double stranded DNA. Each current virus is configured for a particular payload, which may be insufficient for a particular gene therapy. Utilization of configurable delivery devices with the ability to adjust the payload capacity to meet the payload requirements will alleviate such a problem.

Thus, the current efforts to pursue gene therapy would be assisted by utilizing configurable delivery devices to transport the gene and any necessary proteins to specific cells in the body.

V. Chemo Vector Therapy

Utilization of configurable microscopic medical payload delivery devices, referred to in this text as configurable delivery devices CDD, to deliver chemotherapy molecules to specific cell types facilitates a dramatic new approach to managing cancer and inflammatory disorders as well as many other disease states.

By selecting the type of probes that will effectively engage cell-surface receptors on target cells and fixing these probes on the surface of the configurable microscopic medical payload delivery devices, specific types of cells can be targeted with chemicals. See Figure 13. By utilizing configurable delivery devices to deliver chemotherapy molecules to specific cell types, the rate of cell growth and rate of cell replication can be inhibited without provoking unwanted side effects in other cells. A wide variety of cancers and inflammatory disorders are treatable by utilizing this new and unique approach. (See Addendum No. 7)

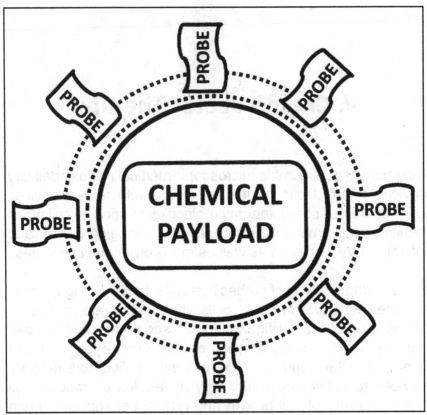

**Figure 13: Configurable Delivery Device
to transport chemical molecules**

Future medical treatment includes the aggressive, widespread utilization of configurable delivery devices (CDD) to deliver chemotherapy molecules directly to specific targeted cell types in the body.

The configurable delivery device transporting chemotherapy molecules represents a very versatile medical treatment delivery device. CDD may be used to deliver chemotherapy molecules to a wide variety of cancer cells and inflammatory cells. Using CDD to deliver chemotherapy molecules directly to targeted cells and only to the targeted cells represents a significant advancement over current chemotherapy treatment techniques in that this strategy avoids many of the unwanted side effects that conventional chemotherapy may be associated with in some individuals. The genetic make-up of individuals is quite varied, resulting in variable responses to chemical and protein agents, which further supports the move to incorporate vehicles to deliver therapeutic agents directly to target cells to minimize complications.

Rheumatoid arthritis is an inflammatory disease affecting millions of people worldwide. The chemotherapy drug methotrexate has been used for over twenty years, and is used quite extensively as a treatment of rheumatoid arthritis. Oral and injectable forms of the methotrexate are used to suppress the growth and cell division of synovial tissues. Oral and injectable methotrexate causes many unwanted side effects. Utilizing configurable microscopic medical payload delivery devices to deliver methotrexate molecules specifically to synovial cells, and only to synovial cells, increases the efficacy of methotrexate and reduces or eliminates the unwanted side effects of methotrexate.

Methotrexate is an antimetabolite of the B vitamin. Methotrexate inhibits dihydrofolate reductase (DHFR). Dihydrofolates must be reduced to tetrahydrofolic acid by the enzyme DHFR in the process of deoxyribonucleic acid synthesis. Methotrexate therefore inhibits synthesis of nucleic acids, which in turn inhibits cellular replication. Actively proliferating cells such as malignant cells, bone marrow, fetal cells, buccal mucosa cells, intestinal mucosa cells, and rheumatoid arthritis activated synovial cells are generally more sensitive to the presence of methotrexate. The rate of cellular proliferation in malignant tissues is generally greater than in normal tissues. Methotrexate generally impairs malignant or inflammatory cell growth without irreversibly damaging normal tissues. In many individuals, treatment with oral or injectable methotrexate does result in significant unwanted side effects, which prevents effective use of the drug in these individuals. Methotrexate is principally excreted from the body by the kidneys.

When utilized to manage an inflammatory arthritis such as rheumatoid arthritis, suppressing folate production suppresses synovial tissue proliferation, which suppresses erosive joint changes. Treatment of rheumatoid arthritis utilizing methotrexate is a strategy of long-term suppression of the disease. Individuals with rheumatoid arthritis will often take methotrexate indefinitely.

Methotrexate generally is categorized as a chemotherapy and also an antimetabolite. Chemotherapies are best known for the use in managing cancers. Methotrexate is but one of numerous chemotherapies available to treat cancer.

Cancer cells generally exhibit a rate of growth and replication that exceeds that of normal healthy cells. Cancer cells whose rate of cell growth and cell division can be slowed down to match that of normal healthy cells would result in such a cancer no longer posing a significant health risk to the body.

Breast cancer is a devastating diagnosis for women and men. The survival rate for breast cancer individuals has risen significantly over the years as treatment strategies have evolved and improved. Still, the diagnosis or even the threat of breast cancer strikes fear in many women and men around the world. If the growth or rate of cell division of breast cancer cells could be reduced to the same rate as normal cells in breast tissue, then the resultant threat that the occurrence of breast cancer causes would be greatly diminished for the individual, family and friends.

Configurable delivery devices could be used to transport a chemotherapy such as methotrexate to breast cells and only the breast cells in an individual diagnosed with breast cancer. Methotrexate would be delivered to all of the breast cells, but since methotrexate tends only to interfere with a cell's replication process, only the cancerous breast cells would be adversely affected. Delivering methotrexate to the breast cells of a nonpregnant woman or a man would neutralize the growth of the cancer and prevent the adverse effects of the cancer. In addition, breast cancer cells that had metastasized beyond the confines of a breast would be managed by this treatment strategy since the CDD would travel to all reaches of the body per the blood stream and the actions of the CDD would be indiscriminant of where in the body the cancerous breast tissue existed.

Various types of chemical molecules could be transported by configurable delivery devices to specific cells to produce a medically beneficial effect. The use of configurable deliver devices will radically change the landscape of medical treatment of cancers and inflammatory arthritis, as well as a broad range of other medical conditions where the introduction of a chemical could exert a positive benefit in a specific cell type.

VI. Oxygen Vector Therapy
and Nutrients

The medical condition where a heart attack or a stroke occurs generally is associated with or the result of a lack of sufficient blood supply to the heart in the case of a heart attack or lack of sufficient blood supply to the brain in the case of a stroke. One of the vital functions of blood is to act as the transport medium, by way of hemoglobin residing in the red cells that circulate in blood, to carry oxygen to the tissues where individual cells can utilize the oxygen for the purpose of aerobic respiration. Other important functions of blood include supplying the body's cells with nutrients, temperature regulation, water and electrolyte balance, and the removal of waste products such as carbon dioxide.

Oxygen becomes critical as demonstrated in the brain, where at a normal body temperature, brain cells cannot be without a sufficient supply of oxygen for more than five minutes before irreversible damage to brain cells begins to occur. Other tissues in the body, including heart cells, demonstrate a chronic need for a sufficient oxygen supply, and when there is not enough oxygen supplied to the tissues of the body, damage occurs to those cells. If a sufficient supply of oxygen is unable to reach cells in the body in a timely fashion, cells at a normal body temperature die for lack of being able to generate a sufficient amount of energy to sustain life.

Oxygen and glucose are two vital consumable elements that provide the viable cells in the body the raw materials to generate energy in the form of adenosine triphosphate (ATP). ATP is the common energy medium used throughout the cell, and in all cells of the body, to power the biologic processes that sustain life in the cell. Both oxygen and glucose are transported by the blood to the cells of the body. Inside the cell, glucose is transformed by the biologic process of glycolysis into pyruvate. To generate the maximum number of ATP molecules from the parent molecule glucose, pyruvate then is metabolized by the tricarboxylic acid cycle and oxidative phosporylation. Oxygen is vital participant in oxidative phosphorylation. When sufficient oxygen is available to the cell, by means of aerobic respiration one glucose molecule can yield 36 ATP molecules. In circumstances where an insufficient amount of oxygen is available to the cell, pyruvate is diverted to an anaerobic respiration process and is converted to lactic acid by the enzyme lactate dehydrogenase. The conversion of pyruvate to lactic acid yields 2 ATP molecules per glucose molecule.

A method of treatment to reduce damage to cells at times when there exists a state where a lack of sufficient aerobic respiration threatens the health of cells, such as a heart attack, stroke or diabetic crisis, is to optimize the overall respiration process or increase the anaerobic respiration process or provide an alternate means of supply the vital nutrients such as oxygen and glucose or the supply of energy molecules in the cells being threatened. The respiration process is comprised of a chain of biologic reactions that occur due to the presence of enzymes that catalyze the reactions. Increasing the number of available enzymes that would participate in the respiration process would help to maximize the utilization of glucose in cells.

For aerobic respiration dependent upon the presence of both oxygen and glucose, increasing only the number of enzymes would potentially force a utilization of all available oxygen and glucose inside the cell, but aerobic respiration would be time limited and would cease once the available oxygen was completely consumed. Two options to optimize cellular respiration inside cells that are threatened by a lack of sufficient oxygen supplied by blood are to increase the efficiency, therefore the output of the anaerobic respiratory process inside the threatened cell or provide an alternative means of supplying the cells with oxygen and glucose or energy molecules. Increasing the endangered cells' oxygen, glucose or other nutrients would enhance the cells' ability to produce the energy it needs to sustain life and increase the survivability and functionality of the cells. Supplying cells cut off from a supply of oxygenated blood with an alternative supply of energy molecules could sustain such threatened cells until the deficiency in the supply of oxygenated blood is corrected.

A method for optimizing the respiratory process inside cells would be to utilize configurable delivery devices as vehicles to transport necessary enzymes, nutrients such as oxygen and glucose molecules and even ATP energy molecules to cells threatened by a lack of oxygen during periods of crisis such as in the event of a heart attack, stroke or diabetic crisis.

The availability of oxygen and glucose to cells of the body has been thought to be one dimensional. In general, cells receive oxygen and glucose from the blood stream. Oxygen enters the body through the respiratory system. Glucose enters the body through the digestive systems. In time of a life-threatening crisis, oxygen is generally administered by nasal canula through the mouth and nose, or if an individual is intubated, oxygen is administered through the intubation tube. During a crisis, glucose can be infused directly into the blood stream through intravenous access to the body.

Life threatening difficulties occur at times when the respiratory system or the heart become dysfunctional, or the blood vessels dilate causing a collapse of the blood pressure. An individual suffering from severe respiratory dysfunction such as what might occur with a massive pulmonary embolism or a shower of embolisms or significant congestion in the lung spaces such as seen with heart failure or infection is not able to acquire oxygen from the air and diffuse this into the blood stream. An individual experiencing a heart attack or a dysfunctional cardiac rhythm may not be able to generate a sufficient enough cardiac output to sustain oxygen being delivered to the heart cells or other cells in the body. Toxins generated by sepsis can cause dilation of the blood vessels which can lead to a loss of vascular resistance which can cause a loss of effective blood circulation, which can result in a lack of sufficient oxygen reaching the cells of the body. In times of crisis, an alternative approach to delivering oxygen and/or glucose directly to critical tissues in an effort to save a life would be a significant advancement in emergency medicine.

As an example, an individual suffers a heart attack while visiting someone in the hospital. The individual collapses because during this heart attack the normal cardiac output of 65% generated by the heart drops to 10%. Some of the cardiac muscle tissues go into spasm due to a lack of oxygen. Only 10% of the volume of blood present in the heart is being pushed out of the heart by every contraction of the ventricular muscles of this victim. In the case of cardiac arrest, the pumping action of the heart muscles cease, the cardiac output goes to zero since the heart is no longer generating beats. Oxygen is a necessity for survival of any tissues. With the heart in cardiac arrest, and the pumping action of heart having ceased, the only cells being oxygenated are most likely the respiratory cells lining the lungs and the trachea. Since the lungs and the trachea cannot exist on their own, blood needs to start re-circulating within five minutes before sensitive tissues such as brain cells begin to suffer irreversible damage due to a lack of oxygen. Longer than five minutes, with the core temperature being normal, and the remainder of the body's tissues begin to become at risk of permanent damage and the body as a whole is at risk for dying.

Other than attempting to oxygenate and circulate blood through means such as administering emergency CPR to victims of a stroke or heart attack, there has been no other method to deliver oxygen and glucose to cells.

Configurable delivery devices could be harnessed at the time of a heart attack or stroke to deliver oxygen and nutrients directly to critical tissues. During a heart attack, a victim's heart could be oxygenated by inserting a needle through the chest wall and delivering a dose of virus-like transport devices that were configured to engage cardiac muscle cells and deliver directly to the distressed muscle cells the oxygen they need to survive. In the case of a stroke, configurable delivery devices could be used as an alternative means to deliver oxygen and nutrients to cerebral cells by being injected into the spinal fluid to access distressed cells in the brain.

Configurable delivery devices make contact with target cells by means of configurable exterior probes. Once the CDD's exterior probes engage the cell-surface receptors of target cells the CDD inserts into the target cells their payload of medically therapeutic protein molecules, nutrient molecules or energy molecules. Medical conditions such as heart attack, stroke, status epilepticus, and diabetic crisis are a result of inadequate aerobic respiration due to a lack of aerobic cellular respiration or proper glucose metabolism. Utilizing configurable delivery devices to transport oxygen, nutrients, energy molecules or medically therapeutic proteins to specific cells in the body, supports cells in the time of crisis to improve survivability and functionality of critical cells.

VII. Dual Vector Therapy:
Device Inside a Device

Systemic Lupus Erythematosus (SLE) is the showcase autoimmune disease. SLE is thought to be caused by a rouge antibody being mistakenly generated by the immune system's B-cells. This rouge antibody attacks normal body tissues with the same vigor as if the antibody was attacking and attempting to destroy an invading pathogen whether it be a virus, a bacteria or a parasite. To this point, this rogue antibody cannot be quantified from serum specimens in a manner useful for practitioners managing patients at the community level. The rouge antibodies of an SLE individual can be seen in certain tissue specimens utilizing a fluorescent microscope when the tissues have been properly stained with a fluorescing dye.

Fifty years ago an individual afflicted with SLE might have been diagnosed with the disorder by examining a bone marrow specimen. Occasionally examination of a bone marrow specimen in an individual with active SLE would demonstrate evidence of an LE cell. An LE cell was the product of one white cell having engulfed another white cell. Though rare to find, discovering an LE cell in the bone marrow or fluid harvested from the chest cavity or seen circulating in the blood was thought to be pathognomonic for the diagnosis of SLE.

The idea that an LE cell exists gives rise to the possibility of utilizing such a concept to create a configurable delivery device that would carry in its core a smaller configurable delivery device as the payload. By positioning one virus inside another virus, the innermost virus could be used to as a delivery device. Such an effort of placing a transport device inside a transport device is termed dual vector therapy.

Some of medicine's most challenging problems could be benefited by having one configurable delivery device carry a second smaller configurable delivery device as its payload to allow:

(1) delivery of select payloads directly to the nucleus or other organelles of a cell,

(2) breaching of the meninges to treat cerebral or spinal conditions, and

(3) delivery of antibiotics, antimetabolites or other medications to cells encapsulated inside a membrane structure such as an abscess.

An example of utilizing dual vector therapy would be to deliver a package of enzymes to the mitochondria inside a cell to bolster ATP production. Dual vector therapy could be utilized to treat various cerebral-spinal protein deficient disorders or make repairs to damaged brain or spinal cord tissues. Infections or cancer cells that have been encapsulated could be treated by utilizing dual vector therapy to insert antibiotics or antimetabolites directly into cells comprising the infection or into cancerous cells.

VIII. Conclusion

The effort described in this text is meant to forge a path from the current 'Whole Body Approach' to medical therapy to a 'Cell Specific Approach' of delivering medical therapies. Viruses provide not only naturally occurring examples of what a Cell Specific Approach can achieve, but nature also provides a variety of examples as to how such an approach can be constructed and manufactured. A Cell Specific Approach to delivering medical therapy reduces unwanted side effects of drugs by lowering the total effective dose required to achieve a meaningful clinical response and delivering the medical therapy directly to the cells that would benefit from such a therapy; shielding non-target cells from the effects of drugs.

Viruses are very efficient at delivering their genome to the host cell that will facilitate generation of copies of the original of viral virion. The efficiency of a virus to infect a host cell and complete its life-cycle has led to the survival of viruses over time. Viruses have a relatively high rate of mutation. Mutation suggests that a virus's payload is amendable to being altered. For purposes of this effort, we propose altering viral payloads, such that a virus-like transport device carries a medical therapy such that the device produces a beneficial effect, rather than being pathogenic by causing harm to individuals.

Cell-surface receptors detect either the presence of hormones, nutrients, various proteins, or the antithesis of the receptor, which often is referred to as a probe. Differing cell types express a unique set of cell-surface receptors. Therefore, specific sets of probes can be utilized to seek out specific cell types. The design and construction of <u>all</u> of the cell-surface receptors utilized in the human body must be stored in the human DNA. Since cells utilize cell-surface receptors for communication purposes, many cell-surface receptors would be useless without the existence of a corresponding probe. The design and construction of all of the cell-cell exterior probes that exist should be present either in human DNA or in viral DNAs.

As demonstrated by the behavior of viruses, a specific cell type can be targeted by mounting on the exterior of a virus the proper set of probes needed to detect and engage the target cell type. Mimicking nature, a configurable delivery device can be constructed to appear similar to the construct of a naturally occurring virus, but where the design deviates is that the surface probes are selected based off of the cell that the configurable delivery device is intended to target. Further, the payload of the configurable delivery device carries is tailored to the disease state the payload is intended to treat by having the payload delivered to a specific type of cell.

Messenger RNA are the protein producing templates of the cell. Deciphering the structure of the mRNA demonstrates three separate regions, each associated with a different role in the molecule's function. Alteration of the 5' region can improve recognition of the mRNA. Changing the coding region can produce protein molecules with enhanced attributes. Varying the 3' region leads to altering the service-life of the molecule, making it possible to vary the length of the survival time of exogenous mRNAs inserted into cells to meet the needs of medical therapy.

Packaging medical therapies inside a configurable vehicle that will transport the therapy directly to a specific cell type, makes a Cell Specific Approach to medical therapy a practical strategy.

Delivery of RNAs, DNAs, proteins, genetic material, chemicals, and nutrients to specific cell types opens up a broad range of new and innovative treatment strategies that can be harnessed to manage many common medical conditions, as well as control or cure many of the most challenging medical diseases.

Postscript 1:
Viruses:
The Workhorses of Evolution

This volume would not be complete without a more definitive description of the role viruses have played in forming life as we know it. The following emerged out of work we have been doing for a number of years. We were not looking to develop a new theory of evolution or even to augment a current one. Our efforts have been directed toward understand the DNA in support of our work to improve medical treatments.

Part of our research into ways to improve the global approach to medicine involved studying the way viruses change the DNA in cells. As this action became clearer, the story of how viruses operate became more intriguing. For example, literature sources tell us that viruses have been on the earth at least as long as life itself, that there are more viruses than forms of life, that viruses are not alive so they can remain dormant for long periods of time, that cells seem to accept and help them reproduce rather than trying to fight them, and that viruses have changed human DNA many times. Alone, these are very intriguing observations. Taken together, they are astounding. Questions such as *Is there a purpose to all of this?* began to arise.

As our investigations continued, a captivating story began to unfold. A story that leads to harmonization of current theories of Evolution rather than supporting one theory over another. One that points to viruses as the missing link: the driving force in the evolution of life. We provide the essence of the story as it unfolded so that readers can make up their own minds.

1. Background

Many theories exist as to how life came about on the earth. Hundreds of books have been written both for and against various theories. Some theories explain life using observations from fossils or from laboratory experiments. Others use information from inspirations, writings and logic. Still others use combinations of these sources. However, what is missing in these theories is the underlying means by which the changes have been made that have resulted in the observed evolution of the life forms. This missing link is critical not only to understanding evolution, but also to understanding how to change medicine to bring about a better life for all.

Our research led us to viruses and some interesting observations. While viruses are a relatively recent discovery, their effect on life forms is not. Our own genome has been changed not once, not 100 times, but more than 450,000 times by viruses[1]. Also changing is our understanding of them and what they can do for us. When originally discovered some 100 years ago, viruses were seen as a bad thing - something to be avoided. Recently, through efforts such as Gene Therapy, the good side of viruses has begun to emerge. Efforts continue in this direction; that is, to understand how can this once dreaded set of elements be used to improve our lives. Our objective in the books in the current series is to take the next step. For example, where Gene Therapy is directed toward replacing genes, our efforts are directed toward modifying the DNA itself so that it provides the RNA needed by specific cells, or to provide that RNA or

1 See for example Human Molecular Biology, Richard J. Epstein, Cambridge University Press, 2003.

other therapeutic material directly to the cells. In this, a detailed understanding of how viruses change cell operations becomes a critical element.

As noted above, we have been working to understand the DNA in support of our efforts to improve medical treatments. As we finished a previous book, *Immortality*,[2] which was written as novel, and began to dig into the DNA across a wide variety of forms of life, a number of questions kept arising. For example, how common are the DNAs of different forms of life? We observed that each species has its own unique DNA (else it would not be a unique species), and we wondered how that could occur. Did it simply happen or was there some rhyme or reason to the development?

The more we searched for answers, the more questions arose, such as:

- Is the order of life simply happenstance?
- What is common among all life forms?
- Are creativity and evolution really different theories?
- Could creativity and evolution be just different parts of the same process?
- Are more than genes provided at conception?
- Are not instructions needed to assemble and operate a life form?
- What changes the DNA?
- How easy is it for a virus to change a cell's DNA?

Genetic researchers have long known about genes that are passed from one generation to the next, and they have recently

2 Immortality, Anthony Scheiber, iUniverse, 2006.

identified the Genetic Code associated with the DNA that relates to the amino acids in proteins. However, at conception, the only thing provided to the new life form is the combined genome from its parents. True, the DNA provided contains the genes. That is, a definition of the parts from which the life form is to be made, but wouldn't the new life form need some assembly instructions? Would not instructions on how to operate different parts of the life form such as legs, arms, kidneys, and liver be required as well as instructions on how to operate all of the organs together in a manner to allow the body itself to function in the intended manner?

We also looked at the different processes that change DNA. Viruses seemed particularly interesting. We examined the Human Immunodeficiency Virus (HIV) and identified more than 14 steps in its replication process. This investigation raised questions as to how and why these steps were even possible. Yet HIV virus replication takes place.

Finally, after going back and forth with these questions, we realized that viruses were the link that answered our questions and brought the different theories of evolution together. We followed that with a considerable amount of analyses. The following contains the highlights of those investigations and discussions.

2. Introduction

We examine three of the theories: the Bible, Darwin's Theory of Evolution, and Intelligent Design. We also look at how a species is defined and to see what fossils tell us.

From Genesis in the Bible[3] we read that God created vegetation on Day 3, fish and birds on Day 5 and animals and humans on Day 6.

---

3 Although many versions of the Bible are available, the bottom line on creation, as presented here, remains the same.

Around the early to middle 1800s, the understanding that offsprings have features in common with their parents began to improve, and concepts emerged as to how life developed on earth. In 1859 Charles Darwin, with the publication of his book *On the Origin of Species*,[4] furthered the understanding of evolutionary biology. Basically his premise is that forms of life change physically because their physical characteristics change in a random way and that natural selection decides which of these changes survive and are passed on to the next generation. Gregor Mendel's work with plants helped to explain hereditary patterns of genetics, which led to an understanding of the mechanisms of inheritance. Ernst Mayr introduced the biological species concept, in which he defined a species as a population or group of populations whose members have the potential to interbreed naturally with one another to produce viable, fertile offsprings. Further, the members of a species cannot produce viable, fertile offsprings with members of other species. That is, members of a species are reproductively isolated from all other species.

George Gaylord Simpson helped to develop the field of fossil research. The study of fossils supports the idea that all living organisms are related. Fossils provide evidence that accumulated changes in organisms over long periods of time have led to the diverse forms of life we see today. A fossil itself reveals the organism's structure and the relationships between present and extinct species. This helped researchers to construct a family tree for most of the life's forms that exist or have existed on earth. And many others have contributed to this growing field.

The theory of Intelligent Design holds that certain features of living things are best explained by an intelligent cause, not an undirected process such as natural selection. According to this theory, one can, through a study and analysis of a system's components, determine whether various natural

---

4 See for example http://www.talkorigins.org/faqs/origin.html

structures are the product of chance, natural law, intelligent design, or some combination thereof. The scientific methods of intelligent design have been applied to many areas including the designs in irreducibly complex biological structures, the complex and specified informational content contained in DNA, the life-sustaining physical architecture of the universe, and the geologically rapid origin of biological diversity in the fossil record during the Cambrian explosion approximately 530 million years ago.[5]

Much work has gone into attempting to merge these as well as other individual ideas into a cohesive understanding of evolutionary theory. For example, efforts have been made to merge Darwin's theory of natural selection, research in heredity, and observations from fossils into a unified explanatory model. But, as we will see in the next section, there are problems with this approach. Perhaps the sum total of all of these theories is still simply a part of the theory of evolution.

3. Issues with the Current Theories of Evolution

Most current theories of evolution contain a common element: that all forms of life stem from the same ancestor. Some indicate that given the right set of circumstances and enough time, evolution leads to the emergence of new species. Furthermore, while mutations from parent to child are to a degree random, natural selection is not. That is, the outcome of natural selection is simply a form of life that can survive better and reproduce more successfully than other forms in the current environment. Thus, the evolutionary process is an inevitable result of imperfect copying by self-replicating organisms that reproduce over many years under the selective pressure of the environment. However, there are a number of issues with these concepts. We will describe seven: gaps in the fossils, lack of continuous evolution, anticipation in evolution, the Cambrian

---

5 More on Intelligent Design can be found in websites such as http://www. intelligentdesign.org/

Explosion, simultaneous worldwide changes, the role of DNA, and the effect of random changes on DNA.

Gaps in the Fossils

Darwin points out gaps in the fossils in chapter 9 of his book, *The Origin of Species*: "But just in proportion as this process of extermination has acted on an enormous scale, so must the number of intermediate varieties, which have formerly existed on the earth, be truly enormous. Why then is not every geological formation and every stratum full of such intermediate links? Geology assuredly does not reveal any such finely graduated organic chain; and this, perhaps, is the most obvious and gravest objection which can be urged against my theory. The explanation lies, as I believe, in the extreme imperfection of the geological record."

What Darwin is saying is that the fossil evidence should show many gradual changes, with one species slowly evolving into the next. In fact, it should be difficult to tell where one species ends and another begins. But that's not what he saw in the fossils available to him.

Darwin, of course, attributed this problem to the imperfection of the fossil evidence. Specifically it was an emerging area, and few fossils had been discovered and examined. He believed that, as the discipline matured and as scientists found more fossils, the gaps would slowly start to fill in.

But that is not what has happened. Paleontologists, those who use fossils to study prehistoric life, have certainly found more fossils, but these fossils have only deepened the problem. As fossils piled up, what paleontologists discovered is not the gradual changes Darwin expected, but stability with, in some cases, sudden appearance followed by equally sudden disappearances. It seems that most fossils representing a species appear all at once, with the species fully formed, and the species changes very little throughout their stay as recorded in the fossil evidence.

Lack of Continuous Evolution

If random events provide the options for natural selection as some theories promote, why do these options not continue today? That is, as we shall describe shortly, if fish came out of the sea and evolved into land animals, why do we not see that same process happening today? Why did Professor Neil Shubin,[6] as described later, need to find a 375-million-year-old half-fish half-animal fossil to show that this was the path to substantiating today's evolutionary theory? If evolution is just the result of random processes and natural selection, why do we not see this happening over and over again throughout the years? Why are we not inundated with fossils of creatures that are part fish and part animal? Something ended that step in the evolutionary process. Given that this same phenomenon seems to have happened to at least most steps in the evolutionary process, as shown by the current state of evolution as well as the fossils, the idea arises of something or someone exercising control over the evolutionary process.

Anticipation in Evolution

Fossils provide a very interesting story of evolution. However, what is missing from the fossils may be as interesting as what is contained in them. Again, we use Professor Shubin's half-fish half-animal creature. What is curious here is that the front part of the creature, the animal half, has on each side of its body,

6 See Your Inner Fish by Neil Shubin, Vintage Books Division of Random House, Inc., 2009.

bone structure corresponding to an arm: upper arm, forearm, wrist elements, and joints. As reported, these elements are very similar to what we see in some animals today. Furthermore, Professor Shubin didn't find 100 or 20 or even 2 fossils with different attempts by nature to get the structure of the arm correct as would be expected with a random process. Finding a 375-million-year-old fossil showing the transition from fish to animal is certainly an extraordinary achievement. But, if this is a random process, one would expect that many fossils are out there showing the results of these attempts. However, that is not what was found. What was found was one containing the bone structure that we see in some animals today. This seems to be more than remarkable. It certainly seems to be more than a random result. It seems to be more the anticipation of the next step in the evolution of this species and certainly begs the question of what would prompt nature to anticipate the next step?

Another way to look at this anticipation is to consider the process itself. That is, consider that some random event started evolution in this direction. Narrow it to only those steps necessary to evolve the front fins of the fish into arms. What Professor Shubin's drawing of the fossil Tiktaalik tends to show is the fish's front fins disappeared and arms began to appear. Consider the many generations of this fish type required to carry out this step. During these years, wouldn't it certainly be harder for the fish to swim, gather food, and mate? This seems counter to the concept of natural selection. On the other hand, the fossil indicates that it did happen. So, asking the question in a different way, what could drive a series of fish to overcome such hardships to permit them to be able to move about on land, a distinctly different environment of which they had no knowledge, given they grew up in the sea?

The Cambrian Explosion

Another problem is the Cambrian Explosion, a period about 545 million years ago when most major animal groups appear for the first time in the fossil records.

The theory of the Cambrian Explosion, as described by the Virtual Fossil Museum,[7] states that "beginning some 545 million years ago, an explosion of diversity led to the appearance over a relatively short period of 5 million to 10 million years of a huge number of complex, multi-celled organisms. Moreover, this burst of animal forms led to most of the major animal groups known today, that is, every extant Phylum.[8] It is also postulated that many forms that would rightfully deserve the rank of Phylum both appeared in the Cambrian only to rapidly disappear. Natural selection is generally believed to have favored larger size, and consequently the need for hard skeletons to provide structural support - hence, the Cambrian gave rise to the first shelled animals and animals with exoskeletons.[9]"

As one can see, such a sudden appearance of such a large number of new, complex, multi-celled organisms is totally counter to Darwin's theory. This raises the question: what kind of process or driving force could have brought this about?

Simultaneous Worldwide Changes

Darwin's observation in chapter 10 of his book in which he wrote,[10] "Scarcely any paleontological discovery is more striking than the fact, that the forms of life change almost simultaneously throughout the world." This is followed by "These observations,

7 http://www.fossilmuseum.net/Paleobiology/CambrianExplosion.htm

8 Author's note: A phylum is division within a kingdom of life. For example, see http://en.wikipedia.org/wiki/Phylum.

9 Author's note: An external skeleton that supports and protects the animal's body.

10 See for example chapter 10 of the book at www.talkorigins.org/faqs/origin/chapter10.html

however, relate to the marine inhabitants of distant parts of the world".

He further wrote "Thus, as it seems to me, the parallel, and, taken in a large sense, simultaneous, succession of the same forms of life throughout the world, accords well with the principle of new species having been formed by dominant species spreading widely and varying; the new species thus produced being themselves dominant owing to inheritance, and to having already had some advantage over their parents or over other species; these again spreading, varying, and producing new species. The forms which are beaten and which yield their places to the new and victorious forms, will generally be allied in groups, from inheriting some inferiority in common; and therefore as new and improved groups spread throughout the world, old groups will disappear from the world; and the succession of forms in both ways will everywhere tend to correspond. "

Having the same change occur "almost simultaneously" around the world would indicate a global power at work, especially since Darwin is referring to ancient times in which travel was extremely limited except for water and air movements. Thus, it would seem that we are looking for a means that is able to change the DNA and that can travel by water or air.

The Role of DNA

As already noted, each species has its own unique DNA. Thus, to create a new form of life requires a new DNA or at least a significant modification of an existing one.[11] Even a small modification of a species' physical character requires more than a simple modification of the DNA. Take the addition of a simple appendage such as a fin to a species that does not have

11 For the moment we are setting aside the possibility that everything required to produce all of the species has been in the genome from the beginning of life itself.

fins. The attachment would need to be made in such a way as to give it the ability to move and the muscles necessary to provide it that motion. Signal paths would be needed from the brain to the muscles so the appropriate elements in the brain can direct its movement. The brain would need to be aware that the fin existed so that it could be used; that is, sensors (nerves) on the fin would need to exist to indicate its position and motion, and to sense pain, heat, and cold. A blood supply would need to be set up and the heart, arteries, and veins would need to be enlarged to carry the extra blood supply. The covering of the fin would need to be identified along with its color so that it blends in with other parts of the species. All of this cannot be left to a random process. It requires a skillful design and development process that would come prior to the natural selection process, which is a testing period.

According to information from the fossils, humans have been around for more than 160,000 years and, to some degree, for more that 4.4 million years given some of the features of 'Lucy'[12] and Ardi.[13] It is interesting to note that the basic human structure and features have not changed very much – externally or internally – for a very long period of time. Further, from the available fossil information, no new species have been generated or emerged from the human race.[14] Fossil evidence does not even seem to suggest attempts to alter the basic structure. What has happened are small tweaks such as the alteration of the CD4 cell-surface receptor on the T-Helper cell of some humans that apparently helped them avoid the bubonic plague in the 14th century and that seems to have made them immune to HIV. However, the assemblage of these tweaks does not make a new species. Both the Bible and fossil

---

12 See for example, "What Was "Lucy"? Fast Facts on an Early Human Ancestor" at http://news.nationalgeographic.com/news/2006/09/060920-lucy.html

13 See for example the 2 October 2009 issue of Science or http://sciencenow.sciencemag.org/cgi/content/full/2009/1001/1

14 Other new species seem to continue to form, but not at the rate seen in the Cambrian Explosion period.

studies end with the creation of humans. In that the theories seem to agree.

In chapter 10 of his book, Darwin wrote "After referring to the parallelism of the Paleozoic forms of life in various parts of Europe, they[15] add, `If struck by this strange sequence, we turn our attention to North America, and there discover a series of analogous phenomena, it will appear certain that all these modifications of species, their extinction, and the introduction of new ones, cannot be owing to mere changes in marine currents or other causes more or less local and temporary, but depend on general laws which govern the whole animal kingdom'". What he might have been referring to here as "general laws" is the master plan for building life forms that is contained in DNA of the species.

Darwin was at a disadvantage because, although DNA was first noticed by Friedrich Miescher in 1869, its connection to genetics and inheritance was not understood until it was observed by Oswald Avery in 1944 and confirmed by Alfred Hershey and Martha Chase in 1952. Thus, Darwin was observing the results of a process that he did not know existed. This caused him to incorrectly suggest that all of the mutations a species might undergo were the result of a random process. If he had the opportunity to understand the vastness and complexity of DNA and that many areas of DNA would have to be modified correctly to provide any significant change to the structure of a species, he would have realized that no random process would be able to produce the changes to the species that were observed in the fossils. Furthermore, such random changes would have shown up in the fossils, and they do not. Thus, this would seem to require a process that changes DNA in a more directed way.

In addition, given the billons of human forms that have been brought to life during this period and the incredible likeness

---

15 The 'they' he is referring to here are MM. de Verneuil and d'Archiac.

that one has to another from outward appearance all the way down to the structure and operation of individual cells, a master plan must exist - some form of a table of traits and a set of instructions on how to build and operate such a complex mechanism. For example, at conception the new form of life is only given a genome. That genome contains two strands of DNA, one from the father and one from the mother. The DNA strands contain the code for the genes that are to be used to build the new form. Since the genes of the mother and father may differ somewhat (for example in eye color), there may be a degree of randomization as to which gene is used by the child: the mother's or the father's. However, it certainly is a considerable stretch of one's imagination to visualize a major change in the new life's characterization coming about due to this random process. That is, if the genes provided to the new life do not contain fins, how would the new life develop fins? As noted above from Mayr, members of one species cannot produce viable, fertile offsprings with members of another species. So interspecies relationships cannot be the driving force behind the development of a new species. Thus, a new explanation is required.

Effect of Random Changes to DNA

The cells contain a sophisticated capability to repair DNA damage from mistakes in replication and environmental effects. Even so DNA mutations occur at an average rate of one base pair per 10^9 to 10^{10} base pairs per generation over all organisms.[16] Thus, humans with a DNA of about 3×10^9 base pairs would have an expected mutation rate of about one base pair per generation. Using 20 years as the length of a generation would lead to about 50,000 changes every million years. A number of that size would certainly be ample to make major changes to the species if it was not for the fact that these are random events. That is, they occur at unconnected random

---

16 Cells, Benjamin Lewin, et al., Jones and Bartlett Publishers, 2007.

points along the DNA. On the other hand, to make a major change in a species, it would be necessary to change not one but a sequence of contiguous base pairs.

Since human DNA has 3×10^9 base pairs and an expected mutation rate of about one base pair per 20 years, 3×10^9 changes would take about 60×10^9 (60 billion) years. To get a particular base pair changed by a truly random process would only take about one-half of that time or 30×10^9 years. On the other hand, a base pair in our DNA has four rather than two states so in a human it would be expected to take even longer for a selected base pair to be switched to the desired state. However, the earth has only existed for about 4.5×10^9 years with life starting about 4×10^9 years ago[17]. Clearly, the probability of random events creating a new species would appear to be virtually zero given the thousands of specific base pairs that would need to be set to specific states to create that species. Thus, this is not a viable concept for how life evolved on earth. [18]

4. What Fossils Tell Us

The fossil information provides a profound stabilizing effect. Diagrams and sequences are everywhere.[19] Authors use fossils to show when certain events happened and how one species evolved into another. Darwin used them in his discussions as noted above.

We are particularly taken by the precision of the fossil information and admire Professor Shubin's efforts as reported in his book *Your Inner Fish*.[20] Professor Shubin reports that he and a colleague spent years searching for a fossil that would

17 See for example, Timeline of Evolution at http://en.wikipedia.org/wiki/Timeline_of_evolution
18 For more on this, see, for example, chapter 6 in The Edge of Evolution by Dr. Michael J. Behe, Free Press, 2007.
19 See for example the "Timeline of Evolution" in Wikipedia.
20 Vintage Books Division of Random House, Inc., 2009

confirm the transition of fish to animals. They knew the date that this particular evolution was thought to have taken place – 375 million years ago – and thus, they knew the date of the fossil for which they were looking. They used this information to pinpoint the best place on earth to search for such a fossil. After six summers they were rewarded by actually finding a fossil of such a fish/animal, which they named Tiktaalik. As described in the book, it has a flat head with two eyes which look forward and its head is free to move independently of its shoulder whereas a fish has an oval head with eyes on each side and the head is fixed to the shoulder. The rear part of Tiktaalik resembles a fish with fins and scales.

What this find shows is the utter precision with which fossils describe how life has evolved on earth. What is disturbing to us is why all of this evolution seems to have happened only once. The fact that Professor Shubin and his colleague were able to determine the timeframe during which the fish-to-animal step in the evolution occurred and then find from that time period a fossil that shows that the transition took place is nothing short of remarkable. The fact that the evolutionary step occurred around 365 million years ago makes the feat astounding.

However, as outstanding as this find was, it is not the fossil that grabs our attention. It is that this step in the evolutionary process stopped, according to the literature, about the same time - 365 million years ago. Why did it stop? Why don't we see this same stage of evolution occurring over the next 10-million-year period, and the next, and the next? Certainly the relatives of the fish that began all of this do not know that this step has taken place. This is not only a question about Professor Shubin's fish, but also for many other individual events in evolution. As pointed out by many researchers who use fossils in their studies, a certain change begins, lasts for a number of years, and then seems to end, some rather abruptly. It would seem that some would continue occurring, but the fossil records do not show this, at least not in the significant way one would expect. Something must stop the changes. That is, once a leg, arm, lungs, or fingers have evolved, there is no need to continue and so that part of the evolutionary process is stopped. But by what means is it stopped? Fossils show us this evolutionary process occurs step by step. Once a step is completed, nature does not repeat it. Our question is Why? How does nature know it's done? What tells the evolutionary process to move on to the next step?

In the natural selection process, random or pseudo-random events generate options that are then evaluated to determine which best support the needs of the evolving species. Could it be that the particular random events that developed each step in evolution are so rare that they only occurred for a period of time? This may be true for some of the steps, but given the large number of steps that evolution has taken and the enormous amount of time over which the process has occurred, it certainly does not answer the question for most of the steps. Fossils show us that the results of the evolutionary process are too precise and too structured for random processes alone to have been the driving force behind it. Something more definitive must be initiating and ending these steps, at least most of them, or we would see them showing up in multiple timeframes, or perhaps virtually continuously, in the fossils.

5. Macroevolution vs. Microevolution

To understand what is happening here, we need to go back to Darwin's original premise: the mutations or changes we see in a species come from the imperfect copying of genes as they are passed from parents to the child. Darwin saw this as a random process, with natural selection deciding which changes survive.

Let us first look at natural selection, which, simply put, is that a life form that can survive better and reproduce more successfully than other forms in a particular environment has a better chance to pass on its genes. This process is driven by the choices given to the new life form and the environment in which it finds itself. This part of Darwin's theory is observable and certainly seems to have proven to be correct.

The other part of his theory, that of how these choices or mutations come about, is a bit harder to understand. There are, in fact, observable mutations. However, what he was not able to see is that, at conception, the only thing given to the new life form is the genome from its parents. While genes do mutate, the fact remains that if a gene does not exist in the DNA that was passed on, it cannot appear in the new life form. What Darwin was seeing was microevolution, like humans growing taller, etc. That is, changes within a species, not the type of changes to a species that develop a new species.

To change one species into another, macroevolution requires, as described above, some very complex changes to the original species' DNA. The absence of fossils would indicate that this is not the result of a random process. If it was, we would see all sorts of spurious changes as the random process was taking place. Even if the random process achieved its destiny it wouldn't know this and would continue to make random changes that would certainly take away from the harmony we see in the tree of species. Fossils indicate that evolutionary steps start, continue for a while, and then stop. They don't continue without end.

The gaps in the fossils and the growing information about them seem to indicate that things definitely happened at certain points in time. This is certainly supported by the large amount of new forms of life that appeared in the period referred to as the Cambrian Explosion.

6. The Missing Link

The theories of evolution certainly have their commonalities. What is missing from each of them is the means or mechanism that caused the changes to come about and move the species from one step to the next. Perhaps if this was better understood the different theories would not appear as different. Perhaps this is the missing link that will bring the different theories into harmony. By missing link we mean a missing element in the theories of evolution as opposed to a missing species or step in the chain that leads to a species such as humans. In this section we use the terms link and element interchangeably. What then is the missing link? What does it do? What are its characteristics? What does it look like? As a first step, let's review the material under Issues.

1. The fossils show that different steps in evolution occurred during specific periods of time. More specifically, the steps appear to start, evolve over a period of time, and then stop. Furthermore, in general, they do not reappear. That is, once a step has been taken, it does not continue to happen, so the missing element must be able to turn a step on and later turn it off. The element must be such that it can prevent that step from occurring again in the future.

2. The gaps in the fossils show that the element must be able to bring into being a new species in a very short period of time. And while we are on the subject of what fossils have shown, it seems that the element must be able to terminate or make extinct a species in a short period of time as well.

3. To be consistent with the Cambrian Explosion period, we see that the element would not only need to be able to act swiftly, in biological time, but it would also need to be able to act on many different species at the same or nearly the same time.

4. From Darwin's observation of simultaneous worldwide changes, we see that the element would need to be transportable by air or water.

5. From the role of DNA, we see that the element would need to be able to make significant changes to the DNA of different life forms.

6. And, from anticipation in evolution, we see that the element must be controllable in the sense that it can be applied according to some plan, scheme, criteria, or wishes of the designer.

That is quite a tall order for a single element. But perhaps there is more than one element.

There is in fact a type of biological element that has existed in nature at least as long as life itself, that can do all of the above. It has many configurations but basically consists of a lipid shell in which it carries its genome. On the outer surface of the shell are probes that can be used to attach the shell to a cell. It is not a living entity. It requires no energy or maintenance, so it can endure in a dormant state for very long periods of time. It can also *act* over extended periods of time. It can *act* swiftly and decisively. Some versions can travel by air and some by water. It is able to use the DNA or RNA that it carries inside its shell to modify the DNA of a cell to which it becomes attached. The element is called a virus.

In the past, viruses have been associated with bad deeds. HIV is an example of a bad virus. However, recently viruses have been shown to have a good side. Viruses are controllable in the sense that the probes they carry on their outside surfaces define the cells to which they can attach and the material they carry inside their shells determine what actions they will attempt once they have attached to their target cell. The size of the virus population is vast because more types of viruses exist than there are forms of life. The extent of the capabilities of this population is yet to be determined as the genomes of only a few have been subjected to any analyses.

Why didn't Darwin see this? Two reasons: first, as noted above, although the DNA was isolated in 1869, 10 years after Darwin published his book, its connection to genetics and inheritance was not understood until 1944. Second, Darwin could not have known about viruses as the first one was not discovered until Dmitri Iwanowsk observed the mosaic tobacco virus in 1892. Although the literature seems void on who discovered that viruses can change the DNA of cells, it obviously would not have received the attention of those studying evolution until after the observations by Avery in 1944.

7. Directed Evolution

As one looks at the universe, our solar system, life on earth, our own bodies, the cells within our bodies and their operations, and the DNA within those cells, one sees an incredible amount of very complex structures, each of which operate in an equally complex way. The precision of these structures and their operations have the attributes of a rather well-laid-out plan. For example, the dependency of lower structures on elements of the upper structures. A cell in the body cannot carry out its function without the body. On the other hand, the upper levels are somewhat dependant on the lower levels. For example, if cells fail, the body may not be able to operate as intended. If sufficient cells fail, the body will cease to operate at all.

Life on earth cannot exist without the sun. If the earth was upright rather than tilted 23.5 degree off the perpendicular to its plane of rotation around the sun, we would have no seasons. If our planet did not spin, but kept a fixed direction to the sun like our moon's relationship to our earth, one side of the earth would always be hot and in daylight while the other side would be cold and dark.

The atmosphere that surrounds our earth contains greenhouse gases, e.g., carbon dioxide, to keep the earth warm and an ozone layer to protect its inhabitants from harmful radiation. If it had a somewhat high concentration of carbon dioxide in its atmosphere, for example like that of Venus, its temperatures would be too high for life as we know it, because heat would get in, but could not get out. Partly because of this, Venus' surface temperature averages 882 °F. If, on the other hand, it had no atmosphere, its surface temperature would vary greatly depending on whether or not the surface faced the sun. For example, the surface temperature of Mercury, which has no atmosphere, varies between -280 and +800 °F.[21]

The earth's oceans help to absorb and retain the sun's heat and energy. Its winds and ocean currents help distribute this heat around the globe. Earth is unique in its ability to maintain sustainable living conditions for its inhabitants because all of its systems and influences are connected to each other, from its atmosphere to its oceans and land, to its seasons, its living inhabitants, and the sun.

In summary, the world we live in, how we live, how our bodies are constructed, and how they function are not the results of random events. Too much design and too much interdependence are evident. For example, when a new life form is created by changing the DNA of a current life form, it follows that this new life must contain a new master plan with the command and control to carry it out. This plan defines how the new life form reproduces, grows, operates, is maintained, and interoperates with its environment for, as we have already seen, without such a plan, and the command and control structures to carry it out, reproduction, growth, operation and maintenance of a life form as well as its interaction with its environment would be chaotic. Currents forms of life do not support that and neither do the fossils.

---

21 Additional information can be found in "The Tilting of the Earth: Shaping Our Seasons and Climates" at http://ecology.com/features/tiltingearth/

Further, it seems that there must be at least two master plans; one at the species level and one at the global level. From above, the master plan for a species must be carried in its DNA. There must be sub plans as well. For example, at least one for each type of cell otherwise they would all operate the same.

We believe that viruses are the key element in bringing about new forms of life. They are the only element that can add to, modify, and/or replace the DNA in non-random, meaningful ways. The modifications do not have to be done all at once; viruses can support gradual evolution. They can turn steps on and off. They can be used to prepare forms of life for new tasks such as getting fish ready to walk on land. When first seen, and for many years thereafter, viruses were thought of as bad elements. However, recently they have been shown to have the potential to do good deeds as well as bad.

A virus is not a living entity. It requires no energy or other support to remain able to carry out its task. It can exist and act over long periods of time. It needs only to be transported from its current location into the structure (body) of a life form. This life form must have the type of cells into which the virus is able to enter and deposit its genome with the general intent of using the cell as a host to replicate the virus.

More types of viruses exist than forms of life. In addition, since the different species share major portions of the DNA, a single virus could potentially change the DNA of many forms of life. Once the DNA of a life form has been adequately changed, the master plan and associated command and control can carry out the functions necessary to reproduce, grow, operate, and maintain that new life form.

The master plan of what things exist, how they interact, what changes are to be made to which forms of life, along with the design and development of the viruses to carry out that master plan are the work of the Creator, who directs the evolution.

8. Virus Cell Interactions

We did not start out to show limitations in existing theories of evolution - quite the opposite. We were studying the operation of the T-Helper cell and the effect of HIV on that operation. As one can easily see, a great deal of information is available on the subject. However, we were greatly troubled by some of the observations about which we read. Specifically, the cell helps, or at least does not resist, the virus changing its DNA. That seemed counter to what we expected. That is, the DNA is the crown jewel of the life form. It specifies everything about that form of life as we have described above. To change it means the life form changes. It could even be killed by the virus. Most forms of life struggle to live, adapting where necessary. The T-Helper cells are part of the human body's immune system, which attempts to keep the body clear of foreign substances. We expected a similar response from the T-Helper cell itself. Instead we found quite the opposite.

In our efforts to understand the effect of HIV on the T-Helper cell's operation, we defined more than 14 steps in the process whereby HIV uses the T-Helper cell as a host for its replication. These steps involve the entrance of the HIV virion and associated molecular structures into the cell's cytoplasm, the transformation of the HIV's RNA into its DNA, the transportation of that DNA to the cell's nucleus where the cell's DNA is kept, the entrance of the HIV DNA into the cell's nucleus and the insertion of the HIV's DNA into the cell's DNA. To us it seemed quite irregular for the cell, which maintains the body's jewels in a specially protected site, to allow a foreign substance into its cytoplasm, let alone into its nucleus where the jewels are kept, and completely absurd to allow this foreign substance to be integrated into its jewels without knowing what changes this foreign substance would make in the cell's operation.

Even worse, the genome carried by the HIV virus does not contain all of the necessary elements to manufacture more HIV viruses. The T-Helper cell not only provides these additional resources, it joins in the process of producing the new HIV viruses generally to the extent of its own demise.

The only reasonable explanation for this seemingly bizarre operation seems to be that the cell was not only expecting the foreign substance, but was expecting it to be integrated into its DNA because that is the way changes have been brought about since the beginning of time. Furthermore, since in the past some changes have been positive (e.g., contributed to the evolution of the life form) and some have been detrimental (e.g., lead to the extinction of the life form), it is not the cell's function to determine what changes the virus' DNA will bring about in the cell's operation, but to allow it to happen. That is, cells have been designed in such a way that viruses can be used to modify their operations. If this were not true, cells would have, at some period in their many millions of years of evolution, developed a means of preventing outside forces, especially foreign substances, from changing their jewels and preventing the cell from continuing to operate in its originally intended manner.

Furthermore, viruses have been around since life itself. There have been in the order of 10 times the number of viruses as there have been life forms.[22] Viruses have been changing our DNA, as well as the DNA of all life forms, for a long time – a very long time. In his book *Human Molecular Biology*,[23] Richard Epstein informs us that the current human genome contains remnants of 450,000 viruses. That is, over the years, our DNA has been modified by at least 450,000 different retroviruses.[24] Some believe that our DNA is more that 50% viral.[25] Another

---

22 Research in Microbiology 154; 245-251, Ackerman, 2003

23 Human Molecular Biology, Richard j. Epstein, Cambridge University Press, 2003.

24 See also Modern Genetic Analyses, Anthony J. F. Griffiths et al., Figure 9-25, W. H. Freeman, 2002.

25 See, for example, Tiny Specks of Misery, both Vile and Useful, New Your Times, 1/8/2008.

recent publication[26] informs us that viruses infect all living things and that most RNA viruses (viruses that carry their genome in RNA form rather that DNA form) can cross species boundaries. The example given is that hosts for the West Nile virus include birds, horses, and humans.

Another point to consider is virus mutation. One might ask how this comes about. The answer is somewhat startling: the viruses are using the machinery of the host cell to mutate. The only place the virus has to modify its DNA or RNA is inside the host cell, so the viruses are using the cell not only to replicate but also to mutate.[27] In addition, if more than one virus infects a single cell, their genes may become intermingled in a process referred to as "reassortment". The result is a new virus - one with a genome consisting of parts from the other or parent viruses. The strain of H1N1 now circulating is an example.

Given that viruses do enter the body and the cells and change the cell's DNA, how do those changes get passed on to the next generation? We will examine this in the next section.

9. How Viruses Can Generate New Species

From the last section we know that viruses have changed our DNA at least 450,000 times. However, viruses have changed the human genome many more times than that. This is because we have two levels of DNA: current and future. The current level is what is being used to develop and maintain one's body. Viruses like HIV, as discussed above, change the current DNA in T-Helper cells. However, that change only affects one's T-Helper cells; it does not get passed on to the next generation. Changes to working cells,[28] like those in one's immune system, do not get passed on. To be transferred to the next generation,

---

26 Principles of Virology, S. J. Flint, et al., ASM Press, 2009.
27 Here we do not distinguish between cause and effect.
28 By this we mean one's non-sperm cells.

the change must be made in or imported into the offsprings. There are a number of ways that this might happen. Consider the following.

A virus could attack the eggs the female carries. This would ensure that the modified genome was provided to all of her offsprings born following the virus attack. Since females in the human species acquire all of their eggs during fetus development, this presents a very significant opportunity for the virus to make changes - both good and bad. That is, if the virus invaded all of the females in a species at a particular point in time, all of the next generation would have the modified genome. On the other hand, if the virus made the eggs infertile, there would be no next generation. Perhaps this gives a clue as to why the female gets all of her eggs at once. Perhaps she is an evolution control point.

In bringing about changes to a species, three conditions stand out in favor of viruses. First, they have been around for a long time so the time limits noted above would seem to provide little if any barrier to their operation. Second, with the time that history tells us was available for evolution, there is no need to focus on a single virus. Indeed, the development of a new form of a species was probably done by a series of viruses over a significant period of time. This seems to be a very reasonable given that there have been more types of viruses than forms of life and that they have existed on earth for a longer period of time. Third, a virus can do its work covertly. That is, it could change the DNA in one's sex cells in such a way that it would not be noticed until the next generation begins to appear. At that point, who would think that an unknown virus did it? Certainly, no one before Avery's observation in 1944.

10. The Integrated Theory

Let us now look at how the different individual theories might fit together into an integrated one. In the above we presented two main thoughts that can be characterized as Command and Control, and Virus-based Evolution. Let's review them and see how they fit in with existing theories.

Command and Control

As noted earlier, the operation of a cell cannot survive without some sort of command and control. Without it a cell would be overproducing one type of protein while under producing another, resulting in chaos. If production is not kept within certain ranges, the cell cannot operate at the intended level. Severe underproduction or overproduction can lead to failure of the cell's operation and cause its death. Furthermore, command and control at the cell level implies the ability to identify each protein as well as the RNA that is used to manufacture it. It also implies that, within each cell, a command and control process keeps the cell working toward its intended objective. This process indicates that a plan exists.

One also notes many features that indicate command and control at work at the body level. At conception, the new life form only receives a genome containing two strands of DNA: one from the mother and one from the father. From this DNA, a new member of the species is formed, and all of the functions necessary to operate it are developed and put into operation. These functions include not only those associated with every cell type, but also those required to integrate the cells into body functions such as those of the heart, liver, eyes, and brain and those needed to connect organs together in such a way that the body operates as a whole.

As the embryo grows to its adult state, it passes through many stages. The steps associated with these stages are not random events, but are highly orchestrated and necessitate significant coordination from the cellular level to the skin that covers the body. So the genome given at conception must contain a master plan - a set of instructions by which to build and operate the new life form. Since the DNA of life forms which have similar characteristics, are very much the same, the master plan associated with each may be much the same with a Table of Traits defining the specifics of how each of what we view as characteristics is to be built and operated. For example, a human has two arms that have specific joints along with elements like muscles, which give rise to its operation. The arms are mirror images of each other all the way down to the bones, joints, muscles, blood flow, etc. These are not random occurrences, but highly orchestrated developmental and operational processes. Since the new life is only given a genome at conception, instructions to build, operate, and maintain it must be contained within the genome.

Virus-based Evolution

A species is defined by its DNA. A new species requires a new DNA, although much of it may be the same as that in one or more other species. The only biological entity that can change an existing DNA in a meaningful way is a virus. The process of changing the DNA can be very slow with many steps taken over a long period of time or it can be rather abrupt. However it is done, it needs to be done with great care and foresight because DNA is an extremely complex and highly coordinated set of instructions. It's certainly not the type of process that could be changed in any random way and still produce a functional life form.

From the above it should be evident that the concept here is not yet another theory of evolution, but rather the description of a means by which each of the existing theories could have been brought about. In that regard, it is a harmonization theory. As described in the following, this concept provides the connections whereby the existing theories can be looked upon as parts of a larger theory. In this discussion we will describe the connections to Darwin's Theory, to the Theory of Creativity, and to the Theory of Intelligent Design.

Darwin's Theory seems to be consistent with the changes that occur over time within a species. The difficulty arises when it is applied to the creation of a new species in that it suffers from a number of problems including gaps in the fossil evidence, speed of development (as in the Cambrian Explosion period), the worldwide simultaneous changes, and the transitions and anticipations seen in some fossils. A new species requires a new DNA or, more likely, a significant modification to an existing DNA. Since DNA dictates the building and operation of the species, it contains a rather complex set of instructions. Random changes to it would create some rather bizarre members of the species, and fossils do not provide evidence of this, at least not to the level one would expect if everything was random. On the other hand, viruses can change DNA as made very clear by the evidence that our genome has already been changed many times as well as by the recent research done on HIV and other viruses. Viruses are not living entities, so they can remain inside and outside of life forms for very long periods of time. This allows them to be available to modify the DNA during whatever period of time is needed or desired. In addition, they can be used in a sequence or applied in combinations. Thus, the virus-based theory fills the gaps in Darwin's theory. Furthermore, fossils indicate the sudden demise of a number of species. Darwin's theory does not deal with that, but virus-based evolution does.

The current Theory of Creation has a number of issues that trouble many people. Much of it seems to boil down to how could the Creator do it and how could he do it in such a short period of time. He could have simply sent out viruses to make the desired changes to a species he chose to use to create the new species. Given the similarities in the DNA across many different species, a small number of viruses could bring about changes across a large number of species in a very short period of time. Also, the modifications could be such that selected species no longer exist. The message here is that viruses provide a great deal of flexibility over the control of life. Viruses may be the way the Creator has chosen to orchestrate life on earth.

The fact that the Bible says that God created man on the 6th day does not mean that it was in what we call a day or that when God does something it is done at the speed to which we are accustom. It is certainly possible that what the Bible refers to as a day we see as millions of years. It is also possible that, at the speed at which God works, he is able to accomplish in a speck of time what we envision happening over millions of years. In any event, virus-based evolution is consistent with the current theory of Creativity in the sense that the Creator willed it. Therefore, it is not, as in Darwin's theory, a random process.

This brings us to the Theory of Intelligent Design. As this theory purports, the world we live in is simply too well-structured, well-organized, and well put together to be the result of a set of random processes. We particularly like the description of a dinner given by one of the theory's followers. He likened the current theory of evolution to taking the ingredients for one of his wife's well laid out dinners and tossing them into the air and having them land in an arrangement acceptable for dinner. Fossils certainly do not support that approach. On the other hand, virus-based evolution is completely consistent with the needs of Intelligent Design. Viruses are the vehicles - the only vehicles - that are able to carry out the intent of the intelligent design in a straightforward and meaningful way.

Thus, we see that virus-based evolution makes the Theory of Intelligent Design consistent with the Theory of Creativity which, as noted above, viruses make consistent with Darwin's Theory. While some might object to the idea that there is a Creator, the developmental and operational complexities of the world we live in from the structure and operation of our environment, to that of life itself, to that of our bodies, and all the way down to the construction and operation of the smallest cells, are not the result of random processes. Therefore, if one does not accept the notion of a Creator, then one needs to explain in detail how all of these interconnected and extremely complex designs have come about in a rather orchestrated way. If one does not believe in creation one might take a bit of time and look at one's own body all the way down to the internal mechanisms of the cells and see if any other explanation fits. Look too not only at the operation of the cells, but also at the interoperability of those cells with other cells and at the large number of interdependent systems involved including the universe itself.

11. Summary and Conclusions

We have very briefly described three theories of evolution: the Bible, Intelligent Design, and Darwin's theory. We have pointed out some of the problems associated with them. In particular the absence of a driving force behind evolution and the command and control necessary to use the driving force to create the highly ordered and integrated structures of the forms of life, both currently living and deceased. We noted that when we look from either direction, that is, downward from our environment or upward from the operation inside of a cell, we see a well-organized, multilevel, integrated, complex, dynamic system. Such a system is not the result of a combination of random processes. Significant design aspects are inherent in the process and they must come about somehow. This leads one to believe that there is a Creator and that the Creator has a vision. Therefore, we see an intelligent design. We believe that the Creator chose to use viruses to build the different forms of life. By creating, activating, and deactivating viruses at different times he can maintain control over all of the forms of life without seeming to do so and with very little effort. Thus, we can clearly see the command and control at the Creator level. The randomness within a species that Darwin saw can be looked upon as giving each member of the species an identity. And with one blast of a virus the Creator can change all of that as well.

As a result of our work we have introduced three new concepts into the theory of evolution. First, viruses are the medium of change and an element of control. To create a new species, a new DNA must be created. A new one can be created by modifying an existing one. Only a virus has the capability to modify a DNA in a meaningful way. Second, cell receptors can be used as a means of cell selection and an element of control. Each cell type has its own specific set of receptors. These receptors can be used by viruses to target specific cell types. Third, in intracellular cooperation, a cell does not object to a virus modifying its DNA.

In short, the importance of viruses in evolution is twofold. First, viruses bring the how and why steps together. Second, viruses are the integrators that bring all of the other theories together. However, for us the primary interest is the viruses' capability to change the operation of cells and bring about substantial changes in the life form. A detailed understanding of the means by which a virus is able to take over a cell's command and control and direct the cell to carry out the objectives of the virus, and of the feedback mechanisms that support the control must be developed. It is this capability that the medical community must understand and harness to provide medicine with the tools needed to lift our mental and physical well being to the next level.

Postscript 2:
Gout:
Eliminating the Uric Acid Load

INTRODUCTION

In the past gout was referred to as a rich man's disease; not that amongst the populace individuals who weren't considered wealthy didn't suffer from gout. Those that could afford wine, red meat and shellfish were thought to be at highest risk of becoming plagued with joints that would intermittently swell and become horrifically painful. Artwork has depicted kings and noblemen with a goblet in their hand, surrounded by a lavish meal, and accompanied by the image of a devil-like figure mischievously striking the gentleman's big toe with the glowing red-hot tip of an iron poker.

By today's standards, gout is considered the most common inflammatory arthritis in the United States. The prevalence of gouty arthritis is approximately 3% with the number of individuals being diagnosed with gout increasing over the last few decades. Patients have reported description of the pain of an inflamed joint from gout as being 'like someone was dancing on their eyeballs' or 'the pain was so bad, it hurts just to look at the joint'. In the past it was considered rare to see a woman with gout, but over the last few decades the number of women presenting with an acute flare of gout has been steadily increasing.

Uric acid is a byproduct of a body's purine metabolism and requires excretion through the kidneys. The renal system in some individuals lacks the capacity to optimally excrete uric acid through the urine. When the concentration of uric acid in the blood stream rises above 6.8 mg/dl the uric acid circulating in the blood may become deposited in different locations around the body. Uric acid crystals tend to be javelin shaped and are negatively birefringent when examined under a polarizing microscope. Buildup of uric acid crystals in the vicinity of the joints leads to gouty arthritis.

The pathophysiology characteristics of the body determine the storage site for excess uric acid to be in the synovial tissues surrounding a joint. A joint is considered to be where the ends of two bones merge. See Figure 14. The surface covering of bone is a soft compressible substance known as cartilage. Synovial tissue wraps around the location were the ends of two bones meet and is referred to as a joint capsule. The synovial tissues produce a viscous fluid comprised of hyaluronic acid. The viscous joint fluid lubricates the surfaces of the bones, reducing friction, facilitating the ease of mobility. Excess uric acid becomes deposited in the synovial tissues of the body, such that any joint in the body could be at risk for flaring from a gout attack.

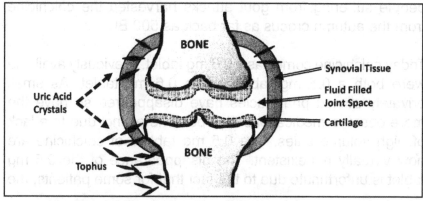

Figure 14: Illustration of a generic joint with uric acid crystals embedded in the synovial tissues surrounding joint

Gout has been a disease of simplicity, mystery and speculative management. The treatment of acute flare-ups of gout attacks have included the use of colchicine, indomethacin or other nonsteroidal anti-inflammatory drugs, narcotics, oral corticosteroids, injectable corticosteroids and injectable ACTH. At times allopurinol has been used to treat an acute attack of gout, which often leads to prolonging an attack rather than shortening the course of symptoms. Cobenecid is a combination product comprised of colchicine and probenecid that has been used at times to treat acute gout.

The management of gouty arthritis is divided into two phases of treatment. The first phase of treatment is generally directed at treating the symptoms of pain and swelling that accompany an acute attack of gout. The second phase of treatment is directed at managing the cause of the gout, the elevation of uric acid in the blood, which results in storage of uric acid crystals in synovial tissues.

ACUTE TREATMENT OF GOUT

The earliest form of treating an acute flare-up of gout has been noted to be colchicine. Colchicine can be obtained from the autumn crocus (*Colchicum autumnale*). It is believed that people suffering from gout attacks harvested the colchicine from the autumn crocus as far back as 500 BC.

Today colchicine comes as a 0.6 mg tablet. Previously available were both a 0.5 mg tablet and a 0.6 mg tablet. As small privately owned pharmacies have disappeared so have the more obscure medications also become extinct due to a lack of high volume sales. The 0.5 mg tablets of colchicine are now virtually nonexistent. The disappearance of the 0.5 mg tablet is unfortunate due to the fact that for some patients, the difference of 0.1 mg between the 0.5 mg tablet and the 0.6 mg tablet meant the difference between experiencing significant diarrhea versus tolerating colchicine.

In its intravenous form, colchicine can be very dangerous and must be used very cautiously and only by physicians intimately familiar with the drug. Colchicine administered into a vein can be toxic to the bone marrow and can suppress the production of blood cells, as well as result in other noxious reactions. The oral form of colchicine is generally safe and well tolerated. See prescribing information for further details. Approximately 20% of patients who take one 0.6 mg dose of oral colchicine twice a day complain of diarrhea and other gastrointestinal disturbances. In those who are very sensitive, the diarrhea can be very debilitating. On the other hand, for those who generally spend their lives with a constipated GI tract, sometimes what some view as a side effect, others experience as an advantage.

Colchicine has often garnished a bad reputation. Most of the ill feelings toward oral colchicine due to misconceptions about the dosing of the drug. Frequently it has been written that when a patient presents with a hot, swollen joint, oral colchicine should be administered every hour until one of three events occur: (1) The gout attack resolves, (2) Eight doses of oral colchicine have been taken, or (3) Violent diarrhea occurs. In practice, if oral colchicine is administered in this manner, for the majority of patients the gout attack does not resolve within eight hours, patients never consume eight tablets in one day, and nearly every one experiences significant diarrhea requiring them to discontinue this regiment of medication. The physician prescribing such a regiment will often become the brunt of a few choice comments about the outcome of this form of treatment strategy. Some clinicians may have distaste regarding colchicine, and may not prescribe the drug, due to .

their patients suffering ill outcomes after having prescribed the drug in what has been considered the traditional manner.

The dosing of colchicine tablets has been based on the traditional manner of dosing drugs based on half-life of the drug. The half-life of a drug is determined by taking the measured peak concentration after administration of the drug and then monitoring how long it takes for half of the peak concentration of the drug to be removed from the blood stream by the body. After the first half-life of the drug, one half of the drug is present in the blood stream. After the second half-life has passed, generally one quarter of the drug remains in circulation in the blood stream. Following the third half-life, approximately one eighth concentration of the drug remains in the blood stream. Unless other information was available, traditionally drugs were dosed using an interval of three half-lives. At the conclusion of three half-lives the amount of drug found circulating in the blood stream should be one eighth concentration of the original peak concentration. At three half-lives, this has traditionally been considered to be the appropriate time to administer a subsequent dose of the drug.

The serum half-life for oral colchicine is approximately twenty minutes; therefore the dosing schedule for colchicine per the traditional method of calculating dosing would be approximately one hour. The problem with choosing such a dosing schedule for colchicine is that the primary action of the drug is not in the blood stream, but in the synovial fluid inside a joint. It is thought that colchicine paralyzes the mobility of the white cells that traverse through the joint fluid. If the mobility of a white cell is disrupted, then the immune cell is unable to seek out and engage uric acid crystals.

The concentration of a drug in the blood stream does not necessarily equate to the concentration of a drug in joint fluid.

This is true of colchicine. Where the half life of colchicine is 20 minutes in the blood stream, the half-life of colchicine is approximately 4 hours in the fluid of a joint. Clinically colchicine often appears to work just as fast and just as well if the drug is dosed 0.6 mg twice a day. The added benefit of taking only two colchicine a day to treat an acute gout attack is the majority of patients don't spend most of the day hobbling around on a painful foot, ankle, or knee in search of a bathroom.

Since oral colchicine may be as old as Hippocrates, the medicinal properties of the drug colchicine had not undergone a FDA approval in the United States until recently. Nongeneric colchicine, referred to as Colcrys, won FDA approval in August of 2009 in the United States as a standalone product for the treatment of gout and familial Mediterranean fever. Studies have suggested that an initial dose of colchicine 1.2 mg followed by 0.6 mg 1 hour later was at least as effective in resolving an acute gout attack in comparison to administering 0.6 mg of colchicine on an hourly basis. Patients with renal or hepatic failure should be under careful surveillance by their doctor, since even oral colchicine may exhibit harmful effects in these clinical situations. The new approach appears to be effective in under half the patients twenty-four hours following the initial treatment. There were reported few side effects from the lower dose of colchicine.

Until recently, the side effects of oral colchicine appeared to be limited to GI distress. There was the concern that if a patient with diabetes and renal insufficiency took colchicine for five years that a reversible drug induced myopathy might occur.

Recent information suggests that there indeed exists significant drug interactions that might induce colchicine toxicity characterized by side effects including but not limited to fever, GI distress, neurotoxicity, myalgias, parasthesias, flaccid tetraparalysis, alopecia, pancytopenia, and death. Coadministration of colchicine with efflux transporter P-glycoprotein inhibitors and/or cytochrome P450 3A4 inhibitors including but not limited to medications such as clarithromycin, cyclosporine, erythromycin, verapamil, diltiazem, aprepitant, fluconazole, and grapefruit juice could possibly be associated with fatal and nonfatal colchicine toxicity. The recommended dose of colchicine for treatment of a gout flare-up in patients taking a moderate CYP 3A4 inhibitor is 1.2 mg of colchicine for one day with a three day lapse before an additional dose be given; but recommendations may be different for each drug given the patient's circumstances, therefore prescribing information should be reviewed prior to administering colchicine. Other potentially significant drug interactions exist with HMG-Co A Reductase inhibitors, other lipid lowering agents and digitalis glycosides. In patients with renal or hepatic impairment colchicine is contraindicated in conjunction with P-gp or strong CYP3A4 inhibitors; life-threatening and fatal colchicine toxicity has been reported with colchicine taken in therapeutic doses; see prescribing information.

The colchicine market has become very dynamic as of recent. October 1, 2010, the Food and Drug Administration ordered a halt to marketing of unapproved colchicine products by December 30, 2010. It is suggested that prescribing information be reviewed for further details and before administering or taking colchicine, especially in light of the new developments that are occurring regarding colchicine.

CHRONIC TREATMENT OF GOUT

Elevation of the uric acid level in the blood leads to deposition of the excess uric acid in different portions of the musculoskeletal system. Outside the blood, uric acid crystallizes in synovial tissues that exist around the joints. The solubility level of uric acid in the blood is considered to be 6.8 mg/dl. A solubility level is likened to when too much sugar is added to ice tea. A little sugar added to a glass of ice tea will become completely dissolved in the solution. Excessive sugar added to a glass of ice tea ends up on the bottom of the glass rather than suspended in the fluid. At the point where sugar added to a glass of ice tea begins to accumulate on the bottom of the glass corresponds to the sugar's saturation level in ice tea. The concentration of uric acid in the blood above the level of 6.8 mg/dl in the blood the uric acid begins to crystallize in the synovial tissues.

Crystallization of uric acid can occur around any joint and often occurs around multiple joints. Crystallization seems to vary around the body and vary between individuals. Most crystallization is microscopic, seen only by means of analyzing synovial tissue with the aid of a microscope. Tophaceous gout is the form of gout whereby collections of uric acid have occurred in the subcutaneous tissues around a joint or at the attachment site of a tendon in a quantity significant enough to produce a mass of crystals under the skin sizeable enough to see or feel by palpation. A subcutaneous deposit of uric acid crystals large enough to see or feel is referred to as a gout tophi. See Figure 15. Super-saturated joints are joints where the tissue comprising the joint capsule is filled to capacity with uric acid crystals. Concentrations of uric acid above the super-saturation state leads to joints primed to shed crystals into the joint space when a joint is placed under stress. The shedding of uric acid crystals into the joint space results in an inflammatory gout attack. Shedding of crystals into the tissues just outside of the joint leads to stockpile crystals in the vicinity of the joint capsule, which results in the formation of a gout tophi.

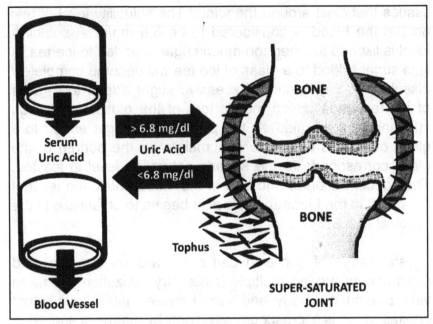

**Figure 15: Uric acid deposited in the
synovial tissues surrounding a joint**

The initial goal of treating a flare-up of gout is generally to manage, as quickly as possible, the pain, swelling and heat of an attack of gout. Once the acute attack has been resolved, treatment of gout as a long-term entity has generally been undertaken in only a fraction of the adults who suffer from gout.

The pathophysiology of chronic gout on one hand has been extensively scientifically documented, but from a clinical perspective, only marginally understood. The need to treat gout as a chronic problem has been an option for the medical provider, and has generally not been considered a necessity. The situations when treatment of chronic gout has been considered important have been when a patient presents with:

(1) a history of kidney stones comprised of uric acid,

(2) destructive changes involving one or more joints as seen on x-ray,

(3) developed palpable nodules thought to be due to significant accumulation of uric acid under the skin, and/or

(4) a patient has suffered a sufficient number of attacks, that the patient was willing to undergo life-long daily treatment for gout.

Part of the reason why gout has not been considered a disease that a healthcare provider should aggressively treat has been that by convention hyperuricemia alone with no history of a gout attack or renal stone is generally considered not a condition that warrants treatment with a uric acid lowering agent. The medical community has thought that long-term use of medications to lower a high serum uric acid level might outweigh the benefits of the drug in a patient who has had no history of joint symptoms. Contributing to this perception was in the late 1980's a decision to remove the measurement of uric acid from routine blood screening panels. Prior to this, routine blood screening detected numerous individuals that had elevated blood uric acid levels, but since these individuals were not reporting gout attacks and therefore would not be considered for treatment, it was thought the cost of the testing and the reporting of elevated uric acid levels was a poor utilization of resources. Serum uric acid testing has remained available to health care providers, but requires a specific request for the test be generated by the ordering physician. Further complicating the decision to treat patients included that some labs have reported uric acid levels as high as 8.8 mg/dl as being the upper limit of normal for uric acid, resulting in a discordance between suspecting a flare-up of gout attack and misinterpretation of the laboratory data.

The decision to remove uric acid testing from routine blood testing procedures may act to haunt the population as time passes. Patients often have very few serum uric acid level data points since uric acid levels are not being routinely checked. The diagnosis of chronic gout is becoming a disease where all parties view such a diagnosis as an unexpected outcome, rather than there being a history that reflects an outcome that might be expected if the history reflected a series of increasingly elevated serum uric acid levels.

As women and men are living longer, tophaceous gout seems to be becoming more prevalent. Twenty years ago it was rare to see a woman present with a gout attack. More recently senior women, as well as men, seem to be appearing in higher frequency with gouty arthritis.

An additional reason why the treatment of chronic gout has been speculative has been that a clear explanation as to why some patients with an elevated serum uric acid level experience a flare-up of gout has not been forthcoming. Since patients frequently present with uric acid levels above the solubility level of 6.8 mg/dl and report they have never experienced a gout attack, the mechanism of triggering a gout attack must therefore involve more than simply having a high serum uric acid level. The exact biologic mechanism that leads to the onset of one or more joints swelling and becoming painful has been inadequately understood.

A gout flare-up, where at least one joint becomes inflamed, is thought to be related to uric acid crystals present in the synovial joint tissue surrounding a joint, migrating into the fluid that occupies and fills the joint space. Gout is a medical condition where when a patient is not experiencing a gout attack, the serum uric acid level is above the saturation level of 6.8 mg/dl, and the excess uric acid is deposited in the synovial tissues that surround a joint, referred to as the joint capsule.

When the uric acid deposits reach a critical point of concentration, such that the synovial tissues of one or more joints has become super-saturated, therefore unable to easily store any further uric acid crystals, the joint is primed to experience a gout attack. If a super-saturated joint is then exposed to either an abrupt rise in serum uric acid or an abrupt decline in serum uric acid, uric acid crystals migrate from synovial tissues into the joint space. Uric acid crystals floating in the fluid occupying the space between two bones are considered to be foreign objects and can trigger a vigorous response by the immune system.

White cells routinely traverse the joint space in search of pathogens. Uric acid crystals floating freely in joint fluid act as an inciting stimulus to the white cells. Examination of synovial fluid harvested from a joint during a gout flare-up often reveals both javelin shaped uric acid crystals and numerous white cells. A comparison of joint fluid analysis from various disease states is provided in Table P2-1.

Joint Inflammation	White Cell Count	Joint Fluid Features	Joint Fluid Appearance
Normal	0-200	No debris	Clear yellow
Osteoar-thritis	200-2000	Possible cartilage debris, occa-sional white cells	Yellow, slightly cloudy
Gout	2000-50,000	Javelin shaped, negatively birefringent uric acid crystals, white cells	Deep yellow, very cloudy, pale to white color depen-dent upon number of white cells pres-ent in the fluid
Bacterial infection	>50,000	Bacteria, nu-merous white cells	Cloudy, dense fluid, white to pale, to gray color, occasional blood

Fungal/ Tuberculosis Infection	4000-100,000	Fungus present, Tuberculosis present	Cloudy, dense fluid, gray, pale white, often bloody
Pseudo-gout	2000-250,000	Rhomboid shaped, positively birefringent calcium pyrophosphate crystals	Deep yellow, very cloudy, pale to white color dependent upon number of white cells present in the fluid
Rheumatoid arthritis	2000-50,000	White cells, occasional Rice bodies	Cloudy yellow to pale white dependent upon the number of white cells present in the fluid
Trauma	Few white cells	Numerous red cells	Bloody joint fluid
Pigmented villonodular synovitis	Few to many white cells	Numerous red cells	Yellow to pale white to bloody joint fluid

TABLE P2-1
Comparison of Joint Fluid Analysis from
Various Medical Conditions.

When an excessive amount of uric acid has accumulated around one or more joints and the patient has joints that are supersaturated with uric acid, the involved joints are in a low threshold state to become inflamed. If the uric acid level in the blood suddenly rises or suddenly decreases, this event can initiate one or more of the supersaturated joints flaring. It is thought that if a person with gout consumes products that increase the serum uric acid, the storage points around the joints become overloaded and uric acid crystals appear in the joint fluid contained inside the capsule of a joint. Consumable products that increase serum uric acid levels include alcohol, red meat and shellfish. Decreasing the water volume in the blood also increases the concentration of uric acid in the blood. Dehydration, caffeine products, and diuretics occurring alone or in combination can initiate a gout flare-up by increasing the concentration of uric acid in the blood, which can lead to one or more joints becoming overloaded with uric acid.

When the uric acid level in the blood declines sharply, it is thought that the uric acid deposited in the synovial fluid reacts by mobilizing. The mobilization of the uric acid crystals is a biochemical phenomenon to return the excess uric acid to the blood stream so that the uric acid can be excreted through the kidneys. As the uric acid crystals are mobilized to leave the synovial tissues, some of the uric acid crystals end up in the joint space and incite a gout flare-up. Typically if an individual prone to gout changes their diet in an effort to lose weight or the diet is altered upon being admitted to a hospital, such circumstances may result in a gout flare-up. It is very common for a patient who is at risk for gout, when hospitalized, not to consume the same variety of foods as they normally would, and suffer with a hot swollen joint 3-4 days following their admission to the hospital.

A third cause of a gout attack is trauma or overuse of a joint. Given the uric acid is stored in synovial tissues, if the capsule of a supersaturated joint is stretched, crushed or otherwise injured, uric acid crystals may migrate from the capsule into the fluid occupying the joint space. The tearing or swelling of synovial tissues due to an injury may cause uric acid crystals to be released thus resulting in a traumatized joint becoming inflamed due a gout attack in addition to the inflammation related to the actual trauma.

White cells transit most of the tissues of the body in search of pathogens or foreign substances. In the case of a joint flare-up due to gout, the white cells transiting through the synovial fluid inside a joint react to new uric acid crystals that form inside the joint. To a white cell, a uric acid crystal floating freely in joint fluid would be likened to a foreign substance that should be removed from the joint. White cells are generally equipped to remove microscopic foreign substances.

In the case of gout, the diameter of a white cell is smaller than the length of the javelin shaped uric acid crystal. Examination of synovial fluid removed from a joint during a gout flare-up under a microscope often demonstrates the appearance of white cells impaled by a uric acid crystal, with the sharp edges of the crystal exiting opposite ends of the white cell. White cells carry vacuoles containing sulfuric acid and hydrochloric acid, as well enzymes and lysozymes. The acids and enzymes are used by the white cells to kill bacteria and viruses. It is thought that when a white cell's outer membrane becomes compromised by a sharp uric acid crystal passing through the outer membrane of the cell, the acids and enzymes spill into the joint fluid which inflames the joint and joint capsule. The presence of the white cell's acids and enzymes in the joint space is what is thought to contribute to an acute joint flare-up.

Any joint can experience an inflammatory flare-up from gout. The joints that flare up most frequently include those in the big toe, the mid foot, the ankle joint, the wrist, the knee and elbow; with the first metatarsal joint and inter-phalange joint of the first toe thought to be the most common. Possibly, the big toe and mid foot suffers from gout attacks most frequently due to a combination of being the most distal location from the heart, encouraging deposition of crystals, regular blunt force trauma from ambulation which repeatedly stretches the joint capsule, along with a chronically high serum uric acid level in concert with a sudden change to that serum uric acid level.

Often, though not true for all of those who experience gout attacks, the inflammation of the joints involved in a flare-up are time-limited. It is thought that once new crystals appear in a joint space and the white cells transiting the joint space generate an inflammatory response to the presence of the crystals, over the subsequent two weeks proteins are formed in the synovial fluid that coat the outer surface of the free floating uric acid crystals. When the exterior of the uric acid crystals become covered with a protein coat additional white cells transiting through the joint space ignore the presence of the crystals, therefore these white cells do not react to the uric acid crystals. When the white cells are no longer attracted to the presence of the crystals, the inflammatory response inside the joint attenuates and eventually resolves. The uric acid crystals floating in the joint fluid dissolve and are re-deposited in the synovial tissues lining the joint.

Colchicine is thought to act to paralyze the white cells transiting the joint fluid such that the white cells are not able to pursue the crystals floating freely in the joint space. Indocin, other nonsteroidal anti-inflammatory medications, and corticosteroids are used to neutralize the production and the effects of prostaglandins that help create joint inflammation. Prostaglandins are diverse hormone-like substances comprised of 20-carbon fatty acid derivatives containing a 5-carbon ring, some of which are responsible for generating inflammation. Treating the acute attack of gout manages the physical ailment the patient experiences, but does not rid the body of the factors that were responsible for the initiation or perpetuation of the gout flare-up.

Long-term treatment of gout should be directed at eliminating the overall excess load of uric acid crystals that the body has accumulated over time. See Figure 16. It has been noted that if the long-term treatment of gout is able to reduce the concentration of uric acid in the blood from a high concentration, such as 10.0 mg/dl down to 5.0 mg/dl, that after 6 to 12 months of continuous treatment patients notice a significant reduction in the frequency of their gout flare-ups. After 18 months to 2 years of continuous treatment and adhering to a diet that restricts the intake of alcohol, red meat and shellfish, most patients with a normal renal function report no further gout attacks. Presently there are three agents on the market in the United States that lower serum uric acid levels. These agents include allopurinol, probenecid and febuxostat; see prescribing information for details regarding these medications.

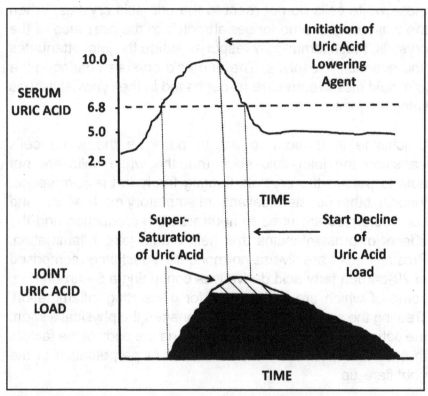

Figure 16: Reducing the uric acid load in the synovial tissues

Long-term treatment has been an important consideration related to excess loads of uric acid deposited in the synovial tissues which can lead to: (1) palpable nodules, (2) gout flare-ups due to strain or exercise of a joint, (3) formation of uric acid kidney stones, and (4) destructive changes to the bone of joint. Patients that accumulate enough uric acid crystals to form palpable nodules can experience a painless destruction of the bone in one or more joints. A case of tophaceous gout left untreated can result in an outcome that has a similar appearance and loss of function as seen with a crippling form of arthritis. Appearance of the nodules alone can be particularly bothersome to patients if the nodules form on the feet, the Achilles tendon, around the knees, elbows or hands.

As an example of the long-term accumulation of uric acid, consider Example 1, a patient who presents to a clinic at age 28 for a physical exam, who has no complaints. Serum uric acid level is checked and found out to be 7.6 mg/dl. At age 28 the patient denies having experienced any joint pain or swelling, so that no medical management is started. At age 30, the uric acid is re-measured and found to be 8.0 mg/dl. At age 39 the serum uric acid is found to be 8.2 mg/dl. At age 41 the serum uric acid was measured to be 7.4 mg/dl. Four years later, now at age 45 a serum uric acid level is again checked and now found to be 8.3 mg/dl. As with all of the previous clinic visits, again the patient denies any episodes of joint swelling or pain. The patient does report that his father has been experiencing episodes of gout attacks. Neither the patient, nor his father, consume alcoholic beverages, except for rare occasions. Kidney function in the form of the serum creatinine is normal. At age 48 the patient notices very infrequent episodes of fleeting pain in the feet, generally lasting less than twelve hours, that are distinctly symptomatic, but last such a short period of time the episodes are not mentioned to the primary care physician and no medical treatment is sought. At age 49 the serum uric acid level is determined to be 7.7 mg/dl. Due to the decline in serum uric acid, the patient believes his condition has improved. See Table P2-2.

Date	1987	1989	1998	2000	2002	2004	2008	2010
Age	28	30	39	41	43	45	49	51
Uric acid	7.6	8.0	8.2	7.4	---	8.3	7.7	8.4
Creatinine	1.2	1.1	0.9	0.9	0.9	1.0	0.9	1.0

TABLE P2-2
Example 1: Serum Uric Acid Levels Over Time.

Just before the patient's fifty-first birthday, he experienced a gout attack involving the left knee. The pain left the patient stranded in a chair at home over the weekend. The patient described the experience as 'if there were razor blades ripping back and forth inside the small confines of the left knee joint preventing any movement of the knee'.

The objective of managing gout is certainly to treat the gout flare-up and sooth the patient's pain. The second objective of managing gout is to eliminate the body's excess uric acid load. To correctly measure an individual's uric acid load one would need to know factors such as (1) concentration of serum uric acid above the saturation level of 6.8 mg/dl, (2) time interval over which serum uric acid level is above the saturation level of 6.8 mg/dl, (3) rate of deposition of uric acid into the soft tissues of the body, (4) creatinine clearance as a measure of renal function and approximation of the rate of uric acid elimination.

Generally, a treating healthcare provider may have only one, or at most only a few serum uric acid levels with which to review when making management decisions regarding gouty arthritis. It should be noted that the serum uric acid level obtained during an acute gout attack has a high likelihood of not being an accurate representation of the serum uric acid that would be measured at other times. A serum uric acid level drawn during an acute gout attack may be deceptively low.

In a study of ten men who were experiencing an acute gout attack, six had a normal uric acid level when their blood specimen was drawn while the gouty arthritis was flared up; while two months after their gout flare-up had resolved all ten men demonstrated uric acid levels higher than the normal range of 6.8 mg/dl. The reason as to why a patient with gout would have a normal uric acid level during a gout flare-up is unclear; unless the event of a normal uric acid level, in a patient who otherwise had an elevated uric acid level, was in fact the stimulus for the attack. Once the synovial tissues of a joint become saturated to a critical mass a relatively sudden rise in serum uric acid or a sudden decline in the serum uric acid may act as the trigger for a gout flare-up. A second reason may be that once the inflammatory reaction begins, serum inflammatory constituents activate the renal tubules to dump serum uric acid thus causing a sudden decrease in the concentration of uric acid present in the serum.

The seemingly paradoxical normal serum uric acid level that occurs during a flare-up of gout tends to cause clinicians to question the diagnosis. Emergency room physicians and clinical healthcare providers find it difficult to make a diagnosis of gout when the serum uric acid level is normal. This is not without merit since flare-ups of pseudogout, Calcium Pyrophosphate Deposition (CPPD) disease, behave much like gout , yet usually presents with a history of normal serum uric acid levels. At this time there is no serum study directly associated with the diagnosis of pseudogout. Calcium pyrophosphate crystals tend to be rhomboid in shape and are positively birefringent when viewed with a polarizing microscope. It has been reported that gout and pseudogout crystals are present simultaneously in ten percent of crystal arthropathy flare-ups. X-rays of the wrists, knees, symphysis pubis, and shoulders are sometimes helpful for searching for evidence of chondrocalcinosis, which may be associated with CPPD. Redrawing a patient's blood 4-6 weeks after a joint flare-up has resolved will generally demonstrate an elevated serum uric acid level in patients with gout.

DETERMINING URIC ACID LOAD
INDIRECTLY BY UTILIZING RATES

The uric acid level load in the body can be roughly estimated by summing up each measured uric acid level in mg/dl that is available for a patient and multiplying by time, from the time of the measurement to the time of the next measurement or the latest date the patient is seen. An estimate of how long it would take to remove the uric acid load from the body is performed by either: (1) dividing by the previously calculated sum by the result of 6.8 mg/dl minus the patient's current serum uric acid level or (2) taking in the case of an ideal response to therapy, which is 1.8 mg/dl, derived by taking 6.8 mg/dl and subtracting 5.0 mg/dl.

Since the exact amount of uric acid, by volume, that the body has stored around the joints is beyond the scope of current clinical testing techniques, an estimate can be arrived at by using rates of acumination of uric acid. The estimated rate of accumulation over time can be then calculated and compared to the rate of excretion of uric acid from the body, while a patient is taking a uric acid lowering agent. An exact amount of how much uric acid a body has stored may not be available, but the rates of accumulation can be estimated and summed over time and this value can be compared to the rate of elimination of uric acid from the body. A length of time necessary to eliminate the uric acid load can be arrived at by dividing the summed estimated rate of accumulation by the rate of elimination. Therefore the indirect method of utilizing rates can replace the direct method of measuring quantity.

In Example 2, uric acid is 8.6 mg/dl in 1990. See Table P2-3. Since there are only two uric acid levels, take the 8.6 mg/dl and subtract 6.8 mg/dl which results in 1. 8 mg/d. Taking the 1.8 mg/dl and multiply by 10 years to represent the interval between the first and second measurement, results in 18 mg/dl. Taking the 18 mg/dl and dividing by the ideal reduction in serum uric acid, which is 1.8 mg/dl/yr, results in ten years. This simple equation suggests if the serum uric acid is 8.6 mg/dl and the serum uric acid remains at this level for ten years, it will take ten years to completely clear the uric acid load from the body if the patient is compliant with the medication, the renal function and diet remain the same, and the patient consumes no alcohol-containing products.

Date	12/31/1990	12/31/2000
Serum Uric Acid	8.6 mg/dl	8.7 mg dl

TABLE P2-3
Example 2: Two Measured Uric Acid Levels.

In Example 3, there are three uric acid levels to be considered. In 1995, the uric acid is measured at 8.4 mg/dl. See Table P2-4. Taking the second measured uric acid level 8.4 mg/dl and subtracting 6.8 mg/dl which results in 1.6 mg/d. Taking the 1.6 mg/dl and multiply by 5 years to represent the interval between the first and second measurement, results in 8 mg/dl. Then taking the third measurement 8.8 mg/dl from 2000 and subtracting 6.8 mg/dl, results in 2 mg/dl. Taking 2 mg/dl and multiplying by 9 years results in 18 mg/dl. Adding the two results together arrives at the sum of 26 mg/dl. Taking the 26 mg/dl and dividing by the ideal reduction in serum uric acid, which is 1.8 mg/dl/yr results in 14.4 years. This calculation suggests if the serum uric acid is 8.4 mg/dl and the serum uric acid remains at this level for five years, then the serum uric acid level changes to 8.8 mg/dl and remains at this level for 9 years, then if medical therapy is introduced and is successful in reducing the serum uric acid level to 5.0 mg/dl and the patient is compliant with eliminating alcoholic beverages from their diet, it will take nearly fourteen and a half years to clear the uric acid load from the body if the renal function and diet remain the same.

Date	1/22/1995	2/1/2000	1/29/2009
Serum Uric Acid	8.4 mg/dl	8.8 mg/dl	8.7 mg/dl
Creatinine	1.2 mg/dl	1.1 mg/dl	1.2 mg/dl

Table P2-4
Example 3: Three Measured Uric Acid Levels.

The actual total accumulation of uric acid in terms of 'true weight' is beyond the scope of this text and may be beyond the scope of present day technology.

Reconsidering the patient in Example 1, Table P2-5 demonstrates the accumulation of uric acid in units of mg/dl include 1.53, 10.9. 2.21. 2.6, 6.88 and 1.05 for a total of 25.17 mg/dl from age 28 to age 51. If the patient is started on either allopurinol or febuxostat, and the serum uric acid level is decreased to approximately 5.0 mg/dl, if the patient is compliant with the medication, if the creatinine is normal, and if the diet is void of alcohol use, is low in shellfish and red meat, then the uric acid load in the body will be decreased by 1.8 mg/dl per year. If the total load of uric acid in the body is 25.17 mg/dl, and medical therapy decreases the uric acid load by 1.8 mg/dl/year, the uric acid load will be substantially eliminated from the body after approximately fourteen years of continuous therapy.

Date Year	Units	1987	1989	1998	2000	2004	2008	2010
Date Month		June	May	June	Jan	May	Dec	Feb
Age	Yrs	28	30	39	41	45	49	51
Creatinine	mg/dl	1.2	1.1	0.9	0.9	1.0	0.9	---
24Hr Urine Uric Acid	mg/dl/vol			322		1010.2		
Uric acid	mg/dl	7.6	8.0	8.2	7.4	8.3	7.7	---
Uric acid -6.8 mg/dl	mg/dl	0.8	1.2	1.4	0.6	1.5	0.9	---
Accumulation Per Interval	mg/dl	0	1.53	10.9	2.21	2.6	6.88	1.05
Accumulation Total Load	mg/dl	0	1.53	12.43	14.64	17.24	24.12	25.17

TABLE P2-5
Example 1: Uric Acid Load Calculated.

If the reduction in uric acid load is as mentioned and applied to the example above, it would take nearly fourteen years of treatment in order to eliminate the estimated uric acid load in terms of mg/dl from the body. If renal function worsens or the diet is rich in consumable products that encourage accumulation of uric acid or if the patient were to consume alcohol products, the elimination of the uric acid load may take longer. If alcohol consumption, in an individual whom is prone to use alcohol products, occurs on a regular basis, the expected reduction in the load of uric acid may not occur.

The above approach represents an approximation of the existing uric acid load in the body. It is beyond the scope of this text to accurately measure the rate of uric acid deposition into individual synovial tissues.

The above calculation does not accurately take into account the elimination rate of the uric acid from the body through the kidneys. Accurately calculating individual rates of elimination of uric acid from the body is beyond the scope of this text, and at the clinical level may beyond the scope of practical medical science. Using 1.8 mg/dl/year at the rate of loss is a gross estimate, which is dependent upon the serum uric acid level being decreased to 5.0 mg/dl and remaining steadily at this level during the treatment program. The approximation is conservative in its estimate of how long it may take to eliminate the uric acid load from the body. The important feature of considering performing such an approximation is that such a calculation would provide a patient, who is afflicted with gout, a basis for being compliant with a chronic uric acid lowering therapy.

QUICK AND EASY CALCULATION

The above calculation may be too cumbersome to be utilized routinely in clinical practice; in addition, since many labs have removed serum uric acid from the set of labs comprising routine blood panels, the information may not be available to a clinician. A more rapid and possible a more meaningful means of estimating the uric acid load in the body is to simply the calculation process. The majority of patients who develop gout recall experiencing their first gout flare-up in their late forties or early fifties. In patients whom develop gout after age 30, a rough estimate of the uric acid load would be to take the patient's age and subtract 30, then multiply this result by the highest known uric acid level on record for the patient and subtract 6.8 mg/dl, then divide this result by 1.4 times 1.8 mg/dl or 2.5 mg/dl. The reason to use a factor such as '1.4' in the estimate is that the accumulation of the uric acid load probably follows a gently sloping exponential curve, rather than a linear curve due to the crystallization of uric acid in the tissues being more robust later in life due to a deterioration in renal function as a result of aging and/or a medical disease.

The estimate is calculated using the following formula:

(Age minus 30) multiplied by (highest uric acid minus 6.8) then divided by (2.5)

In Example 1, if we take 51 years and subtract 30 years, the result would be 21. Then if we took the highest uric acid 8.4 mg/dl and subtract 6.8 mg/dl the result would be 1.6 mg/dl. Taking 21 years and multiplying by 1.6 mg/dl results in 33.6 mg/dl. Then taking 33.6 mg/dl and dividing by 2.5 mg/dl results in 13.6 or approximately 14 years. The result of the rough estimate indicates that if the patient were compliant with uric acid lowering therapy, then the uric acid load stored in the body would be eliminated after 14 years of continuous therapy. The first, more complicated analysis suggested fourteen years and the rough estimate is possibly less accurate, but a much quicker calculation and can be used in the clinic to educate a patient regarding the length of time needed to take chronic therapy in order to substantially lower the uric acid load in their system. Such a clinical calculation tool may undergo revision as additional information regarding rate of uric acid tissue deposition and rate of renal excretion of uric acid become known.

The true clinical value of such a calculation is to demonstrate to a patient that treatment for gout is a long-term strategy rather than a short-term management scheme. Often treatment for gout is discontinued once the patient recognizes that a significant portion of time has passed since the last gout attack occurred, which is often interpreted by the patient as the point when there is no further need to treat gout. Many patients stop treatment after 1-2 years have passed because they fail to have an appreciation for the chronicity of gout. Many patients feel that if their serum uric acid level is normal, then gout has been successfully treated, when they do not understand that a normal uric acid level only facilitates the elimination of uric acid stored in the joints around the body. Patients often do not realize that the serum uric acid level does not represent the 'amount' of uric acid that has been accumulated in the tissues of the joints comprising the body. Unfortunately, at this time there does not exist the means to measure the amount of crystallized uric acid that exists in a patient's body. If gout attacks cease to occur in a person, it is most likely that the patient's uric acid load has been decreased below the super-saturation level; but the overall load of uric acid may remain as a substantial amount unless the treatment program is long enough to eliminate the overall uric acid load. The rationalization for long-term treatment of gout is not only to lower the uric acid load below the super-saturation level, but to reduce the overall uric acid load to zero so that the patient does not suffer the consequences of chronic excessive uric acid load existing in close proximity to the joints.

Any medication where the action of the product is to reduce the concentration of uric acid in the blood stream is likely to cause a person at risk for gout to experience a flaring of one or more of their joints. To prevent a gout flare-up during the initiation of chronic treatment with allopurinol, probenecid or febuxostat often colchicine is utilized. Colchicine at a dose of 0.6 mg one a day or in some cases 0.6 mg twice a day is used to prevent joint flare-ups.

FUTURE OF GOUT

For over forty years no new medication dedicated specifically to the treatment of gout was introduced to the market. Recently both febuxostat and nongeneric colchicine have been made available to health care providers. A number of new products intended to treat and manage gout are predicted to come to the market in the coming years. Anakinra, Rilonacept, canakinumab, and Pegioticase are likely candidates that are currently undergoing testing. See prescribing information when products become available.

SUMMARY

Gout attacks occur, not because they are directly related to an elevated serum uric acid level, but due to a chronically elevated serum uric acid level which leads to an accumulation of uric acid in the synovial tissues of one or more joints that reaches a critical mass termed a super-saturation level. A critical mass of uric acid embedded in synovial tissues that experience a fluctuation in serum uric acid will shed some of the uric acid crystals into the joint space. A joint capsule that is super-saturated with uric acid crystals shedding crystals into the joint space, will activate a vigorous response by the immune system, which results in a flare-up of gout in the one or more of joints that are at critical mass.

Effective chronic treatment of gout is to eliminate the overload of uric acid in the body. A medication such as allopurinol or febuxostat should reduce the serum uric acid level and if taken daily when alcohol products are being avoided, should reduce the overload of uric acid from the synovial tissues surrounding the joints of the body. Low-dose colchicine, if tolerated and able to taken without drug interaction, helps prevent gout flares during the introduction of chronic uric acid lowering therapy.

A simple, rough means of estimating how long it will take to remove the excess uric acid load from the synovial tissues in a patient over 30 years old is to take the patient's age and subtract 30, then multiply this result by the highest known uric acid level on record minus 6.8 mg/dl, then divide this by 2.5 mg/dl. The result provides a teaching tool in terms of a rough estimate to convey to a patient regarding the length of time that treatment needs to be taken in order for the average patient to substantially lower the uric acid load from their body. Patients with renal failure, diets that encourage the accumulation of uric acid and patients with a strong predisposition to gout may require treatment that is substantially longer. Lastly, reducing the uric acid load does not cure the problem. Life-long therapy with a uric acid lowering agent is generally required by patients with a history of gout attacks. It is recommended healthcare providers review current prescribing information before administering any medication and patients review the latest prescribing information prior to taking any medication.

Postscript 3:
Quantum Gene:
Identification of a Gene

WHAT IS A GENE?

The central dogma of microbiology dictates that within the boundaries of the nucleus of a biologically active cell, genes are transcribed to produce messenger ribonucleic acid molecules (mRNAs); these mRNAs migrate to the cytoplasm where they are translated by cellular machinery to produce proteins. One of the great unknowns that has challenged the study of microbiology is the subject of understanding of how the genes, comprising the genome of a species, are organized such that the nuclear transcription machinery can efficiently locate specific transcribable genetic information and instructions that the cell requires to maintain itself, grow and conduct cell replication.

Decoding the means as to how the genetic information contained in the nuclear deoxyribonucleic acid (DNA) of a cell is organized contributes to furthering the efforts to produce an effective gene therapy treatment strategy. Understanding the basis of the genetic instruction code that is stored in a cell's DNA and utilizing such knowledge of labeling and cataloging of genetic information makes inserting biologic instruction into the DNA of cells a practical and effective means of treating a wide variety of challenging medical conditions. It would seem the biologic instructions necessary to build and maintain the human body are individually labeled with some form of unique identification code to assist the nuclear machinery in locating and utilizing the genes when needed.

The human genome is comprised of deoxyribonucleic acid (DNA) separated into 46 chromosomes. A chromosome consists of a DNA double helix bearing a linear sequence of genes, coiled and recoiled around aggregated proteins, termed histones. The number of chromosomes varies from species to species. Most human cells carries twenty two pairs of chromosomes plus two sex chromosomes; two 'x' chromosomes in women and one 'x' and one 'y' chromosome in men. Chromosomes carry genetic information in the form of units which are referred to as genes. Within the DNA, essential bits of information are represented as base pair of nucleotides. The entire human nuclear genome is comprised of 3 billion base pairs (bp) of nucleotides.

The chromosomes are subdivided into genes. Genes represent units of transcribable DNA. It has been estimated that there are 30,000 to 100,000 genes. Transcription of the DNA refers to generating one RNA molecule or a variety of RNA molecules by decoding the genes. Regarding the human genome, currently it is estimated that 5% of the total nuclear DNA is thought to represent genes and 95% is thought to represent redundant non-gene genetic material.

The DNA genome in a cell is comprised of transcribable genetic information and nontranscribable genetic information. Transcribable genetic information represent the segments of DNA that when transcribed by transcription machinery yield RNA molecules, usually in a precursor form that require modification before the RNA molecules are capable of being functional. The nontranscribable genetic information associated with the genes represent segments that act as either points of attachment for the transcription machinery or act as commands to direct the transcription machinery or act as spacers between transcribable segments of genetic information or have no known function at this time. A segment of nontranslatable DNA that is coded as a STOP command, under the proper circumstances, will cause the transcription machinery to cease transcribing the DNA at that point. A segment of DNA coded to signal a REPEAT command, will cause the transcription machinery to repeat its transcription of a segment of genetic information.

The term 'genetic information' refers to a sequence of nucleotides that comprise transcribable portions of DNA and nontranscribable portions of DNA. In the DNA, four different nucleotides comprise the nucleotide sequences. The four different nucleotides that comprise the DNA are adenine, cytosine, guanine, and thymine.

Computer programs, commonly utilized in desk top computers, laptop computers, and mainframe computers, are comprised of a series of software instructions and data. In order for a computer program to run its digital programming in an orderly fashion, each software instruction and each element of data is assigned or associated with a unique identifier such that the software instructions can be carried out in an orderly fashion and each element of data can be efficiently located when there is a need to process the data elements. Similarly, each unit of genetic information, often referred to as a gene, comprising the nuclear DNA of a species genome, must have a unique identifier assigned to it such that the genetic information can be readily located by the transcription machinery and utilized when needed by a cell.

When a gene is to be transcribed approximately forty proteins assemble together into what is referred to as a transcription complex. The transcription complex acts as the transcription machinery to decode the DNA. The transcription complex forms along a segment of DNA, upstream from the start of the transcribable genetic information. The transcription complex transcribes the genetic information to produce RNA. It is vital to the cell that the transcription complex is able to locate a specific gene, amongst the 3 billion base pairs comprising the 46 chromosomes of the human genome, in an orderly and efficient manner. Locating the proper gene in a timely fashion enables a cell to properly operate, survive, grow and replicate.

For purposes of this publication there are several general definitions that apply to the text. A 'ribose' is a five carbon or pentose sugar ($C_5H_{10}O_5$) present in the structural components of ribonucleic acid, riboflavin, and other nucleotides and nucleosides. A 'deoxyribose' is a deoxypentose ($C_5H_{10}O_4$) found in deoxyribonucleic acid. A 'nucleoside' is a compound of a sugar usually ribose or deoxyribose with a nitrogenous base by way of an N-glycosyl link. A 'nucleotide' is a single unit of a nucleic acid, composed of a five carbon sugar (either a ribose or a deoxyribose), a nitrogenous base and a phosphate group. There are two families of 'nitrogenous bases', which include: pyrimidine and purine. A 'pyrimidine' is a six member ring made up of carbon and nitrogen atoms; the members of the pyrimidine family include: cytosine (C), thymine (T) and uracil (U). A 'purine' is a five-member ring fused to a pyrimidine type ring; the members of the purine family include: adenine (A) and guanine (G). A 'nucleic acid' is a polynucleotide which is a biologic molecule such as ribonucleic acid or deoxyribonucleic acid that enable organisms to reproduce. A 'ribonucleic acid' (RNA) is a linear polymer of nucleotides formed by repeated riboses linked by phosphodiester bonds between the 3-hydroxyl group of one and the 5-hydroxyl group of the next. RNAs are single stranded macromolecules comprised of a sequence of nucleotides, these nucleotides are generally referred to by their nitrogenous bases, which include: adenine, cytosine, guanine and uracil. The term 'macromolecule' refers to any very large molecule. RNAs are subset into different types which include messenger RNA (mRNA), transport RNA (tRNA), ribosomal RNA (rRNA) and a variety of small RNAs. Messenger RNAs act as templates to produce proteins. A ribosome is a complex comprised of rRNAs and proteins and is responsible for the correct positioning of mRNA and charged tRNA to facilitate the proper alignment and bonding of amino acids into a strand to produce a protein. A 'charged' tRNA is a tRNA that is carrying an amino acid. Ribosomal RNA (rRNA) represents a subset of RNAs that form part of the physical structure of a ribosome. Small RNAs include snoRNA, U snRNA, and miRNA. The snoRNAs modify precursor rRNA molecules. U snRNAs modify precursor mRNA molecules. The miRNA molecules modify the function of mRNA molecules.

A 'deoxyribose' is a deoxypentose ($C_5H_{10}O_4$) sugar. Deoxyribonucleic acid (DNA) is comprised of three basic elements: a deoxyribose sugar, a phosphate group and nitrogen containing bases. DNA is a macromolecule made up of two chains of repeating deoxyribose sugars linked by phosphodiester bonds between the 3-hydroxyl group of one and the 5-hydroxyl group of the next; the two chains are held antiparallel to each other by weak hydrogen bonds. DNA strands contain a sequence of nucleotides, which include: adenine, cytosine, guanine and thymine. Adenine is always paired with thymine of the opposite strand, and guanine is always paired with cytosine of the opposite strand; one side or strand of a DNA macromolecule is the mirror image of the opposite strand. Nuclear DNA is regarded as the medium for storing the master plan of hereditary information.

A gene is a unit of heredity in a living organism, normally represented as a stretch of DNA that codes an mRNA that when translated codes for a type of protein or for an RNA molecule that serves a function in the cell other than being a template to be translated to produce a protein.

Various standard definitions of a gene exist. Per *Stedman's Medical Dictionary*, 24th edition, copyright 1982: 'The functional unit of heredity. Each gene occupies a specific place or locus on a chromosome, is capable of reproducing itself exactly at cell division, and is capable of directing the formation of an enzyme or other protein. The gene as a functional unit probably consists of a discrete segment of purine (adenine and guanine) and pyrimidine (cytosine and thymine) bases in the correct sequence to code the sequence of amino acids needed to form a specific peptide. Protein synthesis is mediated by molecules of messenger RNA formed on the chromosome with the gene unit of DNA acting as a template, which then pass into the cytoplasm and become oriented on the ribosomes where they in turn act as templates to organize a chain of amino acids to form a peptide. Genes normally occur in pairs in all cells except gametes as a consequence of the fact that all chromosomes are paired except the sex chromosomes (x and y) of the male.'

Per *Dorland's Pocket Medical Dictionary,* 23rd edition, copyright 1982 the definition of 'gene' is 'the biologic unit of heredity, self-producing, and located at a definite position (locus) on a particular chromosome.'

Per the text *Understanding Biology*, Second Edition, Peter Raven, George Johnson, Mosby, copyright 1991: 'Gene: The basic unit of heredity. A sequence of DNA nucleotides on a chromosome that encodes a polypeptide or RNA molecule and so determines the nature of an individual's inherited traits.'

Per *The New Oxford American Dictionary*, Second Edition, copyright 2005: 'Gene: A unit of heredity that is transferred from a parent to offspring and is held to determine some characteristic of the offspring: proteins coded directly by genes. In technical use: a distinct sequence of nucleotides forming part of a chromosome, the order of which determines the order of monomers in a polypeptide or nucleic acid molecule which a cell (or virus) may synthesize.'

Per MedicineNet.com. (*Current as of the time of this publication*): According to the official Guidelines for Human Gene Nomenclature, a 'gene' is defined as "a DNA segment that contributes to phenotype/function. In the absence of demonstrated function a gene may be characterized by sequence, transcription or homology." DNA: Genes are composed of DNA, a molecule in the memorable shape of a double helix, a spiral ladder. Each rung of the spiral ladder consists of two paired chemicals called bases. There are four types of bases. They are adenine (A), thymine (T), cytosine (C), and guanine (G). As indicated, each base is symbolized by the first letter of its name: A, T, C, and G. Certain bases always pair together (AT and GC). Different sequences of base pairs form coded messages. The gene: A gene is a sequence (a string) of bases. It is made up of combinations of A, T, C, and G. These unique combinations determine the gene's function, much as letters join together to form words. Each person has thousands of genes--billions of base pairs of DNA or bits of information repeated in the nuclei of human cells-- which determine individual characteristics (genetic traits).'

Per Wikipedia.com, referenced to: Group of the Sequence Ontology consortium, coordinated by K. Eilbeck, cited in H. Pearson. (2006). Genetics: what is a gene? *Nature*, 441, 398-401 (*Current as of the time of this publication*): A modern working definition of a gene is '*a locatable region of genomic sequence, corresponding to a unit of inheritance, which is associated with regulatory regions, transcribed regions, and or other functional sequence regions.*'

The above definitions of a 'gene' are fairly detailed and at present time generally universally accepted in the science and medical communities as representing the definition of a gene. There is a distinct lack of any previous reference in the medical science literature to a unique identifier associated with genetic material.

Current gene theory is derived from Gregor Mendel (1822-1884), who discovered the basic principles of heredity by breeding garden peas at the abbey where he resided, while teaching at Brunn Modern School. Gregor Mendel built and documented a model of inheritance, often referred to as Mendelian genetics, that has acted as the foundation of modern genetics. Gregor Mendel documented changes in characteristics of the plants he grew and described the physical traits as being related to 'heritable factors'. Over time Mendel's term 'heritable factor' has been replaced by the terms 'gene' and 'allele'. Much of what the current term of a 'gene' describes remains related to and distinctly linked to the physical traits of the live organisms they describe.

Per J. K. Pal, S.S. Ghaskabi, *Fundamentals of Molecular Biology*, 2009: 'The central dogma of molecular biology...states that the genes present in the genome (DNA) are transcribed into mRNAs, which are then translated into polypeptides or proteins, which are phenotypes.' 'Genome, thus, contains the complete set of hereditary information for any organism and is functionally divided into small parts referred to as genes. Each gene is a sequence of nucleotides representing a single protein or RNA. Genome of a living organism may contain as few as 500 genes as in case of Mycoplasma, or as many as an estimated 30,000 genes as in case of human beings.'

Current computer technology utilizes the binary numeric language. Every task a computer performs is related to the language of 'ones' and 'zeros'. Transistors that comprise the inside of computer chips are either turned 'on' representing a 'one' or turned 'off' representing a 'zero'. At the core of all computer programs is the machine language of 'ones' and 'zeros'. The central processing unit (CPU) is the heart of any computer. The most sophisticated CPU in the world only reads and processes the language of 'ones' and 'zeros'. All text, all pictures, all video, all sound and music is diluted down to the form of 'ones' and 'zeros', and consequently all of the computing and storage power of a computer is performed by the computer language of 'ones' and 'zeros'.

In order to keep the computing power of a CPU and associated memory storage devices in synch, all computer instructions and data elements are associated with unique identifiers. In early generations of computers every line of a computer program was identified with a sequential number. As technology progressed, the distinct, sequential numbering system evolved into utilizing names or numbers to label segments of computer code. Instructions and data elements retain unique identification in order to be located, then processed by the CPU in an orderly fashion.

If a computer's CPU processing loses tract of computer instructions or data elements the CPU becomes dysfunctional. Older generations of computers frequently experienced disparity in the sequencing of instructions and data. Once a computer's CPU lost tract of which instruction to process or lost tract of the data it was to process, the computer would shut down; in older computers this often occurred and was referred to as a computer 'crash' and often invoked emotions of frustration. If a computer's CPU shut down, the computer screen would freeze and the input and output devices became disabled. Often the only remedy to bring a frozen computer back to life was to turn off the power to the computer, restart it and reboot it. Today's computers are less likely to exhibit such behavior.

The nucleus of a biologically active cell, arguably possesses the most sophisticated and well organized processing power in the world. To run such a powerful processing unit, a form of biologic computer language would be a necessary foundation with which to transfer and process stored information located in the DNA. Given that the DNA comprising the chromosomes and mitochondrial DNA are both comprised of four different nucleotides including adenine, cytosine, guanine and thymine, and RNA is comprised of four nucleotides including adenine, cytosine, guanine and uracil (uracil in place of thymine), it appears evident the biologic computer language used by a cell's genome is an information language derived from base-four mathematics. Instead of current computer technology utilizing binary computer code comprised of 'ones' and 'zeros', the

DNA and RNA in a biologically active cell utilize an information language comprised of 'zeros', 'one's', two's' and 'threes' to store and transfer information, which in effect represents a base-four language or quaternary language.

The above-mentioned provincial definitions of a 'gene' refer to genes residing in a specific place or locus on a chromosome. Identifying that a gene is present in a particular location is obvious to the human observer, but from a functional standpoint for cell biology this does not necessarily assist a cell in finding or using the information stored in the nucleotide sequence of a particular gene. To rely on location alone, as a means of identifying a gene, would put the function of the entire genome at peril of failure if even a single base pair of nucleotides were added or deleted from the genome or damaged in some manner.

The set of genes acting as the template dedicated to the construct of Eukaryote cells is conserved in nature and utilized across those species utilizing Eukaryote cells as their platform to generate the body tissues for a particular species.

The sharing of genetic information between differing species requires a global numbering system to be present in the genome. With each species the physical location of genes would change, since the size of the genome will be different per species. Physical location of the genetic information becomes irrelevant if position of a gene changes with each species. Since it is known that Nature has shared genetic information between species, some form of a unique identification labeling segments of genes becomes imperative to the proper utilization of such genetic information as needed by each species.

The current understanding of the actual biologic structure of a gene is far more elaborate than the standard definition of a gene leads a casual reader to believe; this knowledge has evolved greatly since Gregor Mendel's work in the 19th century.

A gene appears to be comprised of a number of segments loosely strung together along a particular section of DNA. In general there are at least three global segments associated with a gene which include: (1) the Upstream 5' flanking region, (2) the transcriptional region and (3) the Downstream 3' flanking region. See Figure 17.

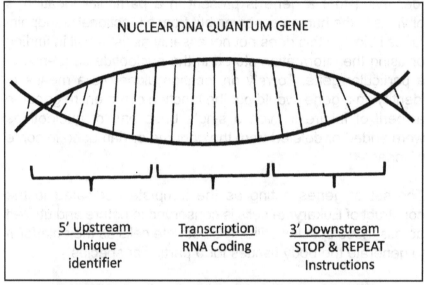

NUCLEAR DNA QUANTUM GENE

5' Upstream	Transcription	3' Downstream
Unique	RNA Coding	STOP & REPEAT
identifier		Instructions

Figure 17: The three global segments of a gene

The Upstream 5' flanking region is comprised of the 'enhancer region', the 'promoter-proximal region', and 'promoter region'.

The 'transcriptional unit' begins at a location designated 'transcription start site' (TSS), which is located in a site called the 'initiator region' (inR), which may be described in a general form as Py_2CAPy_5. See Figure 18. The transcription unit is comprised of the combination of segments of DNA nucleotides to be transcribed into RNA and spacing units known as 'introns' that are not transcribed or if transcribed are later removed post transcription, such that they do not appear in the final RNA molecule. In the case of a gene coding for a mRNA molecule, the transcription unit will contain all three elements of the mRNA, which includes: (1) the 5' noncoding region, (2) the translational region and (3) the 3' noncoding region. Interspersed between these regions are exons, which will not be transcribed and introns that, following transcription, are removed from the precursor form of mRNA prior to the mRNA reaching its final form of maturity. Exons and introns appear to be likened to spacers. The exact role exons and introns play in the transcription process has yet to be determined.

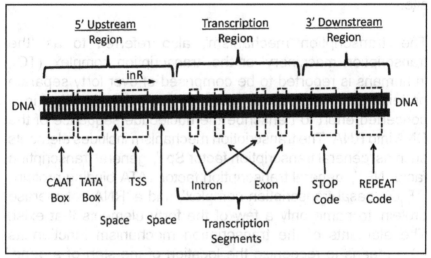

Figure 18: Illustration of the regions surrounding the transcribable region of a gene

The Downstream 3' flanking region contains DNA nucleotides that are not transcribed and may contain what has been termed an 'enhancer region', which may promote the gene previously transcribed to be transcribed again. This region may play a role in selecting the next gene to be transcribed by generating an RNA that points to the next gene.

On either side of the DNA sequencing comprising a gene and its flanking regions, may be inactive DNA which act as boundaries which have been termed 'insulator elements'. The term 'upstream' refers to DNA sequencing that occurs prior to the TSS if viewed from the 5' end to the 3' end of the DNA;

where the term 'downstream' refers to DNA sequencing located after the TSS.

The 'enhancer region' may or may not be present in the Upstream 5' flanking region. If present in the Upstream 5' flanking region, the enhancer region helps facilitate the reading of the gene by encouraging formation of the transcription mechanism. An enhancer may be 50 to 1500 base pairs of nucleotides in length occupying a position upstream from the transcription starting site.

The 'transcription mechanism', also referred to as 'the transcription machinery' or the 'transcription complex' (TC), in humans is reported to be comprised of over forty separate proteins that assemble together to ultimately function in a concerted effort to transcribe the nucleotide sequence of the DNA into RNA. The transcription mechanism includes elements such as 'general transcription factor Sp1', 'general transcription factor NF1', 'general transcription factor TATA-binding protein', 'TF$_{II}$D', 'basal transcription complex', and a 'RNA polymerase protein' to name only a few of the forty elements that exist. The elements of the transcription mechanism function as (1) a means to recognize the location of the start of a gene, (2) proteins to bind the transcription mechanism to the DNA such that transcription may occur or (3) means of transcribing the DNA nucleotide coding to produce a RNA molecule or a precursor RNA molecule.

There are at least three types of RNA polymerase molecules including: RNA polymerase I, RNA polymerase II, and RNA polymerase III. RNA polymerase I tends to be dedicated to transcribing genetic information that will result in the formation of rRNA molecules. RNA polymerase II tends to be dedicated to transcribing genetic information that will result in the formation of mRNA molecules. RNA polymerase III appears to be dedicated to transcribing genetic information that results in the formation of tRNAs, small cellular RNAs and viral RNAs.

The 'promoter proximal region' is located upstream from the TSS and upstream from the core promoter region. The 'promoter proximal region' includes two sub-regions termed the GC box and the CAAT box. The 'GC box' appears to be a segment rich in guanine-cytosine nucleotide sequences. The GC box binds to the 'general transcription factor Sp1' of the transcription mechanism. The 'CAAT box' is a segment which contains the nucleotide sequence 'GGCCAATCT' located approximately 75 base pairs (bps) upstream from the TSS. The CAAT box binds to the 'general transcription factor NF1' of the transcription mechanism.

The 'core promoter' region is considered the shortest sequence within which RNA polymerase II can initiate transcription of a gene The core promoter may include the inR and either a TATA box or a 'downstream promoter element' (DPE). The inR is the region designated Py_2CAPy_5 that surrounds the TSS. The TATA box is located 25 base pairs (bps) upstream from the TSS. The TATA box acts as a site of attachment of the $TF_{II}D$, which is a promoter for binding of the RNA polymerase II molecule. The DPE may appear 28 bps to 32 bps downstream from the TSS. The DPE acts as an alternative site of attachment for the $TF_{II}D$ when the TATA box is not present.

The transcription mechanism or transcription complex appears to be comprised of different elements depending upon whether rRNA is being transcribed versus mRNA or tRNA or small cellular RNA or viral RNA. The proteins that assemble to assist RNA Polymerase I with transcribing the DNA to produce rRNA appear different from the proteins that assemble to assist RNA polymerase II with transcribing the DNA to produce mRNA and from the proteins that assemble to assist RNA polymerase III with transcribing the DNA to produce tRNA, small cellular RNA or viral RNA. A common protein that appears to be present at the initial binding of all three types of RNA polymerase molecules is the TATA-binding protein (TBP). TBP appears to be required to attach to the DNA, which then facilitates

RNA polymerase to bind to the promoter along the DNA. TBP assembles with TBP-associated factors (TAFs). Together TBP and 11 TAFs comprise the complex referred to as $TF_{II}D$.

Upstream from the TATA box is the 'initiator element', which may be considered as part of the 'core promoter' region. The initiator element is a segment of the nuclear DNA that binds the basal transcription complex. The basal transcription complex is comprised of a number of proteins that make initial contact with the DNA prior to the RNA polymerase binding to the transcription mechanism. The basal transcription complex is associated with an activator.

An activator is a protein comprised of three components: a DNA binding domain, a connecting domain, and an activating domain. When the activator's DNA binding domain attaches to the DNA at a specific point along the DNA, the activator's activating domain then causes the other elements of the transcription mechanism to assemble at this location. Generally the assembly of the other proteins occurs downstream from where the activator's DNA binding domain attached to the DNA. There is evidence that the activator is associated with the activity of small RNAs.

The design of the cell is so complex, all of its functions so diverse and intricate that some form of practical order is necessitated. The genes must be ordered in some fashion, especially in a human, where there are at least 30,000 different genes used by the cells. Some estimates put the total number of genes present in the human nuclear DNA genome to be closer to 100,000. If no means of order existed as to how the genes could be identified, then 'random circumstance' would dictate a cell locating a particular portion of genetic information that it requires, at any given time. Randomness tends to favor the occurrence of random events rather than a purposeful order. A 'random circumstance' approach to any living cell would tend to favor failure of the cell rather than survival of the cell.

INTRODUCING THE UNIQUE IDENTIFIER

To allow a cell to utilize the biologic information stored in a gene a 'unique identifier' must be associated with or attached to each gene's specific nucleotide sequence. In the human genome, the cell's transcription mechanism require an organized means to locate and transcribe any given gene's nucleotide sequence amongst the 3 billion nucleotides that reside in the 46 chromosomes that comprise human DNA. Given how the transcription mechanism assembles upstream from the portion of the gene to be transcribed, the nucleotide sequence acting as a unique identifier associated with a specific gene would be positioned upstream from the transcription start site.

The transcription complex (TC) engages the DNA upstream from the genetic information segment the TC transcribes. The unique identifier may be attached directly to the RNA coding segment of genetic material, or there may exist one or more base pairs physically separating the unique identifier and the RNA coding portion of genetic material. Regarding some genes, there may be numerous base pairs separating the unique identifier from the transcribable region of the gene.

A unique identification may exist as (1) a single contiguous segment or (2) two or more segments, with unrelated base pairs of nucleotides present between the segments the two or more segments present along the DNA strand upstream from the RNA coding region. In the case where a unique identification exits as two or more segments, combined, these segments represent the unique identification of the associated quantum gene.

For any form of 'gene therapy' to work efficiently, medically therapeutic genetic material inserted into the native DNA of a cell needs to be associated with a unique identifier. Attaching a unique identifier to medically therapeutic genetic material is essential in making it possible for the components of a transcription complex to, in a timely organized fashion, locate the exogenous medically therapeutic genetic material, assemble around this exogenous genetic material, and decode the information contained therein. If no such unique identifier is used, then utilization of such exogenous transcribable genetic information occurs based on the occurrence of random events rather than dictated by therapeutic design.

Naturally occurring unique identifiers in the nuclear genome may occur in numerous forms. Since humans share 47% of their DNA with bananas and 95% of their DNA with monkeys, a portion of the unique identifiers associated with genes in the nuclear DNA may not be specific to a human. Unique identifiers may have a global utility, with a portion of the genome of any organism being shared amongst numerous species. The rational would be that once Nature developed an adequate fundamental design for a particular facet of biologic organisms, this information may be shared amongst numerous species that would benefit from the design. An example might be the basic design of a eukaryote cell; this information would be shared amongst all life that utilized the eukaryote cell design rather than each successive multi-celled species having to repeatedly re-invent the design of a eukaryote cell. Some unique identifiers may be specific to and help define a particular Phylum, Class, Family, Genus or Species.

To support the theory of evolution, genes need to be present in the DNA and these genes need to be turned on or activated and turned off or deactivated when it is to the advantage to survival of the organism. When a gene is activated, the gene must be able to be identified so that it can be located and used by the organism. Activated genes either in combination or by themselves often express some form of phenotypical feature that acts as a means of recognizing a particular species from another species. When genes are activated and linked to other genes and provide enough genetic information to produce a unique species, activated genes need to be able to be easily identified and located by the processing units in the cell's nucleus so that the genetic information can be easily utilized by the biologic machinery of a cell.

In order for the knowledge base of cellular genetics to progress forward, the definition of a gene must be expanded to include the presence of a 'unique identifier' associated with each gene present within the DNA. The basis for the presence of this unique identifier (UI) associated with each active gene is so that the cell can locate the biologic information stored in the DNA nucleotide sequencing of the gene. An active gene refers to those genes present in the genome that are utilized by a particular species to support conception, development and maintenance of the species.

INTRODUCING THE QUANTUM GENE

Upon adding a unique identifier to a gene, the current term 'gene' is thus expanded to the term 'quantum gene'. The term 'quantal' in biology generally refers to an 'all or nothing' state or response. The term 'quantal' is a derivative of the word quantum. The term 'quantum' means a quantity or amount, and a discrete quantity of energy or a discrete bundle of energy or a discrete quantity of electromagnetic radiation.

A 'quantum gene' (See Figure 19) is comprised of a sequence of nucleotides that represents a 'unique identifier' physically linked to a sequence of nucleotides that represent a discrete quantity of genetic information; these sequences of nucleotides being comprised of some combination of the nucleotides being referred to by their nitrogenous base as adenine (A), thymine (T), cytosine (C), and guanine (G). The genetic information associated with the above-mentioned unique identifier may be comprised of a portion of transcribable genetic information and a portion of nontranscribable genetic information which together define a specific gene, otherwise referred to as a discrete quantity of genetic information.

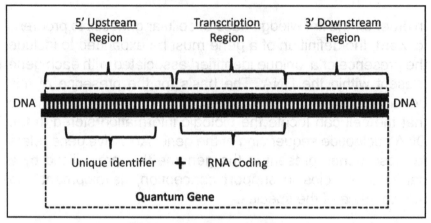

Figure 19: Quantum Gene

Similar to how a gene is described, with regards to a quantum gene, the term 'upstream' refers to DNA sequencing that occurs prior to the transcription start site (TSS) if viewed from the 5' end to the 3' end of the DNA; where the term 'downstream' refers to DNA sequencing located after the TSS.

Similar to the previously described organization of a standard gene found in nuclear DNA, a quantum gene is structured with at least three global segments which include: (1) the Upstream 5' flanking region, (2) the transcriptional unit and possibly instructional units and (3) the Downstream 3' flanking region. The 'unique identifier' is located in the Upstream 5' flanking region. The current standard definition of a gene strictly encompasses the concept that a gene is comprised of a segment of nuclear DNA that when transcribed produces RNA. Therefore, the differences between the current standard definition of a 'gene' and the definition of a 'quantum gene' is that a quantum gene includes both a unique identifier and a segment of nuclear DNA that when transcribed produces RNA. The segment of nuclear DNA that when transcribed produces RNA is comprised of one or more segments of transcribable genetic information that may be accompanied by one or more segments of nontranscribable genetic information. Nontranscribable segments of genetic information include segments that are removed or ignored during the transcription process or segments that act as commands which includes a START code, STOP code or a REPEAT code. When present, a START code signals initiation of the transcription process. When present, a STOP code signals the discontinuation of the transcription process. When present, a REPEAT code signals that the transcription process should repeat the transcription of the segment of DNA that was just transcribed.

Analogous to the standard description of a 'gene', a quantum gene's Upstream 5' flanking region is comprised of the 'enhancer region', the 'promoter-proximal region', and 'promoter region'. The definition of quantum gene adds the presence of the unique identifier to the Upstream 5' flanking region.

Similar to the standard description of a 'gene', a quantum gene's 'transcriptional unit' begins at a location designated TSS, which is located in a site called the 'initiator region' (inR), which may be described in a general form as Py_2CAPy_5. The transcription unit is comprised of the combination of segments of DNA nucleotides to be transcribed into RNA and spacing units known as 'exons' AND 'introns', whereby exons represent segments that are not transcribed and introns represent segments that are transcribed but later removed post transcription, such that they do not appear in the final RNA molecule. In the case of a gene coding for a mRNA molecule, the transcription unit will contain all three elements of the mRNA, which includes: (1) the 5' noncoding region, (2) the translational region and (3) the 3' noncoding region. Interspersed between these regions are exons, which will not be transcribed and introns that if transcribed, are removed from the precursor form of mRNA prior to the mRNA reaching its final form. Exons and introns present in nuclear DNA appear to be likened to spacers interspersed in the nuclear DNA. The exact role exons and introns play in the transcription process is undetermined.

Comparable to the standard description of a gene, with regards to the quantum gene the Downstream 3' flanking region contains DNA nucleotides that are not transcribed and may contain what has been termed an 'enhancer region'. An enhancer region in the Downstream 3' flanking region may promote the quantum gene previously transcribed to be transcribed again or point to the next quantum gene to be transcribed.

On either side of the DNA sequencing comprising a gene and a quantum gene are flanking regions which represent inactive DNA, which act as boundaries which have been termed 'insulator elements'. Insulator elements are areas that are not transcribed to produce RNA. The function of insulator elements, other than acting as boundary markers between differing genes, is unknown.

Embedded in nuclear DNA, quantum genes are comprised of a segment of deoxyribonucleic acid where the portion that represents a unique identifier may be separated from the portion that represents transcribable genetic information by a quantity of base pairs of nucleotides that do not represent a unique identifier and do not represent transcribable genetic information. The purpose of the separation of the portion of the unique identifier from the portion of the genetic information by a quantity of base pairs of nucleotides that do not represent a unique identifier and do not represent genetic information may be to act to facilitate a transcription complex attaching to the quantum gene upstream from the portion of the quantum gene that represents genetic information so that transcription of the biologic information associated with the quantum gene may occur at the designated starting point.

The unique identification or identifier of a quantum gene could be in the form of a nucleotide sequence that represents a name assigned to the quantum gene, or a number assigned to a quantum gene or the combination of a name and number assigned to a quantum gene. Irrespective of whether the unique identifier incorporated in a quantum gene is considered a 'name', or a 'number' or a combination of a name or number, the unique identifier is comprised of a sequence of nucleotides linked to the transcribable genetic information for which it acts as a unique identifier; these sequences of nucleotides being comprised of some combination of the nucleotides being referred to by their nitrogenous base as adenine (A), thymine (T), cytosine (C), and guanine G). It has been estimated that there are as many as 100,000 separate genes stored in the DNA of the 46 chromosomes comprising the human genome. In a base four language, a string of nine nucleotides is needed to code for 256,144 individual genes. If there were over a million quantum genes, then a string of ten nucleotides could be used since ten nucleotides could represent 1,024,576 unique numbers in a base-four number system.

Utilizing a base four number system a string of twenty-five nucleotides would represent the number 1,125,899,906,842,624, which could account for 200,000 different quantum genes in 5 billion different species. (By contrast, the digital technology that acts as the platform for all current computer services, can only represent approximately 17 million different numbers utilizing a string of 25 bits.) Therefore 200,000 different quantum genes could easily be dedicated to producing a biped form of life.

The differing number of species of organisms is recorded to be approximately 1.8 million. There are recorded 4,000 differing bacteria, 80,0000 differing protocitists, 72,0000 differing fungi, 270,000 differing plants, 1,272,0000 differing animal invertebrates and 52,0000 animal vertebrates for a total of 1,750,000 recorded species. The recorded species have been approximated to account for only a small number of actual species that inhabit the planet. It is estimated that 5-14 million different species actually exist on the planet today.

The time the average species is thought to be in existence is estimated to be 10 million years. It is also believed that 99% of the species that have ever existed have already become extinct. Given it is generally accepted that life has existed on earth for 3.5 billion years, it has been estimated that the number of species that has ever existed on the planet is between 200 million and 1 billion. Since a grouping of twenty-five base-four bits offers 5 billion possibilities, given 200,000 possible genes per species, utilizing this base-four mathematics, the genome could account for all of the possible species that have already existed on the planet. Considering that much of the genome required to construct a particular species is potentially shared with other species, especially basic microbiology such as cell constructs, the 200,000 genes allocated to contrive a species may indeed be too high of a number, since the number of genes necessary to produce a particular species may be a much smaller number of genes, thus conserving the unique identifier. This suggests that a unique identifier consisting of a string of twenty-five characters offers an even larger number of possible species beyond 5 billion.

In the human genome 5% of the 3 billion base pairs are considered to represent genes by the current definition of a gene. If 5% of the human genome represents the 100,000 quantum genes in the nuclear DNA, then on average 1500 nucleotides can be dedicated to each gene within this 5% of DNA nucleotides. If 25 nucleotides are dedicated to a unique address or unique identifier, then there remain 1475 nucleotides, on average, to be utilized for coding the biologic information associated with each of the 100,000 quantum genes estimated to exist in the human genome.

By recognizing that a unique identification exists, it may be determined that a portion of the 95% of the human genome not presently considered to represent genes may indeed represent genes that have been unrecognized in their role as a gene. There may be numerous instructions associated with quantum genes that do not have a phenotypical role, but exist as a function role in the construction and maintenance of a cell.

A unique identifier (UI) incorporated in quantum genes could be comprised of a unique number or a unique name or the unique combination of a number and a name. A name might be represented as a single letter or a series of letters. The current convention utilized in science is to apply the four letter alphabet A, C, G, T to represent the four different bases of the nucleotides comprising the DNA, which include adenine, cytosine, guanine, and thymine respectfully. With regards to RNA, the four letter alphabet A, C, G, U is utilized to represent the bases of the nucleotides which include adenine, cytosine, guanine, and uracil. Regarding utilizing a unique identifier for DNA, a name could be comprised of a series of letters derived from the four letters A, C, G, and T. Regarding utilizing a unique identifier for purposes of use within an RNA molecule, a unique identifier could be comprised of a series of letters derived from the four letters A, C, G, and U. The current scientific convention does not recognize a mathematical base-four nomenclature regarding DNA or RNA. The unique identifier could be represented as a number. Names can be translated into numbers and vice versa.

In nuclear DNA, there are several places in the upstream segment of a quantum gene where a contiguous segment of twenty-five, or more, or less, base pairs could exist that acts as the unique identifying code that uniquely identifies the segment of transcribable genetic information. Though a unique identifier having a length of 25 base pairs of nucleotides would serve the purpose of the concept of a unique identifier, a unique identifier may exist as a larger or smaller string of base pairs of nucleotides. The transcription start site (TSS) is present upstream from a segment of transcribable genetic information. There exists a segment of 25 bps upstream from the TSS that occupies the space along the DNA between the TSS and the TATA box. There exists the downstream promoter element (DPE) 28 bps to 32 bps downstream from the TSS. The DPE acts as an alternative site of attachment for the $TF_{II}D$ when the TATA box is not present. Within the 28 bps to 32 bps of DNA separating the DPE from the TSS may also be a convenient location for a unique identifying code to reside and be associated with the genetic information located just downstream. Living cell exist with numerous inherent variability. There exists variation in the arrangement of the elements upstream from the transcribable genetic information, therefore various sites upstream from the transcribable genetic information may function as the unique identifying code for some quantum genes. The unique identifying code may be represented as subsegments of DNA, where subsegments are physically separated from each other, but in combination, the subsegments act in unison to identify a segment of transcribable genetic information.

Computer software programs are comprised of lines of code. See Table P3-1. Each line of code generally represents an instruction or a unit of data. Early computer programming required each line of code to be identified by a unique number. The earliest programming required these unique numbers to be in a sequential order. As computer processors became faster and more powerful, computer programming techniques became less rigid. Large computer programs are often divided into groups of lines of code. A group of lines of code is termed a 'subprogram' and subprograms are often identified by a unique name. The group of instructions comprising a subprogram could then be accessed by the main program by simply referencing the unique name of the subprogram.

Line Number	Program Instruction Statement
001	START
002	INPUT A
003	INPUT B
004	C = A + B
005	PRINT C
006	STOP

TABLE P3-1
Line numbered steps comprising a simple
addition computer program.

Table P3-1 illustrates a computer program comprised of six lines. Each line of the program has a unique line number. The program starts at line 001. Line 002 asks for the variable A to be input. Line 003 asks for the variable B to be input. Once the two variables have been inserted Line 004 represents the command that adds the two variables together. Line 005 prints the result of adding variable A to variable B. Line 006 stops the program.

The term ASCII is an abbreviation for American Standard Code For Information Interchange. The ASCII code was originally developed for teletypewriters but eventually found wide application in personal computers. The initial standard ASCII code used seven-digit binary numbers. By utilizing numbers consisting of various sequences of 0's and 1's, the code could represent 128 different characters.

ASCII was a standard data-transmission code that was used by smaller and less-powerful computers to represent both textual data (letters, numbers, and punctuation marks) and non-input device commands (control characters). Like other coding systems, it converts information into standardized digital formats that allow computers to communicate with each other and to efficiently process and store data.

In 1981, International Business Machines Corporation (IBM) introduced an extended ASCII code, an eight-bit system, for use with its first model of personal computer. Digital computer technology uses a binary code that is arranged in groups of eight rather than of seven bits. Each such eight-bit group is referred to as a byte. By utilizing an eight-bit system, the number of characters the code could represent increased to 256.

The first 32 characters (0-31) of the extended ASCII code are unprintable and are used to control peripheral devices. Printable characters are from binary codes 32 to 127. Numbers from 'zero' to 'nine' are characters 48 to 57. The upper case letters 'A' to 'Z' are characters 65 to 90. The lower case letters 'a' to 'z' are characters 97 to 122. As an example, Table P3-2 demonstrates the decimal numbers '0' to '9' and the associated binary numbers as seen in the extended ASCII code.

ASCII Code	Number	Binary Number
48	0	00110000
49	1	00110001
50	2	00110010
51	3	00110011
52	4	00110100
53	5	00110101
54	6	00110110
55	7	00110111
56	8	00111000
57	9	00111001

Table P3-2
Numbers 0 to 9 represented as their ASCII binary numbers.

As far as the entire scope of digital computer technology is concerned all numbers, letters, characters and instructions are represented as differing strings of ones and zeros. The strings of ones and zeros are linked together to produce numbers, words, text and computer commands. Individual segments of information stored in a computer are tagged with a unique address identifier to facilitate quickly locating the information amongst everything else stored in memory, when the specific information is needed by the computer's central processor.

The core concept of a 'quantum gene' is the association of a 'unique identifier' with a segment of 'translatable DNA'.

Since humans share 47% of their genome with that of the genome of a banana, and 95% of their genome with the genome of a monkey, more than likely genetic instructions are grouped together. This grouping of genetic instructions facilitates the design of segments of a cell not having to be re-invented by each succeeding species.

Table P3-3 illustrates the concept that a biologic genetic program could be organized in the DNA utilizing a unique identifier comprised of a string of 25 characters. Insulin is a protein structure comprised of two proteins each comprised of a differing chain of amino acid molecules. Insulin is generated inside the Beta cells located in the Islets of Langerhans inside the organ known as the pancreas. A set of programming instructions would be required to produce each of the two chains of protein. A more complex set of instructions would be required to construct a Beta cell. Further a more complex set of instructions would be necessary to construct the organ referred to as the pancreas. Any organism sophisticated enough to require a pancreas may carry and utilize the universal set of genes that are needed to construct the pancreas, the Islets of Langerhans, the Beta cells and the insulin protein.

Num- ber	Unique Identifier 25-characters	Tran- script Re- gion	Transcription Instructions
1	3000000000000000001000000	1	Design of Pancreas
2	3000000000000000001100000	2	Design of Islet of Langerhans
3	3000000000000000001110000	3	Design of Beta Cell
4	3000000000000000001110100	4	Insulin Protein 1
5	3000000000000000001110110	5	Insulin Protein 2

TABLE P3-3
Example of how the unique identifier may
be used to organize instructions*.

*all numbers presented as unique identifiers are meant to be for illustra-
tion purposes only

All of the genetic instruction code necessary to build each and every structure comprising the human body could have a unique identifier comprised of 25-characters associated with it to act as a label so that the instruction code can be located when needed. All of the data required to build the various structures of the human body would similarly be labeled and stored in an organized fashion in the DNA of the nucleus. In Figure 20 a series of generic unique identifiers are illustrated along with a series of generic transcribable regions. UI 1 represents a unique identifier for transcribable region 1, while the remaining unique identifiers are associated with other unique transcribable regions.

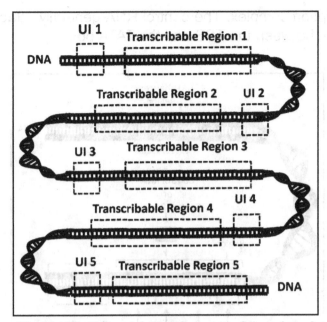

**Figure 20: Unique Identifiers are Associated
with Individual Transcription Regions**

CONTROL RNA AND CONTROL PROTEIN

The concept of a unique identifier is only feasible if there is a means of utilizing the segment of DNA that comprises the unique identifier. The antithesis of the unique identifier would be either in the form of a Control RNA or a Control Protein.

A control RNA is a form of RNA that is coded to attach to the segment of DNA that represents the unique identifier. See Figure 21. By the action of the control RNA attaching to the DNA at the unique identifier, this assists in the assembly of a transcription complex in the 5' Upstream region of the quantum gene so that the translatable region of the quantum gene can be decoded. See Figure 22. Control RNA molecules are small molecules, less than fifty amino acids in length. Control RNA molecules are comprised of a portion that attaches to the unique identifier on the DNA and a segment that acts as a tail, which attracts one or more molecules that assemble into a transcription complex. The control RNA generally attaches to the DNA between the TSS and the TATA box.

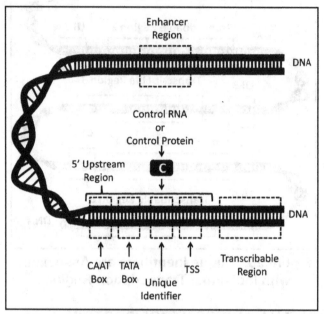

Figure 21: Control RNA or Control Protein binding to the Unique Identifier

Control RNA molecules are derived from decoding the DNA. In order for a stepwise process to occur in an efficient manner, one gene would need to be able to point to a subsequent gene to continue certain processes of building or maintaining biologic structures. While a gene is being transcribed, a portion of the transcription process produces one or more control RNAs. The control RNAs generated when a quantum gene is transcribed, cause other subsequent quantum genes to be transcribed by the nucleus. Control RNAs may even cause the gene that produced the control RNA to be reread, in order to form a looping action, where certain RNAs are required to be continuously produced to maintain either the cell's health or the body's health.

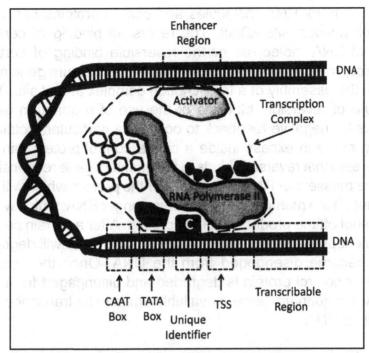

**Figure 22: Presence of Control RNA or Control Protein
activates assembly of a Transcription Complex**

Control proteins provide a means for feedback to the nucleus from the organelle's in the cell's cytoplasm. When a messenger RNA is needed to produce a specific protein, a control protein is generated by an organelle. The control protein migrates from the cytoplasm into the nucleus. Once in the nucleus, the control protein binds to the DNA at the site of the unique identifier that the protein is programmed to interface with. Once bound to the unique identifier of a quantum gene the control protein acts like a control RNA and the binding action stimulates the assembly of a transcription complex in order to facilitate transcription of the transcribable region of the quantum gene.

Both control RNA molecules and control proteins when bound to the unique identifier of a quantum gene can act in a positive manner to activate the assembly of a transcription complex to facilitate transcription of the transcribable region of a quantum gene. Control RNA molecules and control proteins can also exhibit an opposite effect. The reversible binding of certain control RNA molecules or the reversible binding of certain control proteins to the unique identifier of a quantum gene may block the assembly of a transcription complex at that site. The feature of reversible blocking of the use of a quantum gene allows for negative feedback to occur. If a particular protein is being made in excess inside a cell, a control protein can be generated that reversibly binds to the quantum gene responsible for the messenger RNA that codes for the protein, which will act to shut off the manufacture of the messenger RNA, which will in turn shut off the production of the protein. After a certain period of time lapses, the control RNA or control protein will degrade and become disengaged from the DNA. Once the control RNA or control protein is degraded and disengaged from the DNA, the quantum gene is available again to be transcribed to produce RNA.

The above concepts can be utilized to effect very precise and very powerful medical management tools with the least potential side effects. As described earlier in this text, Configurable Delivery Devices (CDD) can be constructed to deliver a variety of medically therapeutic payloads to any specific cell in the body. The options of medical therapeutic payloads that a CDD could transport include RNAs, segments of DNA, proteins, chemicals and nutrients. This segment of text describes the option of utilizing CDDs to deliver control RNAs or control proteins to cells to activate the transcription of quantum genes that are dormant. See Figure 23. With the use of control RNAs and control proteins quantum genes could be transcribed on a selective basis that results in a beneficial medical therapeutic effect for a patient.

In the case where a quantum gene is flawed due to genetic malformation or damage, and cannot be used, a CDD would be able to transport a functional version of the quantum gene to cells that require the quantum gene. Quantum genes can become damaged due to radiation exposure, errors during cell replication and division, and due to harmful effects from viruses. Once a quantum gene has been delivered by a CDD to a cell and inserted into the nuclear DNA, other CDDs can deliver to the cells either control RNAs or control proteins to be used to activate the assembly of transcription complexes in order to facilitate transcription of the delivered quantum genes.

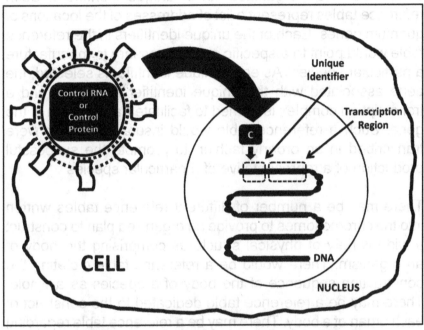

**Figure 23: Control RNA or Control Protein
activates transcription of a quantum gene**

An example of this process would be the treatment of diabetes mellitus. Insulin, a protein, facilitates the transfer of glucose from the blood into cells. Delivering quantum genes, containing the genetic information required to produce insulin, directly to the Beta cells responsible for the production of insulin, then activating transcription of these quantum genes by utilizing control RNAs or control proteins as needed, will significantly improve the medical treatment of diabetes mellitus.

INTRODUCTION OF REFERENCE
TABLES IN THE GENOME

In addition to unique identifiers being present in the 5' Upstream segment of a quantum gene, unique identifiers may comprise an important part of reference tables. To facilitate the physical construction of a species, more than likely there are reference tables present in the chromosomes, these reference tables comprised of an organized list of unique identifiers. Such reference tables represent a list of addresses of the locations of quantum genes. Each of the unique identifiers in the reference table would point to a specific gene necessary to manufacture a particular species. As each unique identifier is selected, the gene associated with the unique identifier is located and a transcription complex is formed to facilitate transcription of the gene. Such a reference table would insure the genes were transcribed in an orderly fashion to promote the successful production of a representative of a particular species.

There may be a number of different reference tables written into the chromosomes to provide an organized plan to construct a wide variety of physical structures comprising the body of an organism. There would be a reference table dictating the construction sequence of the body of a species as a whole. There may be a reference table dedicated to the construct of each organ of a body. There may be a reference table regarding the construction of each of the different cell types comprising a body. There may be a reference table dedicated to the construct of a basic cell design. There may be reference tables defining the construction of each organelle found in a cell. There may also be reference tables assigned to listing a series of unique identifiers that are associated with the maintenance of the body as a whole and/or for each of the different cells comprising a body. Reference tables and the quantum genes they point to are most likely conserved between species. A generic reference table dictating basic construction of a generic cell might appear as the example presented in Table P3-4.

Number	Unique Identifier 25-characters	Transcript Region	Cell Components
1	0000000000000100000000000 AAAAAAAAAAAAAACAAAAAAAAAA	1	Genes to construct cell membrane
2	0000000000000111000000000 AAAAAAAAAAAAAACCCAAAAAAAAA	2	Genes to construct chloroplast
3	0000000000000112000000000 AAAAAAAAAAAAAACCGAAAAAAAAA	3	Genes to construct mitochondria
4	0000000000000113010000000 AAAAAAAAAAAAAACCTACAAAAAAA	4	Genes to construct Golgi Apparatus
5	0000000000000111111000000 AAAAAAAAAAAAAACCCCCCAAAAAA	5	Genes to construct rough endoplasmic reticulum
6	0000000000000111111200000 AAAAAAAAAAAAAACCCCCCGAAAAA	6	Genes to construct smooth endoplasmic reticulum
7	0000000000000111121000000 AAAAAAAAAAAAAACCCCGCAAAAAA	7	Genes to construct flagella
8	0000000000000111131000000 AAAAAAAAAAAAAACCCCTCAAAAAA	8	Genes to construct micro tubular network
9	0000000000000111221000000 AAAAAAAAAAAAAACCCGGCAAAAAA	9	Genes to construct lysosomes
10	0000000000000111223000000 AAAAAAAAAAAAAACCCGGTAAAAAA	10	Genes to construct vacuoles

11	00000000000000200000000000 AAAAAAAAAAAAAAGAAAAAAAAAAA	11	Genes to construct nuclear membrane
12	00000000000000221111000000 AAAAAAAAAAAAAGGCCCCAAAAAA	12	Genes to construct chromosomes
13	00000000000000223111000000 AAAAAAAAAAAAAGGTCCCAAAAAA	13	Genes to construct nucleosides
14	00000000000000223211100000 AAAAAAAAAAAAAGGTGCCCAAAAAA	14	Genes to construct mitotic spin-dles

Table P3-4
Example of how unique identifiers may
organize construction of a cell*.

*all numbers presented as unique identifiers are meant to be for illustration purposes only

The information presented in Table P3-4 is only meant to act as a simplified example of what a reference table for constructing a cell might appear like in the chromosomes. Tables such as this may be widespread throughout the DNA and function to orchestrate the construction of all types of physical elements comprising the body. Reference tables may even be present at the level of providing the proper sequence of steps required to manufacture individual chemical molecules needed by the cell. In Table P3-4, under the heading of 'Unique Identifier 25-characters' is presented both the numerical and the nucleotide sequence for the unique identifier. In this case A=0, C=1, G=2, and T=3.

In and of themselves, reference tables would have no phenotypical characteristics to identify their presence in the

DNA. Reference tables represent a series of commands manifested by pointing to a series of quantum genes that are arranged in an orderly fashion to act as a guide to insure the proper construction of the physical elements comprising a cell. More than likely, reference tables occupy a portion of the DNA that at this time is considered to be meaningless genetic code or as some have described 'useless genetic junk'. Much of the generic code considered to be useless at this time because it does not exhibit the phenotypical features of the currently known genes, is comprised of the instructions necessary to utilize the known body of genes.

GENETIC REFERENCE TABLES: KEY TO EVOLUTION

Unique identifiers make it possible to locate quantum genes in the DNA. Reference tables provide an orderly means for transcribing a group of quantum genes. Speed of transcription becomes an important factor in cell growth and metabolism; and is important to the survival of the entire organism. How fast the nucleus can locate a quantum gene may be just as important as locating and transcribing the gene. Since there are forty-six chromosomes comprising human genetics, knowing which chromosome harbors a particular quantum gene is vital to locating the quantum gene.

There may be one or more reference tables that identify, amongst the forty-six chromosomes, where each quantum gene resides.

Control of transcription of quantum genes may be a hybrid of (1) direction provided by a reference table, but may also be related to (2) instructions present in the end of the transcription region or in the 3' Downstream segment of a quantum gene.

After the transcribable region of a quantum gene has been transcribed, the transcription complex may proceed to transcribe one or more control RNA molecules. The purpose of the control RNA molecules would be to (1) point back to the reference table or (2) point directly to the next gene that is required to be transcribed. Once a control molecule is generated it either traverses the nucleus to the location of the reference table to provide feedback that indicates that the required quantum gene was indeed transcribed and the next quantum gene in the series should be transcribed or the control molecule traverses the genome and directly activates a transcription complex at the site of the next quantum gene. Control RNA molecules may be manufactured as the antithesis of the unique identifier found either in the reference table or in the 5' Upstream region of a quantum gene to facilitate binding of the control RNA to the unique identifier.

The changes that have occurred to the life forms that have inhabited the planet, as documented by paleontologists and geneticists, has been referred to as evolution. Evolution has been thought to be related to alterations in the genes of species, these alterations occurring randomly, but being responsible for the development of new forms of life. Changes in the DNA that has led to evolutionary changes may actually in part be due to functional changes that have occurred within the bounds of the genetic reference tables stored in the genome. If genome reference tables direct the order by which transcription of genes occurs, then an alteration of a genome reference table would change which quantum genes were transcribed or the order of when quantum genes were transcribed.

A master genome reference table may be associated with each species. Genome reference tables represent a list of addresses of the locations of quantum genes. A generic master genome reference table may be refined to specific details associated with most species. This generic master genome reference table may be altered by various external or internal factors that lead to the master genome reference table for each species. This would suggest that genes comprising the DNA may be transcribed or not transcribed. If a quantum gene is necessary for the construction or the maintenance of a species it is transcribable. If a quantum gene is not necessary it is dormant and is never transcribed during the lifecycle of the species.

A species generic master genome reference table would be present in some form for all organisms. Smaller, more truncated forms of the master genome reference table may be present in more primitive organisms. The concept of a generic master genome reference table would help explain why the single celled organism Red Algae possesses 60 chromosomes, while humans possess only 46 chromosomes. As life forms develop into more sophisticated and diverse organisms there may not be a need to conserve all of the genetic instructions from one species to another or from one generation to another.

UNIVERSAL GENOME REFERENCE TABLE

A universal genome reference table would be comprised of quantum genes from all four of the major taxonomy kingdoms. As seen in Table P3-5, all four groupings are represented. Table P3-5 is a very primitive representation of what a universal genome reference table would appear like. An actual universal genome master genome reference table would be much more elaborate and far more detailed. Such an elaborate set of instructions may fill the 95% of the human genome that is currently thought not to represent genes, but instead to represent useless genetic garbage. Basic cell design and structure is present in group one. Construct of fungi and other associated life forms present in group two. Plant design structure present in group three. Animal design and structure present in group four.

Group	Unique Identifier 25-characters	• Instructions to manufacture species
0	0000000000000100000000000 AAAAAAAAAAAAAACAAAAAAAAAAA	Genes to construct cell membrane
0	0000000000000111000000000 AAAAAAAAAAAAAACCCAAAAAAAAA	Genes to construct chloroplast
0	0000000000000112000000000 AAAAAAAAAAAAAACCGAAAAAAAAA	Genes to construct mitochondria
0	0000000000000113010000000 AAAAAAAAAAAAAACCTACAAAAAAA	Genes to construct Golgi Apparatus
0	0000000000000111121000000 AAAAAAAAAAAAAACCCCGCAAAAAA	Genes to construct flagella
0	0000000000000111131000000 AAAAAAAAAAAAAACCCCTCAAAAAA	Genes to construct micro tubular network
0	0000000000000200000000000 AAAAAAAAAAAAAAGAAAAAAAAAAA	Genes to construct nuclear membrane
0	0000000000000221111000000 AAAAAAAAAAAAAAGGCCCCAAAAAA	Genes to construct chromosomes
0	0000000000000223211000000 AAAAAAAAAAAAAAGGTGCCAAAAAA	Genes to construct mitotic spindles
0	0000000000000223211200000 AAAAAAAAAAAAAAGGTGCCGAAAAA	Genes to construct a virus
1	1000000000011223211000000 CAAAAAAAAAACCGGTGCCAAAAAA	Genes to construct hypha
1	1000000000111223211000000 CAAAAAAAAAACCCGGTGCCAAAAAA	Genes to construct spores
2	2000000000012223211000000 GAAAAAAAAAACGGGTGCCAAAAAA	Genes to construct seed
2	2000000000013223211000000 GAAAAAAAAAACTGGTGCCAAAAAA	Genes to construct leaves
3	3000000000111223211000000 TAAAAAAAAAACCCGGTGCCAAAAAA	Genes to construct skeleton
3	3000000000122300001000000 TAAAAAAAAAACGGTAAAACAAAAAA	Construct a heart
3	3000000000222200001000000 TAAAAAAAAAGGGGAAAACAAAAAA	Construct lungs
3	3000000000322200001000000 TAAAAAAAAATGGGAAAACAAAAAA	Construct a kidney

3	3 0 0 0 0 0 0 0 0 0 0 0 0 0 0 0 0 1 0 0 0 0 0 0 T A A A A A A A A A A A A A A A A A C A A A A A A	Genes to construct a pancreas
3	3 0 0 0 0 0 0 0 0 0 3 3 2 2 0 0 0 0 1 0 0 0 0 0 0 T A A A A A A A A A A T T G G A A A A C A A A A A A	Genes to construct a liver
3	3 0 0 0 0 0 0 0 0 0 0 0 0 0 2 2 3 2 1 1 0 0 0 0 0 0 T A A A A A A A A A A A A A G G T G C C A A A A A A	Genes to construct a fin
3	3 0 0 0 0 0 0 0 0 0 0 0 0 0 2 2 3 2 1 1 0 0 0 0 0 0 T A A A A A A A A A A A A A G G T G C C A A A A A A	Genes to construct a leg limb
3	3 0 0 0 0 0 0 0 0 0 0 0 0 0 2 2 3 2 1 1 0 0 0 0 0 0 T A A A A A A A A A A A A A G G T G C C A A A A A A	Genes to construct an arm limb
3	3 0 0 0 0 0 0 0 0 0 0 0 0 0 2 2 3 2 1 1 0 0 0 0 0 0 T A A A A A A A A A A A A A G G T G C C A A A A A A	Genes to construct a tail

Table P3-5
Simplified version of a Universal Genome Reference Table*.

*all numbers presented as unique identifiers are meant to be for illustration purposes only

Each of the four major taxonomy kingdoms of classification including Monera, Protista, Plantae and Animalia may have its own generic master genome reference table comprised of the list of quantum genes that can be selected to support a viable species. Ultimately, most likely there was one original universal genome reference table that described all quantum genes. The universal genome reference table may have been modified into smaller reference tables per Kingdom, Phylum, Family and Order for ease of replication. Diversity amongst life may be related to the switching on and off of genes that are present in generic reference tables. If the genomes of all forms of life were to be combined together and redundant segments reduced to only one copy, the universal master genome reference table could be recompiled together.

The concept of a universal genome reference table would provide an explanation as to why fish in the oceans could over time evolve into legged creatures and birds. A universal master genome reference table coincides with the observations that the basic construct of fins lead to legs and then led to the construct of wings. The genes related to the construct of fins became untranscribable (deactivated), while the genes that led to the construct of legs and wings became transcribable (activated) as necessary. The genes that provide the instructions as to how the physical features are constructed don't necessarily change, the master generic reference tables derived from the universal master genome reference table select combinations of features that provide plant and animal species that are intended to survive given the environmental conditions at the time. Reference tables changing versus genes changing makes for both (1) an organized and adaptable evolutionary process regarding species development, as well as (2) a balanced ecosystem. The concept of reference tables provides the needed explanation of organization leading to a successful viable ecosystem, which has otherwise been explained as the result of sheer randomness.

There is most likely an element of randomness. If the generic master genome reference table produces a species specific reference table which defines certain phenotypic features that are to comprise a species, if that species is produced it is necessary that it survive to pass on its new arrangement of transcribable genes. Many attempts at species specific reference tables have probably been attempted that have never survived, or survived only over the course of a few generations. All known species have appeared and become extinct, except for those in existence today; average life of a species is considered to be 10 million years. The law of survival of the fittest still empowers some species to survive while others become extinct. Species that survive most likely are the product of a species specific reference table that dictates a series of transcribable quantum genes that takes best advantage of the environmental conditions that exist on the planet at the time the species lived on the planet. At least to date, all species eventually die out and become extinct; most likely related to the ever changing environmental factors.

Another observation that generic master genome reference tables helps to explain is that if evolution occurred due purely to random chance, then we should see the development of individual species going forward into more sophisticated forms as well as backwards into less sophisticated or defined forms. That is, random chance works both ways. The number of positive steps forward should equal the number of negative steps backwards. For the most part, life appears to have evolved from a more primitive forms to more sophisticated and complex forms. The utilization of generic master genome reference tables capable of being influenced by external signals such as environmental factors and producing more complex multi-cell organisms, would explain the tendency toward evolution from more primitive forms to more sophisticated life forms.

A generic master genome reference table would also help explain why, following each of the estimated six occurrences when life on the planet experienced a catastrophic event that caused the extinction of ninety percent of the species, that the ecosystem was able to rebuild itself. Evolution, based on random chance would have an extremely difficult time surviving in the face of harsh changes to the habitat. A generic master genome reference table would be able to quickly rearrange the groupings of transcribable quantum genes to produce new life forms that could adapt and flourish in a changing environment.

MASTER GENOME REFERENCE TABLE FOR PLANTS

As mentioned above, the plant kingdom would have its own master genome reference table, which would be further subdivided to provide the necessary instructions to produce all of the individual species of plants. Such a reference table, see Table P3-6, for each plant species would contain instructions to produce a basic cell and instructions to produce each individual component of the plant necessary to produce each specific plant species. The reference table would be stored in the seed of the plant and provide the genetic direction as to how to construct the plant in an orderly step-wise fashion. As in the life of a seed, the reference table could lay dormant for any length of time, until the proper environmental conditions exist necessary to activate the seed.

As a seed is activated, pointers systematically traverse the entries present in the master genome reference table, which in turn facilitates the transcription of transcribable genes or activates other reference tables, which in turn facilitate the transcription of transcribable genes. Mutations, replication errors, selections, viruses or environmental factors may be responsible for certain genes being transcribable versus untranscribable.

Group	Unique Identifier 25-characters	Instructions to manufacture species
0	0000000000000100000000000 AAAAAAAAAAAAAACAAAAAAAAAA	Genes to construct cell membrane
0	0000000000000111000000000 AAAAAAAAAAAAAACCCAAAAAAAAA	Genes to construct chloroplast
0	0000000000000112000000000 AAAAAAAAAAAAAACCGAAAAAAAAA	Genes to construct mitochondria
0	0000000000000113010000000 AAAAAAAAAAAAAACCTACAAAAAAA	Genes to construct Golgi Apparatus
0	0000000000000111131000000 AAAAAAAAAAAAAACCCCTCAAAAAA	Genes to construct micro tubular network
0	0000000000000200000000000 AAAAAAAAAAAAAAGAAAAAAAAAAA	Genes to construct nuclear membrane
0	0000000000000221111000000 AAAAAAAAAAAAAAGGCCCCAAAAAA	Genes to construct chromosomes

0	0000000000000223211100000 AAAAAAAAAAAAAAGGTGCCCAAAAA	Genes to construct mitotic spindles
2	2000000000001223211000000 GAAAAAAAAAAAACGGTGCCAAAAAA	Genes to construct seed
2	2000000000002223211000000 GAAAAAAAAAAAAGGGTGCCAAAAAA	Genes to construct leaves
2	2000000003000223211000000 GAAAAAAAATAAAGGTGCCAAAAAA	Genes to construct flowers
2	2000000000200223211000000 GAAAAAAAAAGAAGGTGCCAAAAAA	Genes to construct roots system
2	2000000000220223211000000 GAAAAAAAAACCAGGTGCCAAAAAA	Genes to construct stem and branches

Table P3-6
Simplified version of a master genome
reference table for plants*.

*all numbers presented as unique identifiers are meant to be for illustration purposes only

MASTER GENOME REFERENCE TABLE FOR ANIMALS

As mentioned above, the animal kingdom would have its own master genome reference table, which would be further subdivided to provide the necessary instructions to produce all of the individual species of animals. Such a reference table, see Table P3-7, for each animal species would contain instructions to produce a basic cell and instructions to produce each individual component of the animal necessary to produce each specific animal species. The reference table would be stored in the genes of the animal and provide the genetic direction as to how to construct the animal in an orderly step-wise fashion.

As an animal species' genome is activated, pointers systematically traverse the entries present in the master genome reference table, which in turn facilitates the transcription of transcribable genes or activates other reference tables, which in turn facilitate the transcription of transcribable genes. Mutations, replication errors, selections, viruses or environmental factors may be responsible for certain genes being transcribable versus untranscribable.

Group	Unique Identifier 25-characters	Instructions to manufacture species
0	0000000000000100000000000 AAAAAAAAAAAAACAAAAAAAAAAA	Genes to construct cell membrane
0	0000000000000112000000000 AAAAAAAAAAAAACCGAAAAAAAAA	Genes to construct mitochondria
0	0000000000000113010000000 AAAAAAAAAAAAACCTACAAAAAAA	Genes to construct Golgi Apparatus
0	0000000000000111121000000 AAAAAAAAAAAAACCCCGCAAAAAA	Genes to construct flagella
0	0000000000000111131000000 AAAAAAAAAAAAACCCCTCAAAAAA	Genes to construct micro tubular network
0	0000000000000200000000000 AAAAAAAAAAAAAGAAAAAAAAAAA	Genes to construct nuclear membrane
0	0000000000000221111000000 AAAAAAAAAAAAAGGCCCCAAAAAA	Genes to construct chromosomes
0	0000000000000223211100000 AAAAAAAAAAAAAGGTGCCCAAAAA	Genes to construct mitotic spindles
3	3000000000000223211000000 TAAAAAAAAAAAAGGTGCCAAAAAA	Genes to construct skeleton
3	3000000000122300001000000 TAAAAAAAAACGGTAAAACAAAAAA	Construct a heart
3	3000000000222200001000000 TAAAAAAAAAGGGGAAAACAAAAAA	Construct lungs
3	3000000000322200001000000 TAAAAAAAAATGGGAAAACAAAAAA	Construct a kidney
3	3000000000000000001000000 TAAAAAAAAAAAAAAAAACAAAAAA	Genes to construct a pancreas
3	3000000000332200001000000 TAAAAAAAAATTGGAAAACAAAAAA	Genes to construct a liver

3	300000000000223211000000 TAAAAAAAAAAAAGGTGCCAAAAAA	Genes to construct a fin
3	300000000000223211000000 TAAAAAAAAAAAAGGTGCCAAAAAA	Genes to construct a leg limb
3	300000000000223211000000 TAAAAAAAAAAAAGGTGCCAAAAAA	Genes to construct an arm limb
3	300000000000223211000000 TAAAAAAAAAAAAGGTGCCAAAAAA	Genes to construct a tail

Table P3-7
Simplified version of a Universal master
genome reference table for animals*.

*all numbers presented as unique identifiers are meant to be for illustration purposes only

HIERARCHY OF GENOME REFERENCE TABLES

As a genome reference table (GRT) is read by a GRT transcription complex one or more control RNA molecules are generated. These control RNA molecules traverse the nucleus and bind to the unique identifier of a specific quantum gene and activate the formation of a transcription complex to transcribe the quantum gene. In this manner, quantum genes are utilized in a precise and organized manner.

Genome reference tables (GRT) provide groups of instructions for various levels of construction of any given organism. The hierarchy of reference tables presented in Table P3-8 demonstrate the various GRTs from higher order to the lower order reference tables. Process specific GRT (#9) involving the least number of instructions or references to quantum genes, therefore represents the lowest order GRT.

	GENOME REFERENCE TABLE	*Includes list of quantum genes to---*
1	Universal Genome Reference Table	***All inclusive genome*
2	Kingdom specific Master GRT	*construct a kingdom*
3	Species specific GRT	*construct a specific species*
4	Organ specific GRT	*construct an organ*
5	Physical Feature specific GRT	*generate limbs & features*
6	Cell specific GRT	*construct cells of each cell design*
7	Organelle specific GRT	*build each organelle*
8	Molecular specific GRT	*produce each molecule*
9	Process specific GRT	*conduct each necessary process*

Table P3-8
Hierarchy of genome reference tables.

Genome Reference Tables are capable of producing variable outcomes. Amongst the list of quantum genes present in any given reference table, not all quantum genes may be read by a GRT Transcription Complex. Influences to the GRT Transcription Complex may cause certain quantum genes to be activated versus other available quantum genes left idle. This may occur as an active process while an organism is alive; or it may be an event that occurs while sex cells are being generated by an organism. Imprinting may occur as a genome is being generated in sex cells. Imprinting may occur to activate or deactivate available instructions present in a reference table.

A GRT at any level of the hierarchy may be comprised of a number of references to quantum genes, but not all of the available references will be utilized by any given species. Imprinting designates which of the available references in a

GRT will be used. In the circumstance where a limp specific GRT exists, it may be comprised of the instructions necessary to produce either an arm, a wing or a fin. Imprinting selects to activate the list of quantum genes necessary to produce an arm, while leaving the quantum genes dedicated to producing a wing or fin deactivated or dormant state.

Certain GRTs, such as lower order GRTs, may not exhibit much variability. The GRTs to produce organelles, molecules, and direct processes may be very well conserved. Higher order GRTs may exhibit the kind of variability to has been necessary to produce the evolutionary process as recorded by science.

The existence of a hierarchy of GRTs facilitates the fact that the earth supports a very well balanced ecosystem. Despite the variety of environmental ranges that exist on the planet, an ecosystem of comprised of various life forms can be found across the globe inhabiting nearly every part of the earth. Despite severe stresses to the earth, some of which have catastrophically eradicated numerous species, the life forms comprising the ecosystems on the planet have adapted to the climate changes and rebuilt complex food chains that have been able to survive. It would appear that the master genome reference tables utilized by kingdoms and species are able to dynamically alter the list of activated quantum genes, selecting or experimenting with dormant quantum genes to select which life forms will survive the best given the prevailing environmental conditions.

VIRUSES INFLUENCING EVOLUTION BY ALTERING REFERENCE TABLES

Viral genomes are generally comprised of either RNA or DNA. The genome of an RNA virus, such as Hepatitis C, which bypasses the nucleus of the host cell, once separated into subunits, mimics messenger RNA and produces the proteins necessary to construct copies of the RNA virus. DNA viruses and RNA viruses such as HIV, which reverse transcribe their genome into DNA may have a genome that either generates messenger RNAs to produce individual proteins, or functions like a reference table that is utilized to activate quantum genes that already exist in the host cell's genome. Viruses that insert their genome into the DNA may simply insert a list of instructions that at some point in the life-cycle of the cell becomes read and therefore activates a series of quantum genes that are required to produce copies of the virus.

Viruses could influence the evolution of species by inserting into the DNA of a species, either new genetic material, variations to existing genetic material or much more powerfully, variations to the reference tables. Viral influence to Genome Reference Tables could affect a block of quantum genes, shutting the quantum genes off or activating a set of quantum genes.

The viral genome's influence could be either directed or indirect. A directed influence would be when the virus inserts new information such as new quantum genes into the genome or inserts genetic material that disrupts the transcription of a quantum gene. An indirect influence which potentially produces a much greater influence of a species, is the insertion of new reference points into a genome reference table or by disrupting reference points. The most powerful affect would be if the viral genome influenced a higher order genome reference table in sex cells and activated or deactivated references to a series of quantum genes. Viral influences could be the cause why the block of genes dedicated to generating a fin in a fish is deactivated and in its place a leg is permanently generated on an amphibian. Viruses may have been responsible for the activation of genome reference tables that produced wings on birds or arms on reptiles and mammals. The influence viruses have had may have produced the illusion of evolution.

Genome reference tables represent a list of addresses of the locations of quantum genes.

DYNAMIC GENOME REFERENCE TABLES EXPLAIN METAMORPHOSIS

Evolution has been considered a slowly progressive alteration of species morphing one form of species into another form of species. Evolution has been thought to be the result of genetic errors suffered by a species' genome that causes the morphing process, that is then subject to survival as dictated by Nature's law of 'Survival of the Fittest'. The perception of time required for a species to morph from one life form to another life time is often considered to take hundreds of thousands of years to maybe even millions of years.

The perceived concept that *'the effort and the time it takes for one species to morph into another species takes extensive time and requires a genetic error to occur'* grossly overlooks the dynamic changes that occur within species that are known to exist on the planet today.

A frog starts out its life cycle in a fertilized egg. The frog emerges from the egg as tadpole. The tadpole swims through the water propelled only be a tail. The tadpole uses internal gills to breath. Metamorphoses occurs with lungs developing, disappearance of the gills, limbs appearing including fore- and hind-limbs, the tail being absorbed and the mouth changing into a froglike mouth. The metamorphosis from tadpole to frog may take two months to two years, depending upon the species.

The frog, other amphibians and various insects such as the butterfly, exhibit dynamic alterations to their overall life form that would be considered features of evolution. To facilitate the changes in these features a series of genome reference tables are read in succession as part of the life-cycle of the frog, that first dictate the physical form of the tadpole, then as the time-line of the frog's lifecycle progresses, generate the features of the adult frog while eliminating features of the tadpole such as the tail and gills. The metamorphosis of a frog and other organisms demonstrates that genome reference tables can be very dynamic, switching the actions of quantum genes on and off, and even switching the actions of reference tables on and off during a species' own lifecycle.

REVIEWING THE ROLE OF THE UNIQUE IDENTIFIER

Utilizing a unique identifier as a means of locating specific genetic material amongst the 3 billion base pairs of nucleotides comprising the human DNA supports the plausible use of gene therapy. Delivering such quantum genes, which contain a unique identifier, to specific cell types provides a means of inserting specific genetic information into the cell's nuclear deoxyribonucleic acid that can be readily located by the cell's nuclear transcription complexes. These medically therapeutic quantum genes are intended to provide a wide variety of medical therapeutic options to clinicians.

The concept of the quantum gene is the key concept that opens the door to exploring the biologic software programming that comprises the DNA. Each gene acts as one or more lines of programming code containing one or more instructions or data files. Small groups of code define the series of enzymes that are necessary for biologic processes to occur. Larger groups of code define the instructions necessary to construct individual organelles inside a cell. Still larger groups of code define the construct of general and specialty cells. Much larger groups of code act as the blueprints to constructing the individual organs that comprise the body. Finally very large groups of biologic code define workings of the human body, acting to coordinate all of the biologic systems that are required to facilitate growth, development and maintenance of the body as a whole.

Identifying the existence of the quantum gene makes possible the understanding of command and control functions that occur at the cellular level. A master biologic program governs the life-cycle of a cell and the life-cycle of every multi-cellular organism. Quantum genes represent the model with which individual phenotypical instruction codes and all of the command and control instruction codes are organized with a unique identifier and the transcribable instruction linked together. Phenotypical instructions are what are identifiable as physical features of a species, while the command and control instructions are those instructions that are necessary to build the phenotypical features, arrange the phenotypical features in an organized manner to define a species, utilize the phenotypical features and maintain the phenotypical features.

Identification of unique identifiers associated with quantum genes leads to new horizons in the treatment of medical conditions. By knowing the unique identifier of a gene, small molecules can be fashioned to interface with the unique identifier of a particular gene with the intention of either activating or deactivating the particular gene. Activating a gene would be accomplished by a small molecule coded for the gene's unique identifier interfacing with the unique identifier of the gene and upon such an interaction, would stimulate the assembly of a transcription complex to transcribe the gene. Deactivating a gene would be accomplished by a small molecule interfacing with the unique identifier of a particular gene that would prevent the assembly of a transcription complex at the site of the gene, thus preventing a gene from being transcribed.

SUMMARY

A quantum gene is a segment of DNA comprised of (1) a unique identifier and (2) a transcribable region that codes for one or more RNAs. The unique identifiers can be used to map out the quantum genes as they exist in the chromosomes. The unique identifiers are utilized to locate quantum genes so that they can be transcribed when needed. Unique identifiers associated with quantum genes are also found as elements comprising reference tables.

Reference tables act to coordinate the construction of cells, organs and the overall architecture of a species. Reference tables consist of a list or series of references to unique identifiers, the function of these elements is to point to quantum genes or point to other reference tables. Reference tables may be comprised of unique identifiers that act to transcribe quantum genes that act as instructions to facilitate the construction of the gross body of the species or reference tables may be comprised of the instructions needed to construct any of the internal components such as organs, cells, organelles, and other various elements of cells. As an example, for the construction of a hand, there may exist a reference table listing the quantum genes necessary to produce the physical structures required to generate a hand.

By the previously mentioned definitions the Universal Master Genome Reference Table may be associated with a master plan for evolution comprised of all of the elements required for all of the species that have lived on the earth, sparing inadvertent genetic mutations that may have occurred. A Generic Master Genome Reference Table represents a subset of the quantum genes that is found in the Universal Master Genome Reference Table, and is related to constructing all of the species of a particular Kingdom. Species specific reference tables are comprised of all of the instructions necessary to construct a specific species. Other reference tables act to generate various organs, features, cells, organelles and elements of cells. Therefore there exists a hierarchy of reference tables in the genome.

As a genome reference table (GRT) is read by a GRT transcription complex one or more control RNA molecules are generated. These control RNA molecules traverse the nucleus and bind to the unique identifier of a specific quantum gene and activate the formation of a transcription complex to transcribe the quantum gene. In this manner, quantum genes are utilized in a precise and organized manner.

Genome reference tables (GRT) provide groups of instructions for various levels of construction of any given organism. The hierarchy of reference tables include:

Universal Genome Reference Table *<All inclusive genome>*,

Kingdom specific Master GRT *<Includes list of quantum genes to construct a kingdom>*

Species specific GRT *<Includes quantum genes for construction of a species>*

Organ specific GRT *<Includes quantum genes for generation of an organ>*

Physical Feature specific GRT *<Includes quantum genes to generate limbs & features>*

Cell specific GRT *<Includes list of quantum genes for each cell design>*

Organelle specific GRT *<Includes quantum genes dedicated to build each organelle>*

Molecular specific GRT *<List of quantum genes to produce each molecule>*, and

Process specific GRT *<List of quantum genes to conduct each necessary process>*.

Genome Reference Tables are capable of producing variable outcomes. Amongst the list of quantum genes present in any given reference table, not all quantum genes may be read by the GRT Transcription Complex. Influences to the GRT Transcription Complex may cause certain quantum genes to be activated versus other available quantum genes left idle. This may occur as an active process while an organism is alive; or it may be an event that occur while sex cells are being generated by an organism. Imprinting may occur as a genome is being generated in sex cells. Imprinting may occur to turn on or off available instructions present in a reference table.

A GRT at any level of the hierarchy may be comprised of a number of references to quantum genes, but not all available references that point to quantum genes will be utilized by any given species. Imprinting designates which of the available references pointing to quantum genes in a GRT will be used. In the circumstance where a limb specific GRT exists, it may be comprised of the instructions necessary to produce either an arm, a wing or a fin. Imprinting selects to activate the list of quantum genes necessary to produce an arm, while leaving the quantum genes dedicated to producing a wing or fin deactivated or dormant state.

Certain GRTs, such as lower order GRTs, may not exhibit much variability. The GRTs responsible for the production of organelles, molecules, and direct processes may be very strictly conserved. Higher order GRTs may exhibit the kind of variability to has been necessary to produce the evolutionary process as recorded by science.

The existence of a hierarchy of GRTs facilitates the fact that the earth supports a very well balanced ecosystem. Despite the variety of environmental ranges that exist on the planet, an ecosystem comprised of various life forms can be found across the globe inhabiting nearly every part of the earth. Despite severe stresses to the earth, some of which have catastrophically eradicated numerous species, the life forms comprising the ecosystems on the planet have adapted to the climate changes and rebuilt complex food chains that have been able to survive. It would appear that the master genome reference tables utilized by kingdoms and species are able to dynamically alter the list of activated quantum genes, selecting or experimenting with dormant quantum genes to select which life forms will survive the best given the prevailing environmental conditions.

The primary objective of the Universal Genome Reference Table is to survive despite potentially catastrophic changes in the environment. The life forms needed to accomplish the primary objective, may take on inconsequential asthenic forms, even if it means the resultant life forms morph into bizarre and possibly unlikely shapes and figures.

The genome of an RNA virus, such as Hepatitis C which bypasses the nucleus of the host cell, once separated into subunits, mimics messenger RNA and produces the proteins necessary to construct copies of the RNA virus. DNA viruses and RNA viruses such as HIV, which reverse transcribe their genome into DNA may have a genome that either generates messenger RNAs to produce individual proteins, or functions like a reference table that is utilized to activate quantum genes that already exist in the host cell's genome. Viruses that insert their genome into the DNA may simply insert a list of instructions that at some point in the life-cycle of the cell becomes read and therefore activates a series of quantum genes that are required to produce copies of the virus.

Viruses could influence the evolution of species by inserting into the DNA of a species, either new genetic material, variations to existing genetic material or much more powerfully, variations to the reference tables. Viral influence to Genome Reference Tables could affect a block of quantum genes, shutting the quantum genes off or activating a set of quantum genes.

Viruses may play an intimate role in altering the DNA and possibly activating and deactivating subprograms creating an illusion of evolution. Where evolution has been thought to be related to random changes to the DNA coupled with the dogma of 'survival of the fittest'; the planet's exquisitely balanced ecosystem suggests a more deliberate effort has been responsible for the various forms of life that comprise the well orchestrated food chains inhabiting the planet. Viruses represent the one subset of entities capable of invading species and altering the DNA of species in a predictably purposeful manner. It is DNA that defines a species. Viruses are capable of manipulating DNA. Viruses may be the factor acting as the essential driver of what we have perceived is evolution.

Unique identifiers can be used as targets for small molecules such as control RNA and control proteins to interface with in order to activate or deactivate genes. Configurable Delivery Devices can be utilized to deliver either quantum genes or control RNA molecules or control proteins or all three to cells that have one or more malformed or damaged quantum genes that require replacement, then activation of the quantum gene. Delivery of the combination of quantum genes and control RNA molecules or control proteins provides a means of inserting needed genetic material into the DNA and then activating it. In some cases, it may be medically beneficial to deactivate certain quantum genes to turn off the transcription of toxic transcribable instructions.

Postscript 4:
Quadsistor:
Quaternary Technology from
Quaternary Medicine

ROOTS OF THE CURRENT BASE-2 TECHNOLOGIES

The fact is that Digital Technology as we know it today has reached its Zenith. As has been predicted, digital electronics will need to be replaced. Lessons learned from genetics, human brain construction and function, and the superiority of a base-four computing system, will logically lead designers of tomorrow's technology to the quadsistor and quaternary technologies.

Digital technology evolved from vacuum tube electronics. Vacuum tube electronics provided a means to amplify signals such a radio waves passing through the air. An antenna would detect a radio wave passing by. At that time radio waves were transmitted in the band of frequencies from roughly 10 kilocycles per second to 100 megacycles per second. Using tubes, inductors, capacitor and resister circuits, specific radio waves traveling through the air at a specific frequency could be selected. Once selected, the weak radio wave captured by the antenna would be passed through a series of vacuum tube amplifiers to boost the power of the radio wave. A signal carried by the radio frequency would be then be fed to a speaker which would create sound by inducing a magnet to vibrate the speaker's membrane.

Simple vacuum tubes were constructed with three wire leads fed into a glass tube. A source lead acted as a source of negatively charged electrons to flow into the vacuum tube. Electrons fed by the source lead formed a cloud around a cathode, a highly negatively charged lead inside the vacuum tube. A second lead, called the anode, was positively charged and acted as a drain for electrons to flow to and then out of the glass tube creating a current. A third lead, called the control grid, influenced the current passing from the cathode to the anode by emitting a small negative charge. The fluctuation of a voltage on the control grid caused considerable changes in the much larger current traveling from the cathode to the anode. As mentioned above, vacuum tubes were readily used to take low intensity radio signals captured by an antenna and amplify the weak signals into a much more robust signal exiting the vacuum tube through the drain lead to either another amplifying vacuum tube or to a speaker. Glass vacuum tubes were bulky in size, fragile, and often overheated or wore out causing equipment failure.

Transistor can be viewed as being modeled from vacuum tube technology. In a transistor, instead of electrons passing through a vacuum from the cathode to the anode, electrons traveled through layers of silicone which act as a conductive medium for electrons. A transistor is designed with a base layer of P-type silicone that is lacking in electrons. A N-type silicone, that carries excessive electrons, is crystallized on the surface of the P-type silicone. When two N-type substrates are separated by a P-type silicone substrate, and are meant to act similar to a variable resistor, one N-type substrate, designated the emitter, acts as a source of electrons and while the second N-type silicone, designated the collector, acts as a drain for electrons. The P-type substrate acts as a gate. See illustration I. of Figure 24. Symbol II. is a conventional symbol for a NPN transistor. The arrow points in the direction of conventional current for a forward biased NPN transistor (forward bias: positive lead of the battery is connected to the transistor's collector lead). Note the arrow in the transistor symbol points in the opposite direction as to the flow of electrons; this is standard for the semiconductor industry. Transistors can be configured to amplify signals, much like a vacuum tube. Transistors may also be utilized as switches. The use of transistors as on/off switches has facilitated the development of electronic circuitry to turn machinery on and off and has acted as the foundation for the development of the binary computer technology that exists today.

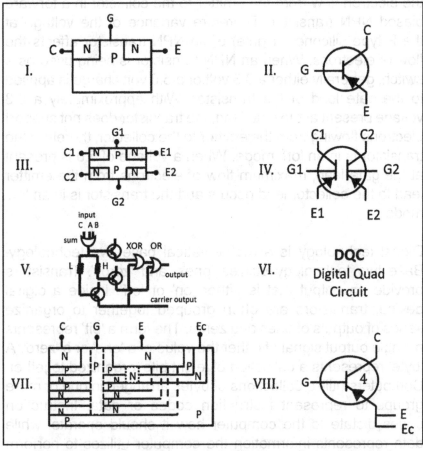

Figure 24: Illustration of a (I) NPN transistor, (III) dual input/output quadsistor, (V) digital quadsistor circuit, and (VII) two dimensional figure of a 3D quadsistor

In a forward biased NPN transistor, the transistor supports the flow of electrons from the Emitter lead to the Collector lead (this is the electron flow). Conventional current regarding silicone devices, as recognized by the electronics industry, is opposite of the flow of electrons. When a positive voltage is placed on the gate lead connected to P-type silicone positioned between the collector lead and the emitter lead, the flow of electrons traveling from the emitter lead to the collector lead is increased. The greater the positive voltage at the gate lead, the greater the electron flow from the emitter to the collector in a forward biased NPN transistor. Therefore variance of the voltage at the P-type silicone (or gate) of an NPN transistor affects the flow of electrons. When an NPN transistor is being used as a switch, generally either a 0.3 volt or a 5.0 volt charge is applied to the gate lead of the transistor. With approximately a 0.3 voltage present at the gate lead, the transistor does not support electrons flowing from the emitter to the collector, therefore the transistor is in an 'off' mode. When a voltage of 5.0 is present at the gate lead, maximum flow of electrons from the emitter lead to the collector lead occurs and the transistor is in an 'on' mode.

Digital technology is a mathematical base two technology. Base two technology utilizes 'ones' and 'zeros'. Transistors provide an output that is either 'on' or 'off'. Inside a digital device, transistors are often grouped together to organize series of outputs of ones and zeros. The term a 'bit' represents a single output signal of either the value of a 'one' or a 'zero'. A 'byte' represents a collection of 'eight bits' organized together. Computers utilize collections of bytes arranged in one or more groups to represent instruction codes or data. Instruction codes dictate to the computer how it should operate, while data represents information the computer utilizes to perform the functions intended for the computer device.

Computer technology started out as computational devices to allow for the addition, subtraction, multiplication and division of a series of numbers. Prior to computers, mathematicians and engineers used the abacus, mathematical tables written in reference texts and later the slide rule. The calculator sped up the act of mathematic calculations but was limited to single calculations. The computer offered the means to program the device to perform an almost infinite number of calculations as needed. Obviously today, the general use of computers has grown far beyond the initial use of the device as a programmable calculator to include gaming, special effects in movies, networking, global communications, large data base analysis to name but a few uses.

Current silicone microchip transistor technology has in effect been created by constructing a base layer of P-type silicone, then layering on top of the P-type silicone varying designs of N-type silicone to create transistors. Current silicone microchip transistor technology generally utilizes only one side of the P-type silicone base layer.

Biology teaches us that DNA utilizes a base-four computer code. The basic building blocks of a species design and function is stored in the species' base-four genetic code contained in the organism's DNA. There are functional points to suggest the human brain functions by the orchestrated efforts of a network of biologic computer processors. The biologic code that acts as the source code for this network of biologic computer processors harbored in the human brain and memory storage is most likely a base-four code. If the DNA and the brain's operating system software are both functioning utilizing base-four, it would appear our best next choice for a technology to replace our current, soon to be outdated digital technology, would be a base-four computer technology.

BASE-FOUR: SEARCH FOR A NEW DIRECTION

Down-sizing computer technology is driving market sales at the moment. The mobile phone is being utilized to not only handle voice communication, but other common functions such as emails, internet access, texting, and streaming live video. In the near future all computer and communications functions may be allocated to the mobile phone, thus replacing home computer systems and land-line phones. The limits to the continued efforts to down-size electronics include (1) power requirements, (2) heat dispersal and (3) physical limit as to how small a transistor can be made.

At present the battle to put additional technology into the mobile phone without increasing the size of the phone is waged against the factors that more electronics means more power consumed, which wears down a battery faster. More electronics means more heat is generated, and more electronics generally means more transistors packed into a smaller space. Switching the current digital technology to a more advanced technology such as a base-four computer system would offer a greater computational capacity, smaller memory requirements and require fewer transistors. Switching from a base-two technology to a base-four technology seemingly would address the need to lower power requirements and reduce the generation of heat, while at the same time boost the proficiency of the device while using fewer transistors.

Where a transistor is considered a base-two electronic device supporting either an 'on' or 'off' state, a quadsistor represents an electronic device that provides four different states. The four states could be labeled 'A', 'B', 'C' and 'D'. Initially, a primitive base four device was contrived to be comprised of two source leads, two drain leads and two input leads, with its intended use to offer four different possible outputs from two different drain leads. See illustration III. of Figure 24. Symbol for the device is present in illustration IV.

The four possible outputs of the device illustrated in illustration III. would include both emitter leads exhibiting a conventional current or being considered 'on', versus both emitter leads not exhibiting a significant conventional current or being considered 'off'; versus one of the two emitter leads exhibiting a conventional current and being considered 'on' while the second emitter lead not exhibiting a significant conventional current and being considered 'off' versus the reverse, where the opposite emitter lead does not exhibit a significant conventional current and is considered 'off' while the other emitter lead does exhibit a substantial conventional and is considered 'on'.

The output of this initial concept for a quadsistor is therefore one of four possibilities including: ON and ON; versus OFF and OFF; versus ON and OFF; versus OFF and ON. With regards to the digital world this might be considered as four possible outputs including: ONE and ONE; versus ZERO and ZERO; versus ONE and ZERO; versus ZERO and ONE. In base-four technology the ZERO and ZERO would be considered 'ZERO' or 'A', the ZERO and ONE output would be considered 'ONE' or 'B', the ONE and ZERO output would be considered 'TWO' or 'C' and the ONE and ONE output would be considered 'THREE' or 'D'.

This initial concept represents a preliminary design phase, and limited due to being constructed with two output leads, rather than one output lead. Two output leads would make it difficult to construct additional circuitry to support the function of this form of a quadsistor. In addition there is no carry over state. A carrier state is needed when designing an 'adder' to facilitate mathematical calculations of two numbers.

Utilizing digital components, a crude base-four circuit can be built. As Illustrated in V. of Figure 24. Illustration V. demonstrates a digital circuit that acts as a base-four computer circuit. Inputs A & B as well as a carrier input 'C' are present at the input or summing unit. The output of the summing unit goes to both the input of an XOR gate and is split between a high resistance resistor and a low resistance resistor. Each resistor is connected to the base of a transistor. The collector output of this transistor connected to the low resistance resistor is fed into the XOR gate. The collector output of the transistor connected to the high resistance resistor is connected to the input of the OR gate. The output of the XOR gate is the second input to the OR gate. The output of the OR gate acts as the output of the digital quadsistor circuit. The collector output of the transistor connected to the low resistance resistor also acts as a carrier output. This carrier output is represented as 2.0v or 'one' in a base-four system comprised of the elements of 0, 1, 2, and 3.

To construct an adding unit, the carrier output of the digital quadsistor circuit can be fed into the input of a second digital quadsistor circuit connected in series. The carrier output of the first digital quadsistor circuit would be connected to the summing unit of the second digital quadsistor summing unit as the 'C' input. The summing unit of the digital quadsistor circuit accepts feds from a carrier as well as two other inputs. More advanced quadsistor units can accept feeds from a single carrier, as well as up to four other carrier inputs to build more sophisticated circuits.

Illustrated in VI. is the heading to represent a quadsistor constructed from digital electronics or Digital Quad Circuit (DQC). Individual base-four units as presented in illustration V. can be strung together in series to produce a base-four adding circuit.

To contrive a functional base-four device utilizing base-four electronics with one output lead, the lead must be able to act as a medium for a signal with four potential values. Current transistors have a single output lead with two potential values, either 'on' or 'off'.

The choice of output signals could be either differing currents, differing voltages, differing frequencies including the light spectrum. Transistors are commonly used to amplify signals or act as on/off switches. A hybrid design transistor might be used to take advantage of both functions of amplifying a signal and acting as a switch. The electronics literature suggests that the quality of a general purpose transistor switch is rather unreliable. More specifically a 0.3 voltage state where the transistor is considered 'off' may not be at 0.3 volts, but some value higher or lower; and the 5.0 voltage state that where the transistor is considered 'on' may not be at 5.0 volts, but a much higher or lower value of voltage. General purpose transistors may only be capable of reliably operating one of these two states of function, a 0.3 volt state or a 5.0 volt state, and not necessarily at reliable voltage states in between.

A high-grade quality transistor could operate with four levels of voltage including a 0.3 volt state, a 2.0 volt state, a 3.5 volt state and a 5 volt state, each voltage associated with a different amplitude of current. Having four states of output offers a means of utilizing transistor technology to represent a zero, a one, a two and a three. Constructing a switching device with four differing outputs is the design objective of a quadsistor.

Current state of computer technology has a long history of generating a vast assortment of electronic circuitry to support the computational function of a computer. Still, the basic premise of early computers was to act as a tool to add numbers together. A new base-four computer technology would need to be able to first fulfill the job of successfully adding numbers together.

To add two base-four numbers together requires both a main-line emitter output lead as well as a carrier emitter output lead. The carrier output is used when the sum of the two input numbers is four or greater. Base-two summation circuitry utilizes a similar two output design with one output indicating a carryover state or a value of '2' when two 'ones' are added together.

To accomplish a base-four silicone device, the concept of our current digital technology needs to be expanded to consider more of a three dimensional design rather than the current N-type silicone substrate added to the surface of a P-type silicone substrate. Thinking three dimensionally, constructing multiple layers of N-type silicone interlaced with P-type silicone layers with channels of N-type and P-type silicone embedded in certain locations offers a means of producing a silicone device with the capacity to add two base-four numbers together, outputting the result utilizing a main-line emitter output lead and a carryover emitter output lead. Illustration VII. of Figure 24 represents a two-dimensional model of a three dimensional quadsistor. Illustration VIII. of Figure 24 represents the electronic symbol for such a base-four quadsistor. Illustration I. of Figure 25 represents a three-dimensional representation of the two-dimensional model in Illustration VIII of Figure 24.

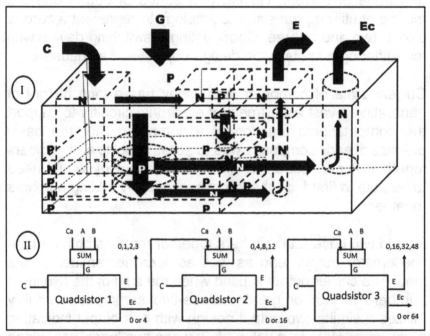

Figure 25: (I)Three dimensional single input dual output quadsistor, and (II) Series of quadsistors

Illustration I. of Figure 25 demonstrates a silicone device that is build with multiple layers of N-type and P-type silicone. When forward biased, such a device would generate a conventional current flowing from the collector lead to the emitter lead. Electron flow would be from the emitter lead to the collector lead. A voltage of 0.3v, 2.0v, 3.5v and 5.0v at the gate lead would generate a conventional current at the emitter lead respective to the corresponding voltages of 0.3v, 2.0v, 3.5v and 5.0v. A voltage of 7.0v at the gate lead would push the conventional current flow to the pathway offered by the first N-type silicone layer below the surface P-type silicone layer. Conventional current flowing through this first lower layer of N-type silicone would produce a conventional current at the emitter-carrier lead and shut off the output current from the emitter lead. A voltage of 8.5v at the gate lead would cause conventional current to pass to the second N-type silicone layer below the surface P-silicone layer. The result of a voltage of 8.5v at the gate would produce the carrier lead outputting a voltage of 2.0 v and a voltage of 2.0v at the emitter lead. A voltage of 10.0v at the gate lead would cause the conventional current to pass to the third N-type silicone layer below the surface P-type silicone layer. The result of 10.0v at the gate lead would produce a carrier lead output of 2.0v and a voltage of 3.5v at the emitter lead. Heat conductive channels can be embedded into the silicon layers to direct undesirable heat out and away from the device.

A quadsistor device such as this is capable of participating in addition, subtraction, multiplication and division utilizing base-four mathematics. Computer logic circuits for digital computers use adding of binary numbers for purposes of addition and subtraction, and adding and shifting binary numbers for purposes of multiplication and division. Similar processes are possible for the purpose of designing logic circuits for addition, subtraction, multiplication and division in a base-four computer. Quadsistors can be linked together to form mathematical circuits. Illustrated in Figure 25, Illustration II., quadsistors can be linked to produce simple addition circuits. Two inputs are placed at A and B, which lead to Gate lead 1 (G1). The summation of the two signals are then output through emitter lead 1 (E1) and emitter carrier lead 1 (Ec1). The output at E1 represents 0,1,2, or 3. The output of the carryover lead Ec1 would represent 4 when the voltage value of the lead is 2.0v. The voltage and therefore current of the carrier is reduced to 2.0v to represent a 'one' rather than a 'four' as input to the next quadsistor in the base-four numeric system. The Ec1 lead connects to the input of the next quadsistor. Inputs C, D and Ec1 are fed into gate number 2 (G2). The output of the second quadsistor E2 and Ec2. The value represented by the E2 lead associated with the second quadsistor is 0, 4, 8, or 12. The output of the carryover lead Ec2 represents the value of 16 when the output voltage of the lead is 2.0v. If a third quadsistor was attached in series, the E3 output would be 0, 16, 32, or 48. The carryover lead Ec3 would represent a value of 64 if the output voltage of the lead were 2.0v. Any number of quadsistors can be strung together as represented by Q3 and Q4.

The limits to state-of-the-art electronics include consumption of power, generation of heat and limits to the miniaturization of digital transistors. Base-4 technology utilizing quadsistors offers a much greater computational and memory storage capacity compared to the current digital technology, which in turn reduces power consumption, heat and number of transistors and other components.

In addition, Base-4 computational algorithms radically change a computer's core logic paradigms and such a system would be capable of interfacing with current digital technology, but be impressively resistant to the community of worldwide hackers. The algorithms for addition, subtraction, multiplication and division in base-four would change in relationship to how such mathematic functions are being conducted in present day computers. The fundamental means of storing and processing data would radically change thus making it more difficult for computer hackers familiar with current technology to successfully attack the newer base-four generations of computers. The need to secure computers from attack is becoming a critical concern. Customers such as the military, the global banking system, and any business concerned about the integrity of its databases and computer operations would be most interested in such a technology to intensify the security of their internal computer networks.

Mobile phones are becoming sophisticated enough to take on the role of certain computer functions as demonstrated by the recent line of smart phones. As the mobile phone morphs into an increasingly more sophisticated programmable device, it becomes increasingly more vulnerable to attacks by viruses, spyware and malware. As the mobile phone becomes progressively more software oriented, thus an increasingly more desirable target for malicious programming, the call for a more advanced technology to protect such devices will become deafening.

Epilogue:
Wrap-Up:
Base-4 Leads to Infinity

The symbol for infinity is the twisted circle that wraps around itself and connects with itself such that whatever traverses the length of the circle makes the loop around the twisted circle continuously for all of eternity, thus infinity. The quest for better electronic technologies will lead us through a loop to the base-4 principles that govern the human body, which in turn will catalyze innovation in medicine and technology for long into the foreseeable future.

The body of this text discussed concepts that biologic viruses, in their natural state, are simply comprised of a protein outer shell and genetic programming code carried in the core. The primary objective of most viruses is to insert into the genetic programming code of a target cell, the viral instructions necessary to redirect the target cell's internal biologic machinery from normal cell function to producing copies of the virus.

This text discusses the concepts of utilizing virus-like devices as transport mediums. By removing a virus's genetic material and replacing or adding probes to the surface of the virus, such a modified form of virus can be used as a proficient transport device. Such deliberately designed transport devices can be utilized to deliver a variety of payloads directly to differing cells in the body to accomplish an almost infinite number of medically necessary tasks.

To accomplish the effort of building viruses to act as transport devices requires further attention to be paid to the primary programming of a virus and of a cell. Both DNA and RNA are comprised of four differing nucleotide elements. By simple observation, this would be considered to represent a base-four instruction code.

Since Gregor Mendel introduced his genetics work, it has been recognized that the genetic code is divided into individual instructions referred to as genes. Genes were discovered and for the most part are still recognized today due to the phenotypic features they produce in an organism. Genes dictate the structural elements of an organism.

To construct the body of an organism requires more than simple recognition of physical features. If one were constructing a specific door in a particular manner based off of a set of instructions, it is not enough to document the door is to be red, swing on hinges and measures a certain height, width and depth, and be of a particular weight. The instructions necessary to convey to builders would need to include the manner of how to construct the door, which would be much more detailed than simply describing the physical features of the door. So it is in nature. The programming instructions required to build a cell, and then combine cells with special features together into a multi-cellular organism such as the human body, requires an instruction code far more detailed than simply describing the physical features of the body or the internal chemical reactions necessary to maintain the body.

Instructions that direct the cells of the body to grow, divide, specialize their function, and cause the cells to act in a coordinated effort with other cells in the body, may not be easily recognized because they may not produce any specific detectable phenotypic feature. In contrast, instructions that are required to produce features rather than the phenotypic nature of features, if tampered with, may simply produce a failure to thrive or even endanger survival of the organism, therefore contributing to the difficulty of recognizing that such instructions exist.

Regardless of whether a section of genetic code represents phenotypic features of an organism or the instructions regarding how an organism is to construct or maintain itself, there must be a plan for organization of such instruction code. Organization of the genetic instruction code is vital to facilitate a series of instructions that will reliably reproduce an organism that is capable of functioning and surviving in its environment, as well as providing the genetic code with a reliable means to locate and utilize the instructions and data files stored in the genetic code of a species in a timely fashion.

Nature, having attached a unique identifier to segments of genetic code representing phenotypic features and instructions provides the means to organize and utilize the information stored in the DNA of organisms.

At the same time that the instruction codes in genetics is being recognized as being comprised of an orderly discrete, labeled individual instructions or groups of instructions which is opening up an entirely new horizon for research, digital technology has successfully reached the pinnacle of its usefulness. Recently it was reported that up to a billion transistors have been packed into a single integrated circuit chip. The limits to advancement in this field include (1) the physical limit as to how small a functional transistor can be constructed, (2) the power requirements of an integrated circuit and the circuitry it supports, (3) the heat generated by all of the transistors packed into an integrated circuit chip.

The physical size of transistors has been steadily reduced over the past few decades, which has facilitated the production of progressively more powerful computer products. There is a physical limit as to how small a transistor can be constructed.

A certain number of atoms are required to define any structure. The limit to miniaturization of digital transistors is predicted to be reached possibly within the next five years. In the general consumer market, this short-coming is stalled by placing two or more processors at work, rather than marketing more sophisticated computer processors.

The consumer market has steadily sought out technology that combines maximum computer power in the smallest package possible. Recent developments in the cell phone industry represent a prime example. Consumers are interested in their mobile phones functioning not only as phones but as computer devices capable of performing a variety of software functions and streaming video. A significant limit to increasing the computer function of any device is its power requirements. Batteries have limits to the amount of power that they can supply to a device. Minimizing power consumption leads to greater computer capacity and longer battery life.

Heat kills electronic devices. Electrons streaming through transistors and connecting wires generates heat. The greater number of transistors in a device, the greater the heat generated by the device. A primary concern when designing any electronic device to keep the generation of heat to a minimum. Heat slows down the function of an electronic device and if the heat reaches too high of a level, the device can become permanently damaged. To accomplish the goal of reducing heat, designers either eliminate sources of heat or increase the efficiency of removing of heat from an electronic device.

The current digital technology has reached its apex, and will need to be replaced with another form of technology. An alternative technology utilizing any mathematical platform besides the current base-two technology will be necessary. Base-three, base-four, base-eight, base-ten are viable alternatives. Given that human genetics is comprised of a base-four coding and there is indication that human brain function is the result of a base-four biologic software, it would seem beneficial to develop future technology in a manner that best interfaces with humans. It would seem that a base-four technology would be the next desired mathematics platform to replace the current base-two standard that has acted as the foundation for technology for the last sixty years.

A natural progression would likely be:

(1) Medical genetic science researchers embark on paralleling the elaborate base-four biologic software program comprising the DNA to how computer technology functions. Each species takes from a collection of master set of biologic programming instructions stored in a master genome reference table, what it needs to generate its body form. Much of the basic programming instructions are shared between differing species within a phylum. Some of the very basic programming instructions are shared amongst all cellular organisms such as cell and organelle design and construction instructions.

(2) The electronics industry targets base-four as the next frontier to explore regarding the development of future computer technologies.

(3) The neurosciences embrace the concept that the human brain's basic circuitry is comprised of a network of microprocessors. The brain's microprocessors are utilizing a base-four biologic software dictated by the base-four genetic code comprising the DNA. Interfacing the next generation of technology with the brain's base-four biologic software would dramatically improve the diagnostic capabilities of clinicians since the brain is constantly monitoring every bodily function in great detail.

(4) The electronics industry begins to develop devices that directly interface with the human's brain biologic software with the intention of being able to retrieve the data the human brain has gathered on bodily systems that are malfunctioning.

(5) The neurosciences develop software patches that are able to overcome deficits in brain function that occur when the brain's processors develop a malfunction.

(6) Development of base-four technology leads to the capacity to decipher the programming code utilized by the genetic code comprising the DNA. Understanding the genetic code allows for screening for defects in the code as well as harmful abnormalities in the genetic code caused by the influence of viruses. Understanding the specifics of the genetic code and recognizing the fundamentals of how viruses function, leads to Medical Vector Therapies that insert genetic patches to repair faulty genetic segments. Genetic patches could remedy diseases, improve bodily functions, and retard the devastating effects of aging.

(7) Understanding the base-four biologic computer code comprising the human genome and viral genomes facilitates practical gene therapy to treat and manage medicine's most challenging disease states.

The future of medicine and technology is intimately intertwined and will run parallel courses. Advancements in either field could be utilized in the future to fuel further evolution in either medicine or technology or both simultaneously. The sooner we recognize how closely the two fields are interrelated, the more rapid the advancement in medicine and technology can progress. Future researchers will be best equipped if they are able to intimately understand both the language of medicine and the language of technology.

We have only just begun to explore ourselves and take advantage of the power of our technology and our brain function have to offer. The full circle is that our base-four genetics dictates our base-four brain function, which interfaces with a base-four computer technology, which in turn assists us better to understand our base-four genetic programming and thus intervening in the genetic programming to positively intercede and efficiently manage or cure some of medicine's toughest challenges.

APPENDIX:
List of Patent Applications

No. 1 CONFIGURABLE MICROSCOPIC MEDICAL PAYLOAD DELIVERY DEVICE TO DELIVER MEDICALLY THERAPEUTIC PAYLOADS TO SPECIFICALLY TARGETED CELL TYPES

No. 2 RNA VECTOR THERAPY

No. 3 RNA VECTOR THERAPY METHOD

No. 4 ADAPTABLE MODIFIED VIRUS VECTOR TO DELIVER MODIFIED MESSENGER RIBONUCLEIC ACID AS A MEDICAL TREATMENT DEVICE TO MANAGE DIABETES MELLITUS AND OTHER PROTEIN DEFICIENT DISEASES

No. 5 ADAPTABLE MODIFIED VIRUS VECTOR TO DELIVER RIBOSOMAL RIBONUCLEIC ACID AS A MEDICAL TREATMENT DEVICE TO MANAGE DIABETES MELLITUS AND OTHER PROTEIN DEFICIENT DISEASES

No. 6 ADAPTABLE MODIFIED VIRUS VECTOR TO DELIVER RIBOSOMAL RIBONUCLEIC ACID COMBINED WITH MESSENGER RIBONUCLEIC ACID AS A MEDICAL TREATMENT DEVICE TO MANAGE DIABETES MELLITUS AND OTHER PROTEIN DEFICIENT DISEASES

No. 7 CHEMO VECTOR THERAPY TO DELIVER CHEMOTHERAPY MOLECULES TO SPECIFIC CELLS TO MANAGE BREAST CANCER, OTHER CANCERS AND INFLAMMATORY DISORDERS

No. 8 QUANTUM UNIFORM INHERITANCE

APPENDIX:
List of Patent Applications

No. 1 CONFIGURABLE MICROSCOPIC MEDICAL PAYLOAD DELIVERY DEVICE TO DELIVER MEDICALLY THERAPEUTIC PAYLOADS TO SPECIFICALLY TARGETED CELL TYPES

No. 2 RNA VECTOR THERAPY

No. 3 RNA VECTOR THERAPY METHOD

No. 4 ADAPTABLE MODIFIED VIRUS VECTOR TO DELIVER MODIFIED MESSENGER RIBONUCLEIC ACID AS A MEDICAL TREATMENT DEVICE TO MANAGE DIABETES MELLITUS AND OTHER PROTEIN DEFICIENT DISEASES

No. 5 ADAPTABLE MODIFIED VIRUS VECTOR TO DELIVER RIBOSOMAL RIBONUCLEIC ACID AS A MEDICAL TREATMENT DEVICE TO MANAGE DIABETES MELLITUS AND OTHER PROTEIN DEFICIENT DISEASES

No. 6 ADAPTABLE MODIFIED VIRUS VECTOR TO DELIVER RIBOSOMAL RIBONUCLEIC ACID COMBINED WITH MESSENGER RIBONUCLEIC ACID AS A MEDICAL TREATMENT DEVICE TO MANAGE DIABETES MELLITUS AND OTHER PROTEIN DEFICIENT DISEASES

No. 7 CHEMO VECTOR THERAPY TO DELIVER CHEMOTHERAPY MOLECULES TO SPECIFIC CELLS TO MANAGE BREAST CANCER, OTHER CANCERS AND INFLAMMATORY DISORDERS

No. 8 QUANTUM UNIT OF INHERITANCE

Patent Applications

No. 1: CONFIGURABLE MICROSCOPIC MEDICAL PAY-LOAD DELIVERY DEVICE TO DELIVER MEDICALLY THERAPEUTIC PAYLOADS TO SPECIFICALLY TARGETED CELL TYPES

INDIVIDUALS REQUESTING PATENT: Dr. Lane B. Scheiber II, MD and Dr. Lane B. Scheiber, ScD

©2010 Lane B. Scheiber II and Lane B. Scheiber. A portion of the disclosure of this patent document contains material which is subject to copyright protection. The copyright owners have no objection to the facsimile reproduction by anyone of the patent document or the patent disclosure, as it appears in the Patent and Trademark Office patent file or records, but otherwise reserves all copyright rights whatsoever.

ABSTRACT

The innovative strategy of treatment described here utilizes configurable microscopic medical payload delivery devices to act as a transport mechanism to deliver medically therapeutic payloads to specific cell types in the body. Utilizing probes on the exterior of the configurable microscopic medical payload delivery devices, these transport devices locate specific types of target cells in the body. Once a specific target cell is encountered and engaged, the configurable microscopic medical payload delivery device inserts its payload into the target cell. These medically therapeutic payloads are intended to improve cell function or the longevity of the cell or eliminate cells that pose a hazard to the general health of the body. By utilizing configurable microscopic medical payload delivery devices as a delivery system, the efficacy of medications and biologic tools are dramatically improved and there is a resultant significant reduction in the occurrence of unwanted side effects.

BACKGROUND OF THE INVENTION

Field of the Invention

This invention relates to any medical device intended to correct a deficiency in the body utilizing a configurable microscopic medical payload delivery device to transport and deliver a medical treatment payload into one or more specific cell types in the body.

Description of Background Art

[0001] Present medical care is attempting to utilize viruses to deliver genetic information into cells. Research in the field of gene therapy has involved certain naturally occurring viruses. Some of the common viral vectors that have been investigated include: Adeno-associated virus, Adenovirus, Alphavirus, Epstein-Barr virus, Gammaretrovirus, Herpes simplex virus, Letivirus, Poliovirus, Rhabdovirus, Vaccinia virus. Naturally occurring virus vectors are limited to the naturally occurring external probes that are affixed to the outer wall of the virus. The external probes fixed to the exterior surface of a virus virion dictates which type of cell the virus can engage and infect. Therefore, as an example, the function of the adenovirus, a respiratory virus, is strictly limited to engaging and infecting specific lung cells. Used as a medical treatment device, the adenovirus can only deliver gene therapy to specific lung cells, which severely limits this vector's usefulness as a deliver device. The therapeutic function of all naturally occurring viral vectors is limited to delivering a DNA or RNA based payload to the cell type the viral vector naturally targets as its host cell.

[0002] Naturally occurring viruses also have the disadvantage of being susceptible to detection and elimination by a body's immune system. Viruses have been infecting humans for hundreds of thousands of years. A human's innate immune system is very efficient at detecting the presence of most naturally occurring viruses when such a virus is inside the body. The human immune system is quite capable of generating a vigorous response to most intruding viruses by attacking and neutralizing the virus virions whenever a viral virion physically exits outside the exterior wall of the virus's host cell. If gene therapy in its current state were to become a clinical therapeutic tool, the naturally occurring viruses selected for gene therapy research will have limited effectiveness due the fact that once the viral vector is introduced into the body, the body's immune system will quickly engage and eliminate the viral vectors, possibly before the vector is able to deliver its payload to its host cell or target cell.

[0003] Cichutek, K., 2001 (US Patent No. 6,323,031 B1) teaches preparation and use of novel lentiviral SiVagm-derived vectors for gene transfer into selected cell types, specifically into proliferatively active and resting human cells.

[0004] Cichutek teaches that it is indeed plausible to re-configure an existing virus and use it as a transport vehicle, though Cichutek's specification and claims are too limited to describe a method that will work for all cell types, if indeed if it will work for any cell type.

[0005] Cichutek describes vectors for 'gene transfer'; in the claims the language that is used is 'genetic information'. Cichutek's Claim 1 of the cited patent states 'A propagation-incompetent SIVagm vector comprising a viral core and a viral envelope, wherein the viral core comprises a simian immunodeficiency virus (SIVagm) viral core of the African vervet monkey Chlorocebus.' Cichutek's does not describe in his claims any further details of the intended payload other than the stating 'SIVagm viral core' in claim 1; in claims 5 & 6 Cichutek describes only 'genetic information'. Transfer of 'genetic information' dramatically limits the useful application of Cichutek's patent in the treatment of medical diseases.

[0006] Cichutek's approach is dependent upon the probes naturally present on the viral vectors reported in the patent, which will direct the viral vectors to only those cells the viruses naturally use as their host cell. Cichutek's approach is very restrictive: limited to gene transfer to only cells the viruses use as their natural host cell.

[0007] Singular type antibodies or ligands can be used for cell to cell communication, but to open an access portal into a cell and insert a payload into the cell requires two different types of antibodies or ligands. As an example, human immunodeficiency virus requires the use of both the gp120 and gp41 probes to open a portal into a T-Helper cell and insert its genome into the T-Helper cell. The gp120 probe engages the CD4+ cell-surface receptor on the T-cell. Once the gp120 probe has successfully engaged a CD4+ cell-surface receptor on the target T-Helper cell, then the HIV virion's gp41 probe can engage either a CXCR4 or a CCR5 cell-surface receptor on the T-Helper cell in order to open up an access portal for HIV to insert its genome into a T-Helper cell. It is well documented in the medical literature that a genetic defect leading to an abnormality in the CXCR4 cell-surface receptor prevents HIV virions from opening an access portal and inserting its genetic payload into such T-Helper cells. This genetic defect offers the subset of people carrying this genetic defect resistance to HIV infection. This example demonstrates the need for at least two types of glycoprotein probes to be present on the surface of a viral vector in order for a viral vector to be capable of opening an access portal and delivering the payload the vector carries into its host cell or target cell.

[0008] A delivery system that offered a defined means of targeting specific types of cells would invoke minimal or no response by the innate immune system when present in the body, and a delivery system that would be capable of inserting into cells a wide variety of differing payloads would significantly improve the current medical treatment options available to clinicians treating patients.

[0009] The solution to arriving at a versatile, workable delivery system that will meet the needs of a number of medical treatments involves three important elements. These elements include:

configurable glycoprotein probes whereby more than one type of glycoprotein probe is to be used to engage and access specific target cell types in order to successfully deliver a payload into a specific cell type,

an exterior envelope comprised of a protein shell or a lipid layer expressing the least number of cell-surface markers, such as the use of a stem cell, to act as the host cell to manufacture the delivery devices,

a configurable core in the vector to enable it to carry and deliver a wide variety of payloads including proteins, chemicals, enzymes, RNAs, DNAs, nutrients, and molecules such as oxygen.

[0010] Viruses are obligate parasites. Viruses simply represent a carrier of genetic material and by themselves viruses are unable to replicate or carry out any form of biologic function outside their host cell. A 'virion' refers to the physical structure of a single complete virus as it exists outside of the host cell. Viruses are generally comprised of one or more nested shells constructed of one or more layers of protein, some with a lipid outer envelope, a genetic payload that represents the instruction code necessary to replicate the virus, and protein enzymes to help facilitate the genetic payload in the function of replicating copies of the virus once the genetic payload has been delivered to a host cell. Located on the outer shell or envelope of a virus are probes. The function of a virus's probes is to locate and engage a host cell's receptors. The virus's surface probes are designed to detect, make contact with and functionally engage one or more receptors located on the exterior of a cell type that will offer the virus the proper environment in which to construct copies of itself. A host cell provides the virus the proper biologic machinery for the virus to successfully replicate itself. Once the virus's genome is inside the host cell, the viral genome takes command of the cell's production machinery and causes the host cell to generate copies of the virus. As the viral copies exit the host cell, these virions set off in search of other host cells to infect.

[0011] Naturally occurring viruses exist in a number of differing shapes. The shape of a virus may be rod or filament like, icosahedral, or complex structures combining filament and polygonal shapes. Viruses generally have their outer wall comprised of a protein coat or an envelope comprised of lipids.

[0012] An outer envelope comprised of lipids may be in the form of one or two phospholipid layers. When the outer envelope is comprised of two phospholipid layers this is termed a lipid bilayer. A phospholipid is a composite molecule comprised of a polar or hydrophilic region on one end and a nonpolar or hydrophobic region on the opposite end. A lipid bilayer covering a virus, like the membrane of a cell, is constructed with the hydrophilic region of one of the phospholipid layers pointed toward the exterior of the virion and the hydrophilic region of the second phospholipid layer pointed inward toward the center of the virus virion; with the hydrophobic regions of each of the two lipid layers pointed toward each other. The outer envelope of some forms of virus may be comprised of an outer lipid layer or lipid bilayer affixed to a protein matrix for support, the protein matrix being located closer to the center of the virus virion than the lipid layer or lipid bilayer.

[0013] Spherical viruses are generally spherical in shape and may be comprised of an outer envelope and one inner shell or an outer envelope and multiple inner shells. Inner shells are approximately spherical in shape; this is because the proteins comprising the protein matrix shell have an irregular shape to their structure. In the case of a spherical virus with an outer envelope and one inner shell, the inner shell is often referred to as a nucleocapsid shell comprised of numerous capsid proteins attached to each other. In the case of a spherical virus being comprised of an outer envelope and multiple inner shells, the outermost inner viral shells may be referred to as comprised of a quantity of matrix proteins, where the innermost shell is referred to as a nucleocapsid and is comprised of a quantity of capsid proteins. The inner protein shells are nested inside each other.

[0014] Viruses carry genetic material in the form of deoxyribonucleic acid (DNA) or ribonucleic acid (RNA) in their nucleocapsid often referred to as the core or capsid. A virus is therefore generally considered to be a DNA virus if its genome is comprised of DNA or the virus is considered a RNA virus if its genome is comprised of RNA. Viruses may also carry enzymes as part of their payload. An enzyme such as 'reverse transcriptase' transforms a RNA viral genome into DNA. Protease enzymes modify the viral genome once it has entered a host cell. An integrase enzyme assists a DNA viral genome with insertion into the host cell's nuclear DNA. The payload is carried inside the virus's nucleocapsid shell.

[0015] The probes attached to the exterior of a virus are constructed to engage specific cell-surface receptors on specific cell types in the body. Only a cell that expresses cell-surface receptors that are capable of being engaged by the probes of a specific virus can act as a host for the virus. Viruses often use two probes to access a host cell. The first probe makes an initial attachment to the host cell, while the action of the virus's second probe often in conjunction with the action of the first probe cause an access portal to be created in the host cell's exterior plasma membrane. Once an access portal is formed, the virus inserts the contents of its payload into the host cell. Once the virus's genome is inside the cytoplasm of the host cell, any enzymes that accompanied the viral genome into the cell, may begin to modify or assist the virus's genome with infecting and taking control of the host cell's biologic functions.

[0016] Probes are attached to the exterior envelope of a virus virion. Probes may be in the form of a protein structure or may be in the form of a glycoprotein molecule. For viruses constructed with a protein matrix as its outer envelope, the probes tend to be protein structures. A portion of the protein structure probe is fixed or anchored in the protein matrix, while a portion of the protein structure probe extends out and away from the protein matrix. The portion of the protein structure probe extending out away from the virus virion is referred to as the 'exterior domain', the portion anchored in the protein matrix is the 'transcending domain'. Some protein probes have a third segment that extends through the envelope and exists inside the virus virion, which is referred to as the 'interior domain'. The exterior domain of a protein structure probe is intended to engage a specific cell-surface receptor on a biologically active cell the virus is targeting as its host cell.

[0017] Viruses that utilize a lipid layer as the outer envelope, are constructed with probes that tend to be glycoproteins. A glycoprotein is comprised of a protein segment and a carbohydrate segment. The carbohydrate segment of the glycoprotein molecule is fixed or anchored in the lipid layer of the outer envelope, while the protein segment extends outward and away from the outer envelope. The protein portion of a glycoprotein probe that extends outward and away from the outer envelope of a virus virion is intended to engage a cell-surface receptor on a biologically active cell the virus is targeting as its host cell.

[0018] Some forms of viruses that utilize a lipid layer as its envelope use protein structure probes. In this case, the portion of the protein structure probe that extends outward and away from the outer envelope is the 'exterior domain', the portion that is anchored in the lipid layer is the 'transcending domain' and again some protein structure probes have an 'interior domain' that exist inside the virion, which may also help anchor the protein structure probe to the virion. The exterior domain of a protein structure probe that extends outward and away from the outer envelope of a virus virion is intended to engage a cell-surface receptor on a biologically active cell the virus is targeting as its host cell.

[0019] When a virus carries a DNA payload and the viral DNA is inserted into the host cell, the viral DNA travels to the host cell's nucleus and is known to become inserted into the host cell's native DNA. In the case where a virus is carrying its genetic payload as RNA, the virus inserts the RNA payload into the host cell and may also insert one or more enzymes to facilitate the RNA being utilized properly to replicate copies of the virus. Once inside the host cell, some species of virus facilitate use of the viral RNA by having the viral RNA converted to DNA. Once the viral RNA has been converted to viral DNA, the viral DNA travels to the host cell's nucleus and is known to become inserted into the host cell's native DNA. Once a virus's genetic material has been inserted into the host cell's native DNA, the virus's genetic material takes command of certain cell functions and redirects the resources of the host cell to generate copies of the virus. Other forms of RNA viruses bypass the need to use the nuclear DNA and simply utilize portions of the viral genome to act as messenger RNA. RNA viruses that bypass the host cell's DNA, cause the cell in general to generate copies of the necessary parts of the virus directly from the virus's RNA genome.

[0020] The human immunodeficiency virus (HIV) has an outer envelope comprised of a lipid bilayer. The lipid bilayer covers a protein matrix consisting of p17^{gag} proteins. Inside the p17^{gag} protein matrix is nested a nucleocapsid comprised of p24^{gag} proteins. Inside the nucleocapsid HIV carries its payload. HIV's genetic payload consists of two single strands of RNA. In addition to the two strands of HIV RNA, there are proteins that are carried in the core of the nucleocapsid along with the two RNA strands. These proteins include 'reverse transcriptase', 'integrase' and 'protease' molecules.

[0021] The T-Helper cell acts as HIV's host cell. HIV locates its host by utilizing at least two different types of probes located on its envelope. The HIV virion utilizes two types of glycoprotein probes affixed to the outer surface of its exterior envelope to engage a T-Helper cell. HIV utilizes a glycoprotein probe 120 to locate a CD4 cell-surface receptor on a T-Helper cell. Once an HIV glycoprotein 120 probe has successfully engaged a CD4 cell-surface receptor on a T-Helper cell a conformational change occurs in the probe and a glycoprotein 41 probe is exposed. The glycoprotein 41 probe's intent is to engage a CXCR4 or CCR5 cell-surface receptor on the same T-Helper cell. Once a glycoprotein 41 probe on the HIV virion successfully engages a CXCR4 or CCR5 cell-surface receptor, the HIV virion opens an access portal through the T-Helper cell's outer membrane.

[0022] Once the HIV virion has opened an access portal through the T-Helper cell's outer plasma membrane, the HIV virion inserts the two positive strand RNA molecules it carries into the T-Helper cell. Each RNA strand is approximately 9500 nucleotides in length. Inserted along with the RNA strands are the enzymes reverse transcriptase, protease and integrase. Once the virus's genome gains access to the interior of the T-Helper cell, the pair of RNA molecules are transformed in the cytoplasm to deoxyribonucleic acid by the reverse transcriptase enzyme. Following modification of the virus's genome to DNA, the virus's genetic information migrates to the host cell's nucleus.

In the nucleus, with the assistance of the integrase protein, HIV's DNA becomes inserted into the T-Helper cell's native DNA. When the timing is appropriate, the now integrated viral DNA is decoded by the host cell's polymerase molecules and the virus's genetic information commands certain cell functions to carry out the replication process to construct copies of the human deficiency virus.

[0023] The outer layer of the HIV virion is comprised of a portion of the T-Helper cell's outer cell membrane. In the final stage of the replication process, as a copy of the HIV capsid, carrying the HIV genome, buds through the host cell's cell membrane the capsid acquires as its exterior envelope, a wrapping of lipid bilayer from the host cell's cell membrane. In the case of HIV, since the surface of the pathogen is covered by an envelope comprised of lipid bilayer taken from the host T-Helper cells, this feature allows the HIV virion the capacity to eluded the immune systems, since the cells comprising the immune system may find it difficult to tell the difference between the surface of an infectious HIV virion and the surface characteristics of a noninfected T-Helper cell.

[0024] The Hepatitis C virus (HCV) is a positive sense RNA virus, meaning a type of RNA that is capable of bypassing the need for involving the host cell's nucleus by having its RNA genome function as messenger RNA. Hepatitis C infects liver cells. The Hepatitis C viral genome becomes divided once it gains access to the interior of a liver host cell. Portions of the subdivisions of the Hepatitis C genome directly interact with ribosomes to produce proteins necessary to construct copies of the virus.

[0025] HCV belongs to the Flaviviridae family and is the only member of the Hepacivirus genus. There are considered to be at least 100 different strains of Hepatitis C virus based on genome sequencing variability.

[0026] HCV is comprised of an outer lipoprotein envelope and an internal nucleocapsid. The genetic payload is carried within the nucleocapsid. In its natural state, present on the surface of the outer envelope of the Hepatitis C virus are probes that detect receptors present on the surface of liver cells. The glycoprotein E1 probe and the glycoprotein E2 probe have been identified to be affixed to the surface of HCV. The E2 probe binds with high affinity to the large external loop of a CD81 cell-surface receptor. CD81 is found on the surface of many cell types including liver cells. Once the E2 probe has engaged the CD81 cell-surface receptor, cofactors on the surface of HCV's exterior envelope engage either or both the low density lipoprotein receptor (LDLR) or the scavenger receptor class B type I (SR-BI) present on the liver cell in order to effect the mechanism to facilitate HCV breaching the cell membrane and inserting its RNA genome payload through the plasma cell membrane of the liver cell into the liver cell. Upon successful engagement of the HCV surface probes with a liver cell's cell-surface receptors, HCV inserts the single strand of RNA and other payload elements it carries into the liver cell targeted to be a host cell. The HCV RNA genome then interacts with enzymes and ribosomes inside the liver cell in a translational process to produce the proteins required to construct copies of the protein components of HCV. The HCV genome undergoes a method of transcription to replicate copies of the virus's RNA genome. Inside the host, pieces of the HCV virus are assembled together and ultimately loaded with a copy of the HCV genome. Replicas of the original HCV then escape the host cell and migrate the environment in search of additional host liver cells to infect and continue the replication process.

[0027] The HCV's naturally occurring genetic payload consists of a single molecule of linear positive sense, single stranded RNA approximately 9600 nucleotides in length. By means of a translational process a polyprotein of approximately 3000 amino acids is generated. This polyprotein is cleaved post translation by host and viral proteases into individual viral proteins which include: the structural proteins of C, E1, E2, the nonstructural proteins NS1, NS2, NS3, NS4A, NS4B, NS5A, NS5B, p7 and ARFP/F protein. Hepatitis C virus's proteins direct the host liver cell to construction copies of the Hepatitis C virus. A membrane associated replicase complex consisting of the virus's nonstructural proteins NS3 and NS5B facilitate the replication of the viral genome. The membrane of the endoplasmic reticulum appears to be the site of protein maturation and viral assembly. Once copies of the Hepatitis C Virus are generated, they exit the host cell and each copy of HCV migrates in search of another appropriate liver cell that will act as a host to continue the replication process.

[0028] Hepatitis C virus life-cycle demonstrates that copies of a virus virion can be generated by inserting RNA into a host cell that functions as messenger RNA in the host cell. The Hepatitis C viral RNA genome functions as messenger RNA, acting as the template in conjunction with the biologic machinery of a host cell to produce the components that comprise copies of the Hepatitis C virion and the Hepatitis C viral RNA provides the biologic instructions to assemble the components into complete copies of the Hepatitis C virions. The Hepatitis C virus life-cycle clearly demonstrates that viral virions can be manufactured by a host cell without involving the nucleus of the cell.

[0029] Deciphering the existence, replication and behavior of viruses provides clear examples of several fundamental concepts, which include: (1) Viruses target specific cells in the body by means of identifying and engaging such target cells utilizing the probes projecting outward from the virus's exterior shell to make contact with cell-surface receptors located on the surface of the target cells, and (2) Viruses are capable of carrying various types of payloads including DNA, RNA and a variety of proteins.

[0030] Current medical therapy generally involves the administration of medications or biologic agents that tend to circulate the body by way of the blood stream and are capable of interacting with nearly all cells comprising the body that make contact with the circulation system. Adverse side effects occur when cells react to the toxic effects of medications or biologic agents. Often unwanted side effects occur due to cell types that are not targeted directly by the medications or biologic agents, being harmed by the presence of the medication or biologic agent circulating in the blood stream or tissues.

[0031] Current gene therapy approach to attempting to deliver a payload to cells in the body use modified forms of existing viruses to act as transport devices to deliver genetic information. This approach is severely limited by restricting the virus virion to target only cells the viral vector naturally seeks out and infects. Current gene therapy approach is further limited by using the pre-existing size of naturally occurring viruses, rather than being able to modify the size of the structure to be able to tailor the volumetric carrying capacity of the payload portion of the modified virus. Further gene therapy is restricted to utilizing naturally occurring viruses to deliver only genetic information; it has not previously been appreciated by those skilled in the art that virus-like transport devices might deliver to variety of specific cell types a wide variety of differing payloads as needed to successfully accomplish a specific medical treatment.

[0032] A dramatic treatment strategy, not previously recognized by those expert in the art, is the development of a transport vehicle that can be fashioned to seek out specific types of cells and deliver to these cells a variety of predetermined payloads as needed to successfully accomplish a specific medical treatment. Transport devices should be versatile enough to deliver a variety of payloads including DNA material, RNA material of various forms, simple proteins, complex proteins, conjugated proteins, globular proteins, polypeptides, chemicals, sugars, nutrients and elements such as oxygen. The RNA payloads include messenger RNA molecules, ribosomal RNA molecules, genetic RNA molecules intended to be converted to DNA, transport RNA molecules, small nuclear RNA molecules. The exterior envelope of a transport should be constructed so as not to alert the immune system of its presence to prevent rejection of the vehicles. Transport vehicles should be capable of being configured to target any specific cell type and engage and deliver their payload only to that specific predetermined cell type. To this point, such device has not been described in the literature.

BRIEF SUMMARY OF THE INVENTION

[0033] Utilization of configurable microscopic medical payload delivery devices is meant to dramatically improve the efficiency and efficacy of medical care. Each configurable microscopic medical payload delivery device (CMMPDD) is intended to deliver specific medications or deliver specific biologic tool directly to specifically targeted cells in the body. By selecting the types of probes that are present on the surface of the configurable microscopic medical payload delivery devices, specific types of cells can be targeted. By delivering specific medications or biologic tools directly to specifically targeted cell types, the efficacy of the medication or the biologic tool is to be significantly improved. By delivering specific medications or biologic tools directly to specifically targeted cell types a reduction in side effects is appreciated due to the cells that are not intended to be exposed to the drug or a biologic tool that the configurable microscopic medical payload delivery devices are carrying, are spared exposure to potential toxic effects of drugs or biologic tools and therefore are not subject to harm.

DETAILED DESCRIPTION

[0034] The future of medical treatment is the widespread utilization of configurable microscopic medical payload delivery devices (CMMPDD) to deliver medications or biologic tools directly to targeted cell types in the body.

[0035] For purposes of this text a medication includes chemical molecule, elements such as oxygen, sugars such as glucose, and other nutrients, which when purposely delivered to cells in the body produces a beneficial medical effect.

[0036] For purposes of this text a 'biologic tool' is a segment of DNA, a segment of RNA molecule, or a protein molecule such as an enzyme.

[0037] For purposes of this text an 'external envelope' refers to the outermost covering of a virus or a virus-like transport device or a configurable microscopic medical payload delivery device. The external envelope may be comprised of a lipid layer, a lipid bilayer, the combination of a lipid layer affixed to a protein matrix or the combination of a lipid bilayer affixed to a protein matrix.

[0038] For purposes of this text an 'internal shell' refers to a protein matrix shell nested inside the external envelope. The inner most protein matrix shell is termed the nucleocapsid. The proteins that comprise the nucleocapsid are termed capsid proteins. In the center or core of the nucleocapsid is where the payload is carried.

[0039] For purposes of this text 'external probes' are molecular structures that are utilized to locate and engage cell-surface receptors on biologically active cells. External probes are generally comprised of a portion which is anchored or fixed in the external envelope and a second portion that extends out and away from the external envelope. External probes may be comprised solely of a protein structure or an external probe may be a glycoprotein molecule.

[0040] For purposes of this text 'glycoprotein molecule' refers to a molecule comprised of a carbohydrate region and a protein region. Glycoprotein molecules that act as probes are generally anchored or fixed to a lipid layer utilizing the carbohydrate portion of the molecule as an anchor. The protein portion of the glycoprotein molecule which extends outward and away from the exterior envelope the glycoprotein has been affixed such that the protein region may function as a probe to locate and attach to the cell-surface receptor it was created to engage.

[0041] The concept of configurable microscopic medical payload delivery devices is modeled after naturally existing viruses. Configurable microscopic medical payload delivery devices in general are spherical in shape; though other shapes may be used as function might warrant the use of a particular shape. The spherical configurable microscopic medical payload delivery devices are comprised of an exterior envelope and one or more inner nested protein shells. A quantity of exterior protein structure probes and/or glycoprotein probes are anchored in the exterior lipid envelope and extend out and away from the exterior lipid envelope. Nesting of protein shells refers to progressively smaller diameter shells fitting snugly inside protein shells of a larger diameter. Inside the inner most protein shell, referred to as the nucleocapsid, is a cavity referred to as the core of the device. The core of the device is the space where the medically therapeutic payload the device carries is located.

[0042] Configurable microscopic medical payload delivery devices are generated to target certain specific cell types in the body. Configurable microscopic medical payload delivery devices target specific cell types by the configuration of probes affixed to the exterior envelope of the CMMPDD. By affixing specific probes to the exterior envelope of the CMMPDD, these probes intended to engage and attach only to specific cell-surface receptors located on certain cell types in the body, the CMMPDD will deliver its payload only to those cell types that express compatible and engagable specific cell-surface receptors. In a similar fashion where the exterior probes of a naturally occurring virus engage specific cell-surface receptors present on the surface of the virus's host cell and only the designated host cell, the CMMPDD's exterior probes are configured to engage cell-surface receptors on a specific type of target cell. In this manner, the payload of medication or biologic tools carried by CMMPDD will be delivered only to specific types of cells in the body. The exterior probes on the surface of a CMMPDD will vary as needed so as to effect the CMMPDD delivery of payloads to cell types as needed to effect a medical treatment.

[0043] The size of configurable microscopic medical payload delivery devices is to depend upon the volume size of the payload the CMMPDD is required to carry and deliver to a target cell. The size of a CMMPDD is dependent upon the diameter of the inner protein matrix shells. The diameter of each inner protein matrix shell is governed by the number of protein molecules utilized to construct the protein matrix shell at the time the protein matrix shell is generated. Increasing the number of proteins that comprise a protein matrix shell, increases the diameter of the protein matrix shell. The external lipid envelope wraps around and covers the outermost protein matrix shell. The larger the volume of the core of the CMMPDD, the greater the physical size payload the CMMPDD is able to carry. The size of the configurable microscopic medical payload delivery device is to be the size of cell (approximately 10^{-4} m in diameter) or less, generally detectable by a light microscope or, as needed, an electron microscope. The size of the CMMPDD is not to be too large such that it would generate a burden to the body by damaging organ tissues through clogging blood vessels, and the maintaining a small enough size that the CMMPDD can be properly disposed of by the body once the CMMPDD has delivered its payload to its target cell. The dimensions of each type of CMMPDD are to be tailored to the mission of the CMMPDD, which takes into account the type of target cell, the size of the payload that is to be delivered to the target cells and the length of time the CMMPDD may engage the target cell.

[0044] Being enveloped in an external lipid layer, configurable microscopic medical payload delivery devices possess the advantage of having their exterior appear similar to the plasma membrane that acts as an outside covering for the cells that comprise the body. By appearing similar to existing plasma membranes, the CMMPDDs appear similar to naturally occurring structures found in the body, affording the CMMPDD the capability to avoid detection by a body's immune system because the exterior of the CMMPDD mimics the cells comprising the body and the surveillance cells of the immune system find it difficult to discern between the CMMPDD and naturally occurring cells comprising the body.

[0045] To carry out the process of manufacturing a configurable microscopic medical payload delivery device, a primitive cell such as a stem cell is selected. The reason for utilizing primitive cells such as stems cells as the host cell, is that the CMMPDD acquires its outer envelope from the host cell and the more primitive the host cell, the fewer in number the identifying protein markers are present on the surface of the CMMPDD. The fewer the identifying surface proteins present on the outer envelope of the CMMPDD, the less likely a body's immune system will identify the CMMPDD as an invader and therefore less likely the body's immune system will react to the presence of the CMMPDD and reject the CMMPDD by attacking and neutralizing the CMMPDD.

[0046] Stem cells used as host cells to manufacture quantities of CMMPDD product are selected per histocompatibility markers present on their surface. Certain histocompatibility markers present on the surface of the final CMMPDD product will be less likely to cause a reaction in a specific patient based on the genetic profile of the patient's histocompatibility markers.

A similar histocompatibility match is done when donor organs are selected to be given to recipients to avoid rejection of the donor organ by the recipient's immune system.

[0047] The selected stem cell used to manufacture configurable microscopic medical payload delivery devices goes through several steps of maturation before it is capable of generating therapeutic CMMPDD product. Messenger RNA would be inserted into the host stem cell that would code for the general physical outer structures of the CMMPDD. Messenger RNA would be inserted into the host that would generate surface probes that would target the surface receptors on specifically target cells. Messenger RNA would be inserted into the host that would be used to generate the therapeutic payload. Similar to how copies of a naturally occurring virus are produced, assembled and released from a host cell, copies of the CMMPDD would be produced, assembled and released from a host cell. Once released from the host cell, the copies of the CMMPDD would be collected, then pooled together to produce a therapeutic dose that would result in a medically beneficial effect.

[0048] The construction of the configurable microscopic medical payload delivery devices is performed by taking stem cells and inserting modified viral genetic programming into the stem cells. Stem cells are chosen as the host cell due to the low number of surface markers, which leads to less antigenicity in configurable microscopic medical payload delivery devices when the configurable microscopic medical payload delivery devices are released by the host cells and wrapped in an outer envelope comprised of the host cells' plasma membrane.

[0049] The stem cells used as host cells are suspended in a broth of nutrients and are kept at an optimum temperature to govern the rate of production of the CMMPDD product. Similar to the natural production of the Hepatitis C virus, the configurable microscopic medical payload delivery devices 'production genome' is introduced into the host stem cells. The configurable microscopic medical payload delivery devices production genome carries genetic instructions to cause the host cells to manufacture the configurable microscopic medical payload delivery devices' outer protein wall, the inner protein matrixes, the surface probes the configurable microscopic medical payload delivery device is to have affixed to its outer envelope and the payload the configurable microscopic medical payload delivery devices are to carry; and the instructions to assemble the various pieces into the final form of the configurable microscopic medical payload delivery devices and the instructions to activate the budding process. The resultant configurable microscopic medical payload delivery devices are collected from the nutrient broth surrounding the host cells and placed together into doses to be used as a treatment for a medical disease.

[0050] The 'production genome' are an array of messenger RNAs that are directly translated by the host cell's internal enzymes. The production genome dictates the characteristics of the final version of the CMMPDD that buds from the host stem cell and is released and is to be utilized as a medical treatment. The production genome is specifically tailored to code for the surface probes that will seek and engage a specific type of target cell. The production genome also carries the instructions to code for the production of the type of payload to be delivered to the specific type of target cell. In the case of a nutrient, the production genome carries the instructions to place a proper amount of nutrient into the CMMPDD. The 'production genome' varies depending upon the configuration of the CMMPDD to effect a specific medical treatment.

[0051] The configurable microscopic medical payload delivery device represents a very versatile delivery device. There are an estimated 100,000 genes located in the human genome. CMMPDD could be used to deliver any of the 100,000 genes to any specific cell type in the body. Regarding RNAs, CMMPDD could be utilized to deliver to specific cell types messenger RNAs, ribosomal RNAs, transport RNAs, small nuclear RNAs. With regards to messenger RNAs, there are at least 210 different cell types in the human body and there are at least 30,000 different proteins that the human body produces. Each of the 30,000 proteins are generated by a cell translating one or more mRNAs responsible for production of a particular protein. The number of different medical treatment options that are possible as a result of delivering messenger RNAs to specific cell types is approximately 6,000,000. A wide variety of proteins could be transported to specific cell types by means of CMMPDD. There are numerous presently existing medications and numerous emerging medications that could be delivered directly to specific cell types per the transport capability of CMMPDD. There are a wide variety of nutrients that could be delivered to specific cells by means of CMMPDD.

[0052] As an example of this method, to treat diabetes mellitus utilizing configurable microscopic medical payload delivery devices to deliver to Beta cells messenger RNA coded to produce insulin, the following production process is followed in the lab: (1) human stem cells are selected. (2) Into the selected stem cells is placed the production genome constructed, in this case, specifically as a means to treat diabetes mellitus. The RNA production genome contains genetic instructions to cause the host stem cells to manufacture the configurable microscopic medical payload delivery devices' outer protein wall, the inner protein matrix, surface probes to include glycoprotein probes that engage the GPR40 cell-surface receptor present on the surface of Beta cells located in the Islets of Langerhans in the pancreas, and the payload, in this case messenger RNA constructed to effect the production of the insulin molecule; and the biologic instructions to assemble the components into the final form of the configurable microscopic medical payload delivery devices; and the biologic instructions to activate the budding process. (3) Upon insertion of the RNA production genome dedicated to producing a messenger RNA coded to produce insulin, into the host stem cells, host stem cells respond by (i) simultaneously translating the different segments of the RNA production genome to produce the proteins that comprise the exterior protein wall, the inner protein matrix molecules, the surface probes to seek out and engage Beta cells, the mRNA payload to produce insulin, and (ii) decoding the RNA instructions to assemble the components into the configurable microscopic medical payload delivery devices. (4) Upon assembly, the configurable microscopic medical payload delivery devices bud through the cell membrane of the host stem cell. (5) At the time of the budding process, the configurable microscopic medical payload delivery devices acquire an outside envelope wrapped over the outer protein shell, this outer envelope comprised of a portion of the plasma membrane from the host stem cell as the configurable microscopic medical payload delivery devices exit the host cell. (6) The resultant configurable microscopic medical payload delivery devices are collected from the nutrient broth surrounding the host stem cells. (7) The configurable microscopic medical payload delivery devices are washed in sterile solvent to remove contaminants. (8) The configurable microscopic medical payload delivery devices are removed from the sterile solvent and suspended in a hypoallergenic liquid medium. (9) The configurable microscopic medical payload delivery devices are separated into individual quantities to facilitate storage and delivery to physicians and patients. (10) The configurable microscopic medical payload delivery devices transported in the hypoallergenic liquid medium is administered to a diabetic patient per injection in a dose that is tailored to receiving patient's requirement to produce sufficient amount of insulin to control the blood sugar. (11) Upon being injected into the body, the configurable microscopic medical payload delivery devices migrate to the Beta cells located in the Islets of Langerhans by means of the patient's blood stream. (12) Upon the configurable microscopic medical payload delivery devices reaching the Beta cells, the configurable microscopic medical payload delivery devices engage the cell-surface receptors located on the Beta cells and insert the payload they carry into the Beta cells. The payload, in this case being messenger RNA coded to produce insulin, is translated by the cell's ribosomes to produce insulin molecules. The increase in insulin production by Beta cells successfully manages diabetes mellitus.

Conclusions, Ramification, and Scope

[0053] Accordingly, the reader will see that the configurable microscopic medical payload delivery device to deliver medically therapeutic payloads to specifically targeted cell types provides advantages over existing art by being a delivery device that (1) is constructed to seek out and engage specific types of cells by design based on medical need, (2) is versatile enough in its construction to deliver a wide variety of possible payloads to specific cell types, and (3) is constructed with a surface envelope that will avoid detection by the innate immune system so as not to activate the immune system to its presence; for these reasons this represents a new and unique medical delivery device that has never before been recognized nor appreciated by those skilled in the art.

[0054] Although the description above contains specificities, these should not be construed as limiting the scope of the invention but as merely providing illustrations of some of the presently preferred embodiments of the invention.

[0055] Thus the scope of the invention should be determined by the appended claims and their legal equivalents, rather than by the examples given.

CLAIMS: Reserved.

No. 2: RNA VECTOR THERAPY

INDIVIDUALS REQUESTING PATENT: Dr. Lane B. Scheiber, ScD and Dr. Lane B. Scheiber II, MD

©2010 Lane B. Scheiber and Lane B. Scheiber II. A portion of the disclosure of this patent document contains material which is subject to copyright protection. The copyright owners have no objection to the facsimile reproduction by anyone of the patent document or the patent disclosure, as it appears in the Patent and Trademark Office patent file or records, but otherwise reserves all copyright rights whatsoever.

ABSTRACT

The innovative treatment strategy described here utilizes configurable microscopic medical payload delivery devices to act as a transport vector to deliver a wide variety of cellular ribonucleic acid molecules to specific types of cells in the body. Utilizing probes on the exterior of the transport devices, the transport devices locate a specific type of cell in the body. Once a specific target cell type has been encountered, the configurable microscopic medical payload delivery devices insert their payload of cellular ribonucleic acid molecules into the target cells. By delivering cellular ribonucleic acid molecules into specific cells a wide variety of protein deficiencies are correctable, gene expression is capable of being modulated, and telomere synthesis is enhanced.

BACKGROUND OF THE INVENTION

Field of the Invention

This invention relates to any medical device intended to treat medical conditions utilizing a configurable microscopic medical payload delivery device to insert cellular ribonucleic acid molecules into one or more specific type of cells in the body to improve cell function.

Description of Background Art

[0001] Cellular ribonucleic acid (RNA) molecules are divided into two major functional categories which are 'protein coding RNAs' and 'non-coding RNAs'. Protein coding RNAs, usually referred to as messenger RNAs, undergo the process of translation in the cytoplasm of the cell and produce proteins by ribosomes decoding the genetic information carried in the coding region of the messenger RNA. Non-coding RNAs perform a wide variety of tasks both in the nucleus and in the cytoplasm of a cell.

[0002] Present medical research is attempting to utilize viruses to deliver genetic information into cells. Research in the field of gene therapy has involved certain naturally occurring viruses. Some of the common viral vectors that have been investigated include: Adeno-associated virus, Adenovirus, Alphavirus, Epstein-Barr virus, Gammaretrovirus, Herpes simplex virus, Letivirus, Poliovirus, Rhabdovirus, Vaccinia virus. Naturally occurring virus vectors are limited to the naturally occurring external probes that are affixed to the outer wall of the virus. The external probes fixed to the outside wall of a virus virion dictate which type of cell the virus can engage and infect. Therefore, as an example, the function of the adenovirus, a respiratory virus, is strictly limited to engaging and infecting specific lung cells. Used as a medical treatment device, the adenovirus can only deliver gene therapy to specific lung cells, which severely limits this vector's usefulness as a deliver device. The therapeutic function of all naturally occurring viral vectors is limited to delivering a DNA or RNA payload to the cell type the viral vector naturally targets as its host cell.

[0003] Naturally occurring viruses also have the disadvantage of being susceptible to detection and elimination by a body's immune system. Viruses have been infecting humans for hundreds of thousands of years. A human's immune system is very efficient at detecting the presence of most naturally occurring viruses when such a virus is inside the body. The human immune system is quite capable of generating a vigorous response to most intruding viruses, attacking and neutralizing virus virions whenever a virus virion physically exists are outside the exterior wall of the virus's host cell. If gene therapy in its current state were to become a clinical therapeutic tool, the naturally occurring viruses selected for gene therapy research will have limited effectiveness due the fact that once the viral vector is introduced into the body, the body's the immune system will quickly engage and eliminate the viral vectors, possibly before the vector is able to deliver its payload to its host cell or target cell.

[0004] Cichutek, K., 2001 (US Patent No. 6,323,031 B1) teaches preparation and use of novel lentiviral SiVagm-derived vectors for gene transfer into selected cell types, specifically into proliferatively active and resting human cells.

[0005] Cichutek teaches that it is indeed plausible to re-configure an existing virus and use it as a transport vehicle, though Cichutek's specification and claims are too limited to describe a method that will work for all cell types, if indeed if it will work for any cell type.

[0006] Cichutek describes vectors for 'gene transfer'; in the claims the language that is used is 'genetic information'. Cichutek's Claim 1 of the cited patent states 'A propagation-incompetent SIVagm vector comprising a viral core and a viral envelope, wherein the viral core comprises a simian immunodeficiency virus (SIVagm) viral core of the African vervet monkey Chlorocebus.' Cichutek's does not describe in his claims any further details of the intended payload other than the stating 'SIVagm viral core' in claim 1; in claims 5 & 6 Cichutek describes only 'genetic information'. Transfer of 'genetic information' dramatically limits the useful application of Cichutek's patent in the treatment of medical diseases.

[0007] Cichutek's approach is dependent upon the probes naturally present on the viral vectors reported in the patent, which will direct the viral vectors to only those cells the viruses naturally use as their host cell. Cichutek's approach is very restrictive, limited to gene transfer to only cells the viruses use as their natural host cell.

[0008] Singular type antibodies or ligands can be used for cell-to-cell communication, but to open an access portal into a cell and insert a payload into the cell requires two different types of antibodies or ligands. As an example human immunodeficiency virus requires the use of both the gp120 and gp41 probes to open a portal into a T-Helper cell and insert its viral genome into the T-Helper cell. The gp120 probe engages the CD4+ cell-surface receptor on the T-cell. Once the gp120 probe has successfully engaged a CD4+ cell-surface receptor on the target T-Helper cell, then the HIV virion's gp41 probe can engage either a CXCR4 or a CCR5 cell-surface receptor on the T-Helper cell in order to open up an access portal for HIV to insert its viral genome into a T-Helper cell. It is well documented in the medical literature that a genetic defect leading to an abnormality in the CXCR4 cell-surface receptor prevents HIV virions from opening an access portal and inserting its genetic payload into such T-Helper cells. This genetic defect in the CXCR4 cell-surface receptors offers the subset of people carrying the genetic defect resistance to HIV infection. This example demonstrates the need for at least two types of glycoprotein probes to be present on the surface of a viral vector in order for a viral vector to be capable of opening an access portal and delivering the payload the vector carries into its host cell or target cell.

[0009] A delivery system that offered a defined means of targeting specific types of cells would invoke minimal or no response by the innate immune system and the adaptable immune system when present in the body, and a delivery system that would be capable of inserting into cells a wide variety of ribonucleic acid molecules would significantly improve the current medical treatment options available to clinicians treating patients.

[0010] The solution to arriving at a versatile, workable delivery system that will meet the needs of a number of medical treatments involves three important elements. These elements include:

(1) configurable external probes whereby more than one type of protein structure probe or more than one type of glycoprotein probe is to be used to engage and access specific target cell types in order to successfully deliver a payload into a specific cell type,

(2) an exterior envelope comprised of a protein shell or lipid layer expressing the least number of cell-surface markers, such as the use of a stem cell to act as the host cell to manufacture the delivery devices,

(3) configuring the core of the vector to enable it to carry and deliver a wide variety of cellular ribonucleic acid molecules.

For purposes of this text, the use of the terms 'specific target cell type', 'target cell', 'specific cell type', 'specific cell', 'specific type of cell' are equivalent and interchangeable; the configuration of cell-surface receptors that a specific cell type has located on and protruding from its outer cell membrane determines the cell type.

[0011] Viruses are obligate parasites. Viruses simply represent a carrier of genetic material and by themselves viruses are unable to replicate or carry out any form of biologic function outside their host cell. A 'virion' refers to the physical structure of a single complete virus as it exists outside of the host cell; a more archaic term for 'viral virion' was 'virus particle'.

Viruses are generally comprised of one or more nested shells constructed of one or more layers of protein, some with a lipid outer envelope, a genetic payload that represents the instruction code necessary to replicate the virus, and protein enzymes to help facilitate the genetic payload in the function of replicating copies of the virus once the genetic payload has been delivered to a host cell. Located on the outer shell or envelope of a virus are probes. The function of a virus's external probes is to locate and engage a host cell's receptors. The virus's surface probes are designed to detect, make contact with and functionally engage one or more receptors located on the exterior of the type of cell that will offer the virus the proper environment in which to construct copies of itself. A host cell provides the virus the proper biologic machinery for the virus to successfully replicate itself. Once the virus's genome is inside the host cell, the viral genome takes command of the cell's production machinery and causes the host cell to generate copies of the virus. As the viral copies exit the host cell, these virions set off in search of other host cells to infect.

[0012] Naturally occurring viruses exist in a number of differing shapes. The shape of a virus may be rod or filament like, icosahedral, or complex structures combining filament and polygonal shapes. Viruses generally have their outer wall comprised of a protein coat or an envelope comprised of lipids.

[0013] An outer envelope comprised of lipids may be in the form of one or two phospholipid layers. When the outer envelope is comprised of two phospholipid layers this is termed a lipid bilayer. For purposes of this text the term 'lipid' includes 'phospholipid' molecules. A phospholipid is a composite molecule comprised of a polar or hydrophilic region on one end and a nonpolar or hydrophobic region on the opposite end. A lipid bilayer covering a virus, like the membrane of a cell, is constructed with the hydrophilic region of one of the phospholipid layers pointed toward the exterior of the virion and the hydrophilic region of the second phospholipid layer pointed inward toward the center of the virus virion; with the hydrophobic regions of each of the two lipid layers pointed toward each other. The outer envelope of some forms of virus may be comprised of an outer lipid layer or lipid bilayer affixed to a protein matrix for support, the protein matrix being located closer to the center of the virus virion than the lipid layer or lipid bilayer.

[0014] Spherical viruses are generally spherical in shape and may be comprised of an outer envelope and one inner shell or alternatively an outer envelope and multiple inner shells. Inner shells are approximately spherical in shape; this is because the proteins comprising the protein matrix shell have an irregular shape to their structure, but when constructed together form a shape that resembles a sphere. In the case of a spherical virus with an outer envelope and one inner shell, the inner shell is often referred to as a nucleocapsid shell comprised of numerous capsid proteins attached to each other. In the case of a spherical virus being comprised of an outer envelope and multiple inner shells, the outermost inner viral shells may be referred to as comprised of a quantity of matrix proteins, where the innermost shell is referred to as a nucleocapsid and is comprised of a quantity of capsid proteins. The inner protein shells are nested inside each other. The cavity created by the innermost shell or nucleocapsid is referred to as the 'core' or 'center of the virus'. Any payload carried by the virus virion is generally carried in the core or center of the virion.

[0015] Viruses carry genetic material in the form of deoxyribonucleic acid (DNA) or ribonucleic acid (RNA) as their payload. DNA or RNA genome payloads are carried in the cavity of the nucleocapsid referred to as the core. A virus is therefore generally considered to be a DNA virus if its genome is comprised of DNA or the virus is considered a RNA virus if its genome is comprised of RNA that acts as genetic instructions to generate copies of the virus. Viruses may also carry enzymes as part of their payload. An enzyme such as 'reverse transcriptase' transforms a RNA viral genome into DNA. Protease enzymes modify the viral genome once it has entered a host cell. An integrase enzyme assists a DNA viral genome with insertion into the host cell's nuclear DNA. The entire genetic payload is carried inside cavity created by the virus's nucleocapsid shell.

[0016] The probes attached to the exterior of a virus are constructed to engage specific cell-surface receptors on a specific type of cell in the body. Only a cell that expresses cell-surface receptors that are capable of being engaged by the probes of a specific virus can act as a host for the virus. Viruses generally use two probes to access a host cell. The first probe makes an initial attachment to the host cell, while the action of the virus's second probe often in conjunction with the action of the first probe cause an access portal to be created in the host cell's exterior plasma membrane. Once an access portal is formed, the virus inserts the contents of its payload into the host cell utilizing the open access portal. Certain types of virus may be engulfed whole by a target cell. Once the virus's genome is inside the cytoplasm of the host cell, any enzymes that accompanied the viral genome into the cell, may begin to modify or assist the virus's genome with infecting and taking control of the host cell's biologic functions.

[0017] Probes are attached to the exterior envelope of a virus virion. Probes may be in the form of a protein structure or may be in the form of a glycoprotein molecule. For viruses constructed with a protein matrix as its outer envelope, the probes tend to be protein structures. A portion of the protein structure probe is fixed or anchored in the protein matrix, while a portion of the protein structure probe extends out and away from the protein matrix. The portion of the protein structure probe extending out away from the virus virion is referred to as the 'exterior domain', the portion anchored in the protein matrix is the 'transcending domain'. Some protein probes have a third segment that extends through the envelope and exists inside the virus virion, which is referred to as the 'interior domain'. The exterior domain of a protein structure probe is intended to engage a specific cell-surface receptor on a biologically active cell the virus is targeting as its host cell.

[0018] Viruses that utilize a lipid layer as the outer envelope, are constructed with probes that tend to be glycoproteins. A glycoprotein is comprised of a protein segment and a carbohydrate segment. The carbohydrate segment of the glycoprotein molecule is fixed or anchored in the lipid layer of the outer envelope, while the protein segment extends outward and away from the outer envelope. The protein portion of a glycoprotein probe that extends outward and away from the outer envelope of a virus virion is intended to engage a cell-surface receptor on a biologically active cell the virus is targeting as its host cell.

[0019] Some forms of viruses that utilize a lipid layer as its envelope use protein structure probes. In this case, the portion of the protein structure probe that extends outward and away from the outer envelope is the 'exterior domain', the portion that is anchored in the lipid layer is the 'transcending domain' and again some protein structure probes have an 'interior domain' that exist inside the virion, which may also help anchor the protein structure probe to the virion. The exterior domain of a protein structure probe that extends outward and away from the outer envelope of a virus virion is intended to engage a cell-surface receptor on a biologically active cell the virus is targeting as its host cell.

[0020] When a virus carries a DNA payload and the viral DNA is inserted into the host cell, the virus's DNA travels to the host cell's nucleus and is known to become inserted into the host cell's own native DNA. In the case where a virus is carrying its genetic payload as RNA, the virus inserts the RNA payload into the host cell and may also insert one or more enzymes to facilitate the RNA being utilized properly to replicate copies of the virus. Once inside the host cell, some species of virus facilitate use of the viral RNA by having the RNA converted to DNA. Once the viral RNA has been converted to DNA, the virus's DNA travels to the host cell's nucleus and is known to become inserted into the host cell's native DNA. Once a virus's genetic material has been inserted into the host cell's native DNA, the virus's genetic material takes command of certain cell functions and redirects the resources of the host cell to generate copies of the virus. Other forms of RNA viruses bypass the need to use the nuclear DNA and simply utilize portions of the viral genome to act as messenger RNA. RNA viruses that bypass the host cell's DNA, cause the cell in general to generate copies of the necessary parts of the virus directly from the virus's RNA genome.

[0021] The human immunodeficiency virus (HIV) is a RNA virus and has an outer envelope comprised of a lipid bilayer. The lipid bilayer covers a protein matrix consisting of p17^{gag} proteins. Inside the p17^{gag} protein is nested a nucleocapsid comprised of p24^{gag} proteins. Inside the nucleocapsid HIV carries its payload. HIV's genetic payload consists of two single strands of RNA and several enzymes. The enzymes that accompany HIV's genome include 'reverse transcriptase', 'integrase' and 'protease' molecules.

[0022] The T-Helper cell acts as HIV's host cell. The HIV virion utilizes two types of glycoprotein probes affixed to its exterior envelope to locate and engage a T-Helper cell. HIV utilizes a glycoprotein probe 120 to locate a CD4 cell-surface receptor on a T-Helper cell. Once an HIV glycoprotein 120 probe has successfully engaged a CD4 cell surface-receptor on a T-Helper cell a conformational change occurs in the glycoprotein 120 probe and a glycoprotein 41 probe is exposed. The glycoprotein 41 probe's intent is to engage a CXCR4 or CCR5 cell-surface receptor on the same T-Helper cell. Once a glycoprotein 41 probe on the HIV virion successfully engages a CXCR4 or

CCR5 cell-surface receptor, the HIV virion opens an access portal through the T-Helper cell's outer membrane.

[0023] Once the HIV virion has opened an access portal through the T-Helper cell's outer plasma membrane, the HIV virion inserts two positive strand RNA molecules and the associated enzymes it carries into the T-Helper cell. Each RNA strand is approximately 9500 nucleotides in length. Inserted along with the RNA strands are the enzymes reverse transcriptase, protease and integrase. Once the virus's genome gains access to the interior of the T-Helper cell, in the cytoplasm the pair of RNA molecules are transformed to deoxyribonucleic acid by the reverse transcriptase enzyme. Following modification of the virus's genome to DNA, the virus's genetic information migrates to the host cell's nucleus. In the nucleus, with the assistance of the integrase protein, the HIV's DNA becomes inserted into the T-Helper cell's native nuclear DNA. When the timing is appropriate, the now integrated viral DNA is decoded by the host cell's polymerase molecules and the virus's genetic information commands certain cell functions to carry out the replication process to construct copies of the human immunodeficiency virus.

[0024] The outer layer of the HIV virion is comprised of a portion of the T-Helper cell's outer cell membrane. In the final stage of the replication process, as a copy of the HIV virion, carrying the HIV genome, buds through the host cell's cell membrane the outer protein shell acquires as its exterior envelope, a wrapping of lipid bilayer from the host cell's cell membrane. In the case of HIV, since the surface of the pathogen is covered by an envelope comprised of lipid bilayer taken from the host T-Helper cells, this feature allows the HIV virion the capacity to elude the two immune systems, since the detectors comprising the innate immune system and the adaptable immune system may find it difficult to distinguish between the surface of an infectious HIV virion and the surface characteristics of a noninfected T-Helper cell.

[0025] The Hepatitis C virus (HCV) is a positive sense RNA virus, meaning a type of RNA that is capable of bypassing the need for involving the host cell's nucleus by having its RNA genome function as messenger RNA. Hepatitis C infects liver cells. The Hepatitis C viral genome becomes divided once it gains access to the interior of a liver host cell. Portions of the subdivisions of the Hepatitis C genome directly interact with ribosomes to produce proteins necessary to construct copies of the virus.

[0026] HCV belongs to the Flaviviridae family and is the only member of the Hepacivirus genus. There are considered to be at least 100 different strains of Hepatitis C virus based on genome sequencing variability.

[0027] HCV is comprised of an outer lipoprotein envelope and an internal nucleocapsid. The genetic payload is carried within the nucleocapsid. In its natural state, present on the surface of the outer envelope of the Hepatitis C virus are probes that detect receptors present on the surface of liver cells. The glycoprotein E1 probe and the glycoprotein E2 probe have been identified to be affixed to the surface of HCV. The E2 probe binds with high affinity to the large external loop of a CD81 cell-surface receptor. CD81 is found on the surface of many cell types including liver cells. Once the E2 probe has engaged the CD81 cell-surface receptor, cofactors on the surface of HCV's exterior envelope engage either or both the low density lipoprotein receptor (LDLR) or the scavenger receptor class B type I (SR-BI) present on the liver cell in order to effect the mechanism to facilitate HCV breaching the cell membrane and inserting its RNA genome payload through the plasma cell membrane of the liver cell into the liver cell. Upon successful engagement of the HCV surface probes with a liver cell's cell-surface receptors, HCV inserts the single strand of RNA and other payload elements it carries into the liver cell targeted to be a host cell. The HCV RNA genome then interacts with enzymes and ribosomes inside the liver cell in a translational process to produce the proteins required to construct copies of the protein components of HCV. The HCV genome undergoes a method of transcription to replicate copies of the virus's RNA genome. Inside the host, pieces of the HCV virus are assembled together and ultimately loaded with a copy of the HCV genome. Replicas of the original HCV then escape the host cell and migrate the environment in search of additional host liver cells to infect and continue the replication process.

[0028] The HCV's naturally occurring genetic payload consists of a single molecule of linear positive sense, single stranded RNA approximately 9600 nucleotides in length. By means of a translational process a polyprotein of approximately 3000 amino acids is generated. This polyprotein is cleaved post translation by host and viral proteases into individual viral proteins which include: the structural proteins of C, E1, E2, the nonstructural proteins NS1, NS2, NS3, NS4A, NS4B, NS5A, NS5B, p7 and ARFP/F protein. Hepatitis C virus's proteins direct the host liver cell to construction copies of the Hepatitis C virus. A membrane associated replicase complex consisting of the virus's nonstructural proteins NS3 and NS5B facilitate the replication of the viral genome. The membrane of the endoplasmic reticulum appears to be the site of protein maturation and viral assembly. Once copies of the Hepatitis C Virus are generated, they exit the host cell and each copy of HCV migrates in search of another appropriate liver cell that will act as a host to continue the replication process.

[0029] Hepatitis C virus life-cycle demonstrates that copies of a virus virion can be generated by inserting RNA into a host cell that functions as messenger RNA in the host cell. The Hepatitis C viral RNA genome functions as messenger RNA, acting as the template in conjunction with the biologic machinery of a host cell to produce the components that comprise copies of the Hepatitis C virion and the Hepatitis C viral RNA provides the biologic instructions to assemble the components into complete copies of the Hepatitis C virions. The Hepatitis C virus life-cycle clearly demonstrates that viral virions can be manufactured by a host cell without involving the nucleus of the cell.

[0030] Deciphering the existence, replication and behavior of viruses provides clear examples of several fundamental concepts, which include: (1) Viruses target specific cells in the body by means of identifying and engaging such target cells utilizing the probes projecting outward from the virus's exterior shell to make contact with cell-surface receptors located on the surface of their host cells, and (2) Viruses are capable of carrying a variety of different types of payloads including DNA, RNA and a variety of proteins.

[0031] Current gene therapy approach to attempting to deliver a payload to cells in the body use modified forms of existing viruses to act as transport devices to deliver genetic information. This approach is severely limited by restricting the virus virion to the target only cells the viral vector naturally seeks out and infects. Current gene therapy approach is further limited by using the pre-existing size of naturally occurring viruses, rather than being able to modify the size of the structure to be able to tailor the volumetric carrying capacity of the payload portion of the modified virus. Further, gene therapy is restricted to utilizing naturally occurring viruses to deliver only genetic information; it has not previously been appreciated by those skilled in the art that virus-like transport devices might deliver to a variety of specific cell types a wide variety of differing payloads.

[0032] Ribonucleic acids are inherent to a cell and RNAs are used by some viruses to act as the virus's genome to generate copies of the virus. RNAs inherent to a cell are referred to as 'cellular RNAs' and include protein coding RNAs and non-coding RNAs (ncRNA). Protein coding RNAs, generally referred to as messenger RNAs, code for proteins and undergo translation to produce protein molecules. Non-coding RNA represent a variety of functional RNA molecules that do not undergo translation to produce a protein. Non-coding RNAs are highly abundant and functionally important for the cell. Non-coding RNAs have also referred by such terms as non-protein-coding RNAs (npcRNA) or non-messenger RNA (nmRNA) or small non-messenger RNA (snmRNA) or functional RNAs (fRNA). The non-coding RNAs include: transfer RNAs (tRNA), ribosomal RNAs (rRNA), small nuclear RNAs (snRNA), small nucleolar RNAs (snoRNA), signal recognition particle RNA (SRP RNA), antisense RNA (aRNA), micro RNA (miRNA), small interfering RNA (siRNA), Y RNA, telomerase RNA. RNA found in naturally occurring viruses are referred to as 'viral RNA'.

[0033] Transfer RNAs (tRNA), are RNAs that carries amino acids and deliver them to a ribosome. Ribosomal RNAs (rRNA), are RNAs that couple with ribosomal proteins and participate in translation of mRNA to produce protein molecules. Small nuclear RNAs (snRNA) are RNAs involved in splicing and other nuclear functions. Small nucleolar RNAs (snoRNA) are RNAs involved in nucleotide modification. Signal recognition particle RNA (SRP RNA) are RNAs are involved in membrane integration. Antisense RNA (aRNA) are RNAs involved in transcription attenuation, mRNA degradation, mRNA stabilization, and translation blockage. Micro RNA (miRNA) are RNAs involved in gene regulation and have been implicated in a wide range of cell functions including cell growth, apoptosis, neuronal plasticity, insulin secretion. Small interfering RNA (siRNA) are RNAs involved in gene regulation, often interfering with the expression of a single gene. Y RNA are RNAs involved in RNA processing and DNA replication. Telomerase RNA are RNAs involved in telomere synthesis. The primary purpose of 'viral RNA' is to make copies of the virus that carries of a genome RNA.

[0034] Messenger RNA molecules are comprised of three regions (or segments). These three regions include: (1) a 5' untranslatable region, (2) a coding region and (3) a 3' untranslatable region. The 5' untranslatable region acts as the initiation point for a ribosome to attach to the mRNA. The 'coding region' acts as the template from which a protein is constructed. An 'untranslatable region' represents a segment of a messenger RNA molecule that does not code for a protein and is not used to yield a protein and therefore 'translation' does not occur in such a region. The 3' untranslatable region is associated with the degradation of the usefulness of the mRNA. Different mRNAs have different service life expectancies. The half-life of the naturally occurring mRNA that acts as the template responsible for the production of the protein 'glucokinase' is two hours. The half-life of the naturally occurring mRNA that acts as the template to produce the protein 'alcohol dehydrogenase' is ten hours. The half-life of the naturally occurring mRNA that acts as the template to produce the protein 'glucuronidase' is thirty hours. By modifying the nucleotides that comprise the 3' untranslatable unit of an mRNA, the service half-life of the mRNA may be altered to be lengthened or shortened depending upon the need for the quantity of protein and timeframe over which the mRNA is required to produce the protein coded in the protein template of the mRNA's coding region.

[0035] RNA found in naturally occurring viruses are referred to as 'viral RNA'. The primary function of 'viral RNA' is dedicated to making copies of the virus that carries the RNA genome. Cellular RNAs are inherent to a cell and do not include 'viral RNAs'. Modifications to messenger RNA molecules occur naturally due to errors that occur in the DNA and errors that occurring during the transcription phase and maturation phase of generating messenger RNA. Modifications to ribonucleic acid molecules may occur purposely to produce a medical therapeutic response.

[0036] Modified ribonucleic acid molecules are naturally occurring cellular ribonucleic acid molecules that have purposely undergone modification to the nucleotide sequence to enhance the performance of the naturally occurring cellular ribonucleic acid molecule. Naturally occurring cellular ribonucleic acid molecules can purposely have their nucleotide sequence modified in the 3'untranslatable region, the coding region or the 5' untranslatable region or modification may be made in any combination of the three regions to enhance the performance of the modified ribonucleic acid molecule above and beyond that of the naturally occurring ribonucleic acid molecule. Naturally occurring cellular ribonucleic acid molecules that purposely have a quantity of their nucleotides altered to produce a medical benefit are termed 'modified ribonucleic acids', versus naturally occurring cellular ribonucleic acid molecules that undergo mutation due to an error that occurs in production of the molecule would be termed 'mutant ribonucleic acids'.

[0037] Research has demonstrated that natural proteins can be altered to produce medically beneficial effects. The parathyroid hormone (PTH) is one example. Intact PTH is produced by cells in the parathyroid glands. There are four parathyroid glands present in the neck, generally in the vicinity of the thyroid gland. The term 'para-' means 'next to', so early anatomists identified the four glands 'parathyroid glands' because they were generally found 'next to' the thyroid gland in the neck. Parathyroid hormone is released in response to the cells of the parathyroid gland sensing a decline in the level of serum calcium. Parathyroid hormone, in its natural state, acts to stimulate osteoclast cells present in bone to release calcium from bone, thereby acting as a mechanism to return the serum calcium level to the normal range whenever the serum calcium drops below the normal range. On the other hand, it has been quite well demonstrated that if (1) the amino acid chain of the parathyroid hormone is shortened and (2) the shorter parathyroid hormone molecule is pulsed, by injecting it into the body once a day, the action of this modified parathyroid hormone molecule is opposite of the intact parathyroid hormone. One such form of a shorter length parathyroid hormone molecule is termed 'teriparatide'. Teriparatide (1-34) has the identical sequence from 1 to the 34th N-terminal amino acid of the 84-amino acid endogenous human parathyroid hormone. The skeletal effects of the modified protein molecule act on bone cells to preferentially cause osteoblastic activity over osteoclastic activity, which results in storage of calcium into bone, rather than a release of calcium from bone if the teriparatide is administered once a day. Teriparatide has been a recognized and widely used treatment of osteoporosis since at least as far back as the year 2000.

[0038] Purposely modifying the 'coding region' of a messenger RNA modifies the protein the messenger RNA produces when ribosomes attach to and translate such a modified messenger RNA. As demonstrated by the case of modifying the naturally occurring parathyroid hormone by administering a molecule that is comprised of fewer amino acids than the original PTH molecule, modifying proteins the messenger RNAs produce may provide health care providers with an entirely new and widely spanning armamentarium of medically beneficial therapies.

[0039] The 5' untranslatable region of a messenger RNA molecule is used to identify the messenger RNA and utilized as a point of attachment by ribosomes to the messenger RNA molecule. Modifying the 5' untranslatable region of a messenger RNA by altering the nucleotide sequence in the 5' untranslatable region makes it easier to identify a modified messenger ribonucleic acid molecules in a fashion that the modified messenger ribonucleic acid molecules can be more easily or readily engaged by ribosomes. Altering the nucleotide sequence of the 5' untranslatable region of a modified messenger ribonucleic acid molecule to create a unique identifier, facilitates ribosomes to preferentially engage the modified messenger ribonucleic acid molecule to preferentially produce the protein for which the modified messenger ribonucleic acid molecule is acting as a template.

[0040] Modifying the nucleotide sequence of messenger ribonucleic acid molecules in the 3' untranslatable region extends or shortens the service life of said modified messenger ribonucleic acid molecules, compared to naturally occurring messenger ribonucleic acid molecules. Service life refers to the quantity of time a messenger RNA molecule, present in the cytoplasm, will be able to undergo translation before it is degraded by cellular enzymes. By modifying the nucleotide sequence of a messenger RNA molecule to extend its service life, this allows additional time for ribosomes to decode the information present on the modified messenger ribonucleic acid molecules. Modifying the naturally occurring messenger ribonucleic acid molecule in the 3' untranslatable region in a fashion to cause the molecule to resist degradation by cellular enzymes without compromising the functionality of the modified messenger ribonucleic acid molecules increases production of proteins by ribosomes which results in an enhanced medically therapeutic treatment.

[0041] A dramatic, not previously recognized by those expert in the art is the need to develop a transport vehicle that can be fashioned to seek out specific types of cells and deliver to these cells cellular ribonucleic acid molecules to treat medical conditions related to a protein deficiency. By providing cellular RNAs to these specific target cells a wide variety of cellular functions can be enhanced including gene expression, protein production, and telomere synthesis. The exterior envelope of a transport should be constructed so as not to alert the immune system to its presence to prevent rejection of these vehicles. Transport vehicles should be capable of being configured to target any specific type of cell and engage and deliver their payload only to that specific type of cell. To this point, no such device or process has been conceived.

BRIEF SUMMARY OF THE INVENTION

[0042] Utilization of configurable microscopic medical payload delivery devices to deliver ribonucleic acid molecules to specific types of cells facilitates a dramatic new approach to managing a wide variety of medical conditions. By selecting the type of probes that will effectively engage cell-surface receptors on target cells and fixing these probes on the surface of the configurable microscopic medical payload delivery devices, specific types of cells can be targeted. By utilizing configurable microscopic medical payload delivery devices to deliver cellular ribonucleic acid molecules to specific cell types, medical conditions including protein deficient states, genetic deficiencies, conditions related to over expression of genes previously incapable of being treated, are now treatable utilizing this new and unique approach.

DETAILED DESCRIPTION

[0043] The future of medical treatment includes the aggressive, widespread utilization of configurable microscopic medical payload delivery devices (CMMPDD) to deliver a wide variety of ribonucleic acid molecules directly to targeted cell types in the body.

[0044] This patent introduces the concepts: (1) configurable microscopic medical payload delivery devices can carry ribonucleic acid molecules inherent to the cell as the payload, and (2) glycoprotein probes present on the exterior of the configurable microscopic medical payload delivery devices include specific glycoprotein probes or protein structure probes affixed to the exterior, these glycoprotein probes or protein structure probes intended to seek out and engage cell-surface receptors attached to the exterior of whichever cell the configurable microscopic medical payload delivery devices is intended to deliver its payload of cellular RNAs to in order to produce a predetermined medically beneficial effect.

[0045] For purposes of this text, the use of the terms 'specific target cell type', 'target cell', 'specific cell type', 'specific cell', 'specific type of cell' are equivalent and interchangeable; the configuration of cell-surface receptors that a specific cell type has located on and protruding from its outer cell membrane determines the cell type.

[0046] For purposes of this text an 'external envelope' refers to the outermost covering of a virus or a virus-like transport device or a configurable microscopic medical payload delivery device. The external envelope may be comprised of a lipid layer, a lipid bilayer, the combination of a lipid layer affixed to a protein matrix or the combination of a lipid bilayer affixed to a protein matrix. A protein matrix is equivalent to a protein shell and may be referred to as a protein matrix shell. The terms protein matrix, protein shell, protein matrix shell are equivalent to the term capsid, where the term capsid is meant to represent 'a protein coat or shell of a virus particle, surrounding the nucleic acid or nucleoprotein core'. For purposes of this text, the term 'particle' is equivalent to the term 'virion'; further the term 'virus particle' is equivalent to 'viral virion'.

[0047] For purposes of this text an 'internal shell' refers to a protein matrix shell nested inside the external envelope. Multiple inner shells may exist, with those of smaller diameter concentrically nested inside those of a larger diameter. The innermost protein matrix shell is termed the nucleocapsid. The proteins that comprise the nucleocapsid are termed capsid proteins. In the cavity created by the nucleocapsid, referred to as the center or core of the nucleocapsid, is where the payload of ribonucleic acid molecules is carried.

[0048] For purposes of this text 'external probes' are molecular structures that are utilized to locate and engage cell-surface receptors on biologically active cells. External probes are generally comprised of a portion which is anchored or fixed in the external envelope and a second portion that extends out and away from the external envelope. The portion of the external probe that extends out and away from the external envelope is intended to make contact and engage a specific cell-surface receptor located on a biologically active cell. External probes may be comprised solely of a protein structure or an external probe may be a glycoprotein molecule.

[0049] For purposes of this text 'glycoprotein molecule' refers to a molecule comprised of a carbohydrate region and a protein region. Glycoprotein molecules that act as probes are generally anchored or fixed to a lipid layer utilizing the carbohydrate portion of the molecule as an anchor. The protein portion of the glycoprotein molecule which extends outward and away from the exterior envelope the glycoprotein has been affixed such that the protein region may function as a probe to locate and attach to the cell-surface receptor it was created to engage.

[0050] The concept of configurable microscopic medical payload delivery devices is modeled after naturally existing viruses. Configurable microscopic medical payload delivery devices in general are spherical in shape; though other shapes may be used as function might warrant the use of a particular shape. The spherical configurable microscopic medical payload delivery devices are comprised of an exterior envelope and one or more nested inner protein shells. A quantity of exterior protein structure probes and/or glycoprotein probes are anchored in the exterior envelope and a portion extends out and away from the exterior envelope. Nesting of protein shells refers to progressively smaller diameter shells fitting snugly inside protein shells of a larger diameter. Inside the innermost protein shell, referred to as the nucleocapsid, is a cavity referred to as the core of the device. The core of the device is the space where the medically therapeutic payload the device carries is located. The payload of the device is comprised of ribonucleic acid molecules.

[0051] Configurable microscopic medical payload delivery devices (CMMPDD) target specific types of cells in the body. Configurable microscopic medical payload delivery devices engage specific types of cells by the configuration of probes affixed to the exterior envelope of the CMMPDD. By fixing specific probes to the exterior envelope of the CMMPDD, these probes intended to engage and attach only to specific cell-surface receptors located on certain cell types in the body, the CMMPDD will deliver its payload to only those cell types that express compatible and engagable specific cell-surface receptors. In a similar fashion where the exterior probes of a naturally occurring virus engage specific cell-surface receptors present on the surface of the virus's host cell and only the designated host cell, the CMMPDD's exterior probes are configured to engage cell-surface receptors on a specific type of target cell and only those cells. In this manner, the payload of cellular RNAs carried by CMMPDD will be delivered only to specific types of cells in the body. The configuration of the exterior probes on the surface of a CMMPDD varies as needed so as to effect the CMMPDD delivery of specific cellular RNA payloads to specific types of cells as needed to effect a particular predetermined medical treatment.

[0052] The size of the configurable microscopic medical payload delivery devices is dependent upon the diameter of the inner protein matrix shells and this is dictated by the volume size of the payload the CMMPDD is required to carry and deliver to a target cell. The diameter of each inner protein matrix shell is governed by the number of protein molecules utilized to construct the protein matrix shell at the time the protein matrix shell is generated. Increasing the number of proteins that comprise a protein matrix shell increases the diameter of the protein matrix shell. When applicable, as dictated by the capacity the CMMPDD is to be utilized to function as, an external lipid envelope wraps around and covers the outermost protein matrix shell. The larger the volume of the core of the CMMPDD, the greater the physical size of the payload the CMMPDD is able to carry. The size of the configurable microscopic medical payload delivery device is to be generally the size of cell (approximately 10^{-4} m in diameter) or less, generally detectable by a light microscope or, as needed, an electron microscope. The size of the CMMPDD is not to be too large such that it would generate a burden to the body by damaging organ tissues through clogging blood vessels or the glomeruli in the kidneys. The dimensions of each type of

CMMPDD are to be tailored to the mission of the CMMPDD, which takes into account factors such as the type of target cell, the size of the payload that is to be delivered to the target cells and the length of time the CMMPDD may have to engage the target cell.

[0053] The payload of the configurable microscopic medical payload delivery devices include cellular RNAs, which include protein coding RNAs and non-coding RNAs. Protein coding RNAs include messenger RNAs. The non-coding RNAs include: transfer RNAs (tRNA), ribosomal RNAs (rRNA), small nuclear RNAs (snRNA), small nucleolar RNAs (snoRNA), signal recognition particle RNA (SRP RNA), antisense RNA (aRNA), micro RNA (miRNA), small interfering RNA (siRNA), Y RNA, telomerase RNA.

[0054] Being enveloped in an external lipid layer, configurable microscopic medical payload delivery devices possess the advantage of having their exterior appear similar to the plasma membrane that acts as an outside covering for the cells that comprise the body. By appearing similar to existing plasma membranes, the CMMPDDs appear similar to naturally occurring structures found in the body. CMMPDD are afforded the capability to avoid detection by a body's immune system because the exterior of the CMMPDD mimics the cells comprising the body and the surveillance elements of the immune system find it difficult to discern between the CMMPDD and naturally occurring cells comprising the body.

[0055] To carry out the process of manufacturing a configurable microscopic medical payload delivery device, a primitive cell such as a stem cell is selected. The reason for utilizing primitive cells such as stems cells as the host cell, is that the CMMPDD acquires its outer envelope from the host cell and the more primitive the host cell, the fewer in number the identifying protein markers are present on the surface of the CMMPDD. The fewer the identifying surface proteins present on the outer envelope of the CMMPDD, the less likely a body's immune system will identify the CMMPDD as an intruder and therefore less likely the body's immune system will react to the presence of the CMMPDD and reject the CMMPDD by attacking and neutralizing the CMMPDD.

[0056] Stem cells used as host cells to manufacture quantities of CMMPDD product are selected per histocompatibility markers present on their surface. Certain histocompatibility markers present on the surface of the final CMMPDD product will be less likely to cause a reaction in a specific patient based on the genetic profile of the patient's histocompatibility markers. A similar histocompatibility match is done when donor organs are selected to be given to recipients to avoid rejection of the donor organ by the recipient's immune system.

[0057] The selected stem cells used to manufacture configurable microscopic medical payload delivery devices goes through several steps of maturation before it is capable of generating therapeutic CMMPDD product. RNA inserted into the host stem cell code for the general physical outer structures of the CMMPDD. RNA inserted into the host generate surface probes that target the cell-surface receptors on a specific target cell type. RNA is inserted into the host that is used to generate the payload of ribonucleic acid molecules. Similar to how copies of a naturally occurring virus, such as the Hepatitis C virus or HIV, are produced, assembled and released from a host cell, copies of the CMMPDD are produced, assembled and released from a stem cell functioning as a de facto host cell. Once released from the host cell, the copies of the CMMPDD are collected, then pooled together to produce a therapeutic dose that results in a medically beneficial effect.

[0058] The stem cells used as host cells are suspended in a broth of nutrients and are kept at an optimum temperature to govern the rate of production of the CMMPDD product. Similar to the natural production of the Hepatitis C virus, the configurable microscopic medical payload delivery devices 'production genome' is introduced into the host stem cells. The configurable microscopic medical payload delivery devices production genome carries genetic instructions to cause the host cells to manufacture the configurable microscopic medical payload delivery devices' outer protein wall, the inner protein matrixes, the surface probes the configurable microscopic medical payload delivery device is to have affixed to its outer envelope, the ribonucleic acid molecules the configurable microscopic medical payload delivery devices are to carry, and the instructions to assemble the various pieces into the final form of the configurable microscopic medical payload delivery devices along with the instructions to activate the budding process. The resultant configurable microscopic medical payload delivery devices are collected from the nutrient broth surrounding the host cells and placed together into doses to be used as a treatment for a protein deficiency state.

[0059] The 'production genome' are an array of RNAs, which include messenger RNAs that are directly translated by the host cell's ribosomes. The production genome dictates the characteristics of the final version of the CMMPDD that buds from the host stem cell and is released and is to be utilized as a medical treatment. The production genome is specifically tailored to code for the surface probes that will seek and engage a specific type of target cell. The production genome also carries the instructions to code for the production of the type of ribonucleic acid molecules to be delivered to the specific type of target cell. The 'production genome' varies depending upon the configuration of the CMMPDD and the specific type of ribonucleic acid molecules the CMMPDD will transport to effect a specific predetermined medical treatment in a specific type of cell.

[0060] The configurable microscopic medical payload delivery device transporting ribonucleic acid molecules represents a very versatile medical treatment delivery device. CMMPDD is used to deliver a number of different ribonucleic acid molecules to a wide variety of cells in the body.

[0061] The construction of a naturally occurring virus can be likened to the act of following a programmed script to produce a specific result. It is known that the genetic code that a virus carries dictates the production of copies of the virus. It is known that specific segments of the viral genetic code represent instructions that dictate the construction of different parts of the virus so that copies of the virus can be made inside the host cell. It is well documented that there exist different subtypes of most viruses, based off of mutations that have occurred to the viral genome over time; these mutations to the viral genome producing variants in the construction of the virus. Configurable microscopic medical payload delivery devices which carry RNA are constructed much like a naturally occurring virus virion would be constructed in a host cell. Altering the production RNA alters the configuration of the external probes or alters the configuration of the size of the inner shells or alters the type of RNA the CMMPDD will carry or alters any combination of the three.

[0062] As an example of this method, to treat diabetes mellitus the following production process is followed in the lab: (1) Human stem cells are selected. (2) Into the selected stem cells is placed the RNA production genome constructed, in this case, specifically as a means to treat diabetes mellitus. The RNA production genome contains genetic instructions to cause the host stem cells to manufacture the CMMPDDs' outer protein wall, the inner protein matrix, surface probes to include a quantity of glycoprotein probes that engage the GPR40 cell-surface receptor present on the surface of Beta cells located in the Islets of Langerhans in the pancreas, and the messenger RNA payload to facilitate the production of the insulin molecule; and the biologic instructions to assemble the components into the final form of the CMMPDD and the biologic instructions to activate the budding process. (3) Upon insertion of the RNA production genome into the host stem cells, host stem cells' protein production cellular machinery responds by simultaneously translating the different segments of the RNA production genome to produce the proteins that comprise the exterior protein wall, the inner protein matrix molecules, the surface probes, the mRNA payload to produce insulin and decode the instructions to assemble the components into the CMMPDDs. (4) Upon assembly, the CMMPDDs bud through the cell membrane of the host stem cell. (5) At the time of the budding process, the CMMPDDs acquire an outside envelope over the outer protein shell, this outer envelope comprised of a portion of the plasma membrane from the host stem cell the CMMPDD exits. (6) The resultant CMMPDDs are collected from the nutrient broth surrounding the host stem cells. (7) The CMMPDD product is washed in a sterile solution to remove unwanted elements of the nutrient broth. (8) The configurable microscopic medical payload delivery devices are removed from the sterile solution wash and suspended in a sterile hypoallergenic liquid medium. (9) The CMMPDD are separated into individual quantities to facilitate storage and delivery to physicians and patients. (10) The CMMPDD product carried in the sterile hypoallergenic liquid medium is administered to a diabetic patient per injection in a dose that is tailored to receiving patient's requirement to produce sufficient amount of insulin to control the blood sugar. (11) Upon being injected into the body, the CMMPDD product migrates to the Beta cells located in the Islets of Langerhans by means of the blood stream. (12) Upon the CMMPDD product reaching the Beta cells, the probes on the surface of the CMMPDDs engage the cell-surface receptors located on the Beta cells and inserts the RNA payload, including mRNA, into the Beta cells. The mRNA payload is translated by the cell's ribosomes to produce insulin molecules. The increase in insulin production by Beta cells successfully treats diabetes mellitus.

[0063] In a similar fashion, configurable microscopic medical payload delivery devices can be fashioned to deliver a payload of a specific type of ribonucleic acid molecule to any type of cell in the body. Different cell types express different cell-surface markers on the exterior of their plasma membrane. The differing configurations of cell-surface markers on differing types of cells distinguish one cell type from another cell type. By configuring the exterior probes that extend from the surface of the configurable microscopic medical payload delivery device to seek out and engage specific cell-surface receptors present on a specific cell type, payloads of any messenger ribonucleic acid molecule or any non-coding ribonucleic acid molecule can be delivered to specific cells in the body.

Conclusions, Ramification, and Scope

[0064] Accordingly, the reader will see that the configurable microscopic medical payload delivery device to deliver cellular ribonucleic acid molecules to specific targeted cell types provides advantages over existing art by (1) being a delivery device that seeks out specific types of cells, (2) by being a delivery device that is versatile enough to deliver a variety of cellular ribonucleic acid molecules to accomplish various medical treatments and (3) by being a delivery device constructed with a surface envelope that will avoid detection by the innate immune system and the adaptable immune system so as not to activate the immune system to its presence; for these reasons this represents a new and unique medical delivery device that has never before been recognized nor appreciated by those skilled in the art.

[0065] Although the description above contains specificities, these should not be construed as limiting the scope of the invention but as merely providing illustrations of some of the presently preferred embodiments of the invention.

[0066] Thus the scope of the invention should be determined by the appended claims and their legal equivalents, rather than by the examples given.

CLAIMS: Reserved.

No. 3: RNA VECTOR THERAPY METHOD

INDIVIDUALS REQUESTING PATENT: Dr. Lane B. Scheiber, ScD and Dr. Lane B. Scheiber II, MD

©2010 Lane B. Scheiber and Lane B. Scheiber II. A portion of the disclosure of this patent document contains material which is subject to copyright protection. The copyright owners have no objection to the facsimile reproduction by anyone of the patent document or the patent disclosure, as it appears in the Patent and Trademark Office patent file or records, but otherwise reserves all copyright rights whatsoever.

ABSTRACT

The innovative treatment method described here utilizes configurable microscopic medical payload delivery devices to act as a transport vector to deliver a wide variety of cellular ribonucleic acid molecules to specific types of cells in the body. Utilizing probes on the exterior of the transport devices, the transport devices locate a specific type of cell in the body. Once a specific target cell type has been encountered, the configurable microscopic medical payload delivery devices insert their payload of cellular ribonucleic acid molecules into the target cells. By delivering cellular ribonucleic acid molecules into specific cells a wide variety of protein deficiencies are correctable, gene expression is capable of being modulated, and telomere synthesis is enhanced.

BACKGROUND OF THE INVENTION

Field of the Invention

This invention relates to any medical method intended to treat medical conditions utilizing a configurable microscopic medical payload delivery device to insert ribonucleic acid molecules into one or more specific cell types in the body to improve cell function.

Description of Background Art

[0001] Cellular ribonucleic acid (RNA) molecules are divided into two major functional categories which are 'protein coding RNAs' and 'non-coding RNAs'. Protein coding RNAs, usually referred to as messenger RNAs, undergo the process of translation in the cytoplasm of the cell and produce proteins by ribosomes decoding the genetic information carried in the coding region of the messenger RNA. Non-coding RNAs perform a wide variety of tasks both in the nucleus and in the cytoplasm of a cell.

[0002] Present medical research is attempting to utilize viruses to deliver genetic information into cells. Research in the field of gene therapy has involved certain naturally occurring viruses. Some of the common viral vectors that have been investigated include: Adeno-associated virus, Adenovirus, Alphavirus, Epstein-Barr virus, Gammaretrovirus, Herpes simplex virus, Letivirus, Poliovirus, Rhabdovirus, Vaccinia virus. Naturally occurring virus vectors are limited to the naturally occurring external probes that are affixed to the outer wall of the virus. The external probes fixed to the outside wall of a virus virion dictate which type of cell the virus can engage and infect. Therefore, as an example, the function of the adenovirus, a respiratory virus, is strictly limited to engaging and infecting specific lung cells. Used as a medical treatment device, the adenovirus can only deliver gene therapy to specific lung cells, which severely limits this vector's usefulness as a deliver device. The therapeutic function of all naturally occurring viral vectors is limited to delivering a DNA or RNA payload to the cell type the viral vector naturally targets as its host cell.

[0003] Naturally occurring viruses also have the disadvantage of being susceptible to detection and elimination by a body's immune system. Viruses have been infecting humans for hundreds of thousands of years. A human's immune system is very efficient at detecting the presence of most naturally occurring viruses when such a virus is inside the body. The human immune system is quite capable of generating a vigorous response to most intruding viruses, attacking and neutralizing virus virions whenever a virus virion physically exists are outside the exterior wall of the virus's host cell. If gene therapy in its current state were to become a clinical therapeutic tool, the naturally occurring viruses selected for gene therapy research will have limited effectiveness due the fact that once the viral vector is introduced into the body, the body's the immune system will quickly engage and eliminate the viral vectors, possibly before the vector is able to deliver its payload to its host cell or target cell.

[0004] Cichutek, K., 2001 (US Patent No. 6,323,031 B1) teaches preparation and use of novel lentiviral SiVagm-derived vectors for gene transfer into selected cell types, specifically into proliferatively active and resting human cells.

[0005] Cichutek teaches that it is indeed plausible to re-configure an existing virus and use it as a transport vehicle, though Cichutek's specification and claims are too limited to describe a method that will work for all cell types, if indeed if it will work for any cell type.

[0006] Cichutek describes vectors for 'gene transfer'; in the claims the language that is used is 'genetic information'. Cichutek's Claim 1 of the cited patent states 'A propagation-incompetent SIVagm vector comprising a viral core and a viral envelope, wherein the viral core comprises a simian immunodeficiency virus (SIVagm) viral core of the African vervet monkey Chlorocebus.' Cichutek's does not describe in his claims any further details of the intended payload other than the stating 'SIVagm viral core' in claim 1; in claims 5 & 6 Cichutek describes only 'genetic information'. Transfer of 'genetic information' dramatically limits the useful application of Cichutek's patent in the treatment of medical diseases.

[0007] Cichutek does not claim the use of specific glycogen probes to target specific types of cells. Cichutek's approach is dependent upon the probes naturally present on the viral vectors reported in the patent, which will direct the viral vectors to only those cells the viruses naturally use as their host cell. Cichutek's approach is very restrictive, limited to gene transfer to only cells the viruses use as their natural host cell.

[0008] It is questionable that Cichutek's approach as described in the specification and claims is feasible. Cichutek's claim 4, states 'The SIVagm vector of claim 1, wherein the viral envelope further comprises a single chain antibody (scFv) or a ligand of a cell surface molecule.' By use of the words 'a' and 'or' in the claim, the claim is limited in the singular, meaning Cichutek claims a single chain antibody or a singular ligand. Singular type antibodies or ligands can be used for cell-to-cell communication, but to open an access portal into a cell and insert a payload into the cell requires two different types antibodies or ligands. As an example human immunodeficiency virus requires the use of both the gp120 and gp41 probes to open a portal into a T-Helper cell and insert its viral genome into the T-Helper cell. The gp120 probe engages the CD4+ cell-surface receptor on the T-cell. Once the gp120 probe has successfully engaged a CD4+ cell-surface receptor on the target T-Helper cell, then the HIV virion's gp41 probe can engage either a CXCR4 or a CCR5 cell-surface receptor on the T-Helper cell in order to open up an access portal for HIV to insert its viral genome into a T-Helper cell. It is well documented in the medical literature that a genetic defect leading to an abnormality in the CXCR4 cell-surface receptor prevents HIV virions from opening an access portal and inserting its genetic payload into such T-Helper cells. This genetic defect in the CXCR4 cell-surface receptors offers the subset of people carrying the genetic defect resistance to HIV infection. This example demonstrates the need for at least two types of glycoprotein probes to be present on the surface of a viral vector in order for a viral vector to be capable of opening an access portal and delivering the payload the vector carries into its host cell or target cell.

[0009] A delivery system that offered a defined means of targeting specific types of cells would invoke minimal or no response by the innate immune system and the adaptable immune system when present in the body, and a delivery system that would be capable of inserting into cells a wide variety of ribonucleic acid molecules would significantly improve the current medical treatment options available to clinicians treating patients.

[0010] The solution to arriving at a versatile, workable delivery system that will meet the needs of a number of medical treatments involves three important elements. These elements include:

configurable external probes whereby more than one type of protein structure probe or more than one type of glycoprotein probe is to be used to engage and access specific target cell types in order to successfully deliver a payload into a specific cell type,

an exterior envelope comprised of a protein shell or lipid layer expressing the least number of cell-surface markers, such as the use of a stem cell to act as the host cell to manufacture the delivery devices, configuring the core of the vector to enable it to carry and deliver a wide variety of ribonucleic acid molecules.

For purposes of this text, the use of the terms 'specific target cell type', 'target cell', 'specific cell type', 'specific cell', 'specific type of cell' are equivalent and interchangeable; the configuration of cell-surface receptors that a specific cell type has located on and protruding from its outer cell membrane determines the cell type.

[0011] Viruses are obligate parasites. Viruses simply represent a carrier of genetic material and by themselves viruses are unable to replicate or carry out any form of biologic function outside their host cell. A 'virion' refers to the physical structure of a single complete virus as it exists outside of the host cell; a more archaic term for 'viral virion' was 'virus particle'. Viruses are generally comprised of one or more nested shells constructed of one or more layers of protein, some with a lipid outer envelope, a genetic payload that represents the instruction code necessary to replicate the virus, and protein enzymes to help facilitate the genetic payload in the function of replicating copies of the virus once the genetic payload has been delivered to a host cell. Located on the outer shell or envelope of a virus are probes. The function of a virus's external probes is to locate and engage a host cell's receptors. The virus's surface probes are designed to detect, make contact with and functionally engage one or more receptors located on the exterior of a cell type that will offer the virus the proper environment in which to construct copies of itself. A host cell provides the virus the proper biologic machinery for the virus to successfully replicate itself. Once the virus's genome is inside the host cell, the viral genome takes command of the cell's production machinery and causes the host cell to generate copies of the virus. As the viral copies exit the host cell, these virions set off in search of other host cells to infect.

[0012] Naturally occurring viruses exist in a number of differing shapes. The shape of a virus may be rod or filament like, icosahedral, or complex structures combining filament and polygonal shapes. Viruses generally have their outer wall comprised of a protein coat or an envelope comprised of lipids.

[0013] An outer envelope comprised of lipids may be in the form of one or two phospholipid layers. When the outer envelope is comprised of two phospholipid layers this is termed a lipid bilayer. For purposes of this text the term 'lipid' includes 'phospholipid' molecules. A phospholipid is a composite molecule comprised of a polar or hydrophilic region on one end and a nonpolar or hydrophobic region on the opposite end. A lipid bilayer covering a virus, like the membrane of a cell, is constructed with the hydrophilic region of one of the phospholipid layers pointed toward the exterior of the virion and the hydrophilic region of the second phospholipid layer pointed inward toward the center of the virus virion; with the hydrophobic regions of each of the two lipid layers pointed toward each other. The outer envelope of some forms of virus may be comprised of an outer lipid layer or lipid bilayer affixed to a protein matrix for support, the protein matrix being located closer to the center of the virus virion than the lipid layer or lipid bilayer.

[0014] Spherical viruses are generally spherical in shape and may be comprised of an outer envelope and one inner shell or alternatively an outer envelope and multiple inner shells. Inner shells are approximately spherical in shape; this is because the proteins comprising the protein matrix shell have an irregular shape to their structure, but when constructed together form a shape that resembles a sphere. In the case of a spherical virus with an outer envelope and one inner shell, the inner shell is often referred to as a nucleocapsid shell comprised of numerous capsid proteins attached to each other. In the case of a spherical virus being comprised of an outer envelope and multiple inner shells, the outermost inner viral shells may be referred to as comprised of a quantity of matrix proteins, where the innermost shell is referred to as a nucleocapsid and is comprised of a quantity of capsid proteins. The inner protein shells are nested inside each other. The cavity created by the innermost shell or nucleocapsid is referred to as the 'core' or 'center of the virus'. Any payload carried by the virus virion is generally carried in the core or center of the virion.

[0015] Viruses carry genetic material in the form of deoxyribonucleic acid (DNA) or ribonucleic acid (RNA) as their payload. DNA or RNA genome payloads are carried in the cavity of the nucleocapsid referred to as the core. A virus is therefore generally considered to be a DNA virus if its genome is comprised of DNA or the virus is considered a RNA virus if its genome is comprised of RNA that acts as genetic instructions to generate copies of the virus. Viruses may also carry enzymes as part of their payload. An enzyme such as 'reverse transcriptase' transforms a RNA viral genome into DNA. Protease enzymes modify the viral genome once it has entered a host cell. An integrase enzyme assists a DNA viral genome with insertion into the host cell's nuclear DNA. The entire genetic payload is carried inside cavity created by the virus's nucleocapsid shell.

[0016] The probes attached to the exterior of a virus are constructed to engage specific cell-surface receptors on specific cell types in the body. Only a cell that expresses cell-surface receptors that are capable of being engaged by the probes of a specific virus can act as a host for the virus. Viruses generally use two probes to access a host cell. The first probe makes an initial attachment to the host cell, while the action of the virus's second probe often in conjunction with the action of the first probe cause an access portal to be created in the host cell's exterior plasma membrane. Once an access portal is formed, the virus inserts the contents of its payload into the host cell utilizing the open access portal. Certain types of virus may be engulfed whole by a target cell. Once the virus's genome is inside the cytoplasm of the host cell, any enzymes that accompanied the viral genome into the cell, may begin to modify or assist the virus's genome with infecting and taking control of the host cell's biologic functions.

[0017] Probes are attached to the exterior envelope of a virus virion. Probes may be in the form of a protein structure or may be in the form of a glycoprotein molecule. For viruses constructed with a protein matrix as its outer envelope, the probes tend to be protein structures. A portion of the protein structure probe is fixed or anchored in the protein matrix, while a portion of the protein structure probe extends out and away from the protein matrix. The portion of the protein structure probe extending out away from the virus virion is referred to as the 'exterior domain', the portion anchored in the protein matrix is the 'transcending domain'. Some protein probes have a third segment that extends through the envelope and exists inside the virus virion, which is referred to as the 'interior domain'. The exterior domain of a protein structure probe is intended to engage a specific cell-surface receptor on a biologically active cell the virus is targeting as its host cell.

[0018] Viruses that utilize a lipid layer as the outer envelope, are constructed with probes that tend to be glycoproteins. A glycoprotein is comprised of a protein segment and a carbohydrate segment. The carbohydrate segment of the glycoprotein molecule is fixed or anchored in the lipid layer of the outer envelope, while the protein segment extends outward and away from the outer envelope. The protein portion of a glycoprotein probe that extends outward and away from the outer envelope of a virus virion is intended to engage a cell-surface receptor on a biologically active cell the virus is targeting as its host cell.

[0019] Some forms of viruses that utilize a lipid layer as its envelope use protein structure probes. In this case, the portion of the protein structure probe that extends outward and away from the outer envelope is the 'exterior domain', the portion that is anchored in the lipid layer is the 'transcending domain' and again some protein structure probes have an 'interior domain' that exist inside the virion, which may also help anchor the protein structure probe to the virion. The exterior domain of a protein structure probe that extends outward and away from the outer envelope of a virus virion is intended to engage a cell-surface receptor on a biologically active cell the virus is targeting as its host cell.

[0020] When a virus carries a DNA payload and the viral DNA is inserted into the host cell, the virus's DNA travels to the host cell's nucleus and is known to become inserted into the host cell's own native DNA. In the case where a virus is carrying its genetic payload as RNA, the virus inserts the RNA payload into the host cell and may also insert one or more enzymes to facilitate the RNA being utilized properly to replicate copies of the virus. Once inside the host cell, some species of virus facilitate use of the viral RNA by having the RNA converted to DNA. Once the viral RNA has been converted to DNA, the virus's DNA travels to the host cell's nucleus and is known to become inserted into the host cell's native DNA. Once a virus's genetic material has been inserted into the host cell's native DNA, the virus's genetic material takes command of certain cell functions and redirects the resources of the host cell to generate copies of the virus. Other forms of RNA viruses bypass the need to use the nuclear DNA and simply utilize portions of the viral genome to act as messenger RNA. RNA viruses that bypass the host cell's DNA, cause the cell in general to generate copies of the necessary parts of the virus directly from the virus's RNA genome.

[0021] The human immunodeficiency virus (HIV) is a RNA virus and has an outer envelope comprised of a lipid bilayer. The lipid bilayer covers a protein matrix consisting of $p17^{gag}$ proteins. Inside the $p17^{gag}$ protein is nested a nucleocapsid comprised of $p24^{gag}$ proteins. Inside the nucleocapsid HIV carries its payload. HIV's genetic payload consists of two single strands of RNA and several enzymes. The enzymes that accompany HIV's genome include 'reverse transcriptase', 'integrase' and 'protease' molecules.

[0022] The T-Helper cell acts as HIV's host cell. The HIV virion utilizes two types of glycoprotein probes affixed to its exterior envelope to locate and engage a T-Helper cell. HIV utilizes a glycoprotein probe 120 to locate a CD4 cell-surface receptor on a T-Helper cell. Once an HIV glycoprotein 120 probe has successfully engaged a CD4 cell surface-receptor on a T-Helper cell a conformational change occurs in the glycoprotein 120 probe and a glycoprotein 41 probe is exposed. The glycoprotein 41 probe's intent is to engage a CXCR4 or CCR5 cell-surface receptor on the same T-Helper cell. Once a glycoprotein 41 probe on the HIV virion successfully engages a CXCR4 or CCR5 cell-surface receptor, the HIV virion opens an access portal through the T-Helper cell's outer membrane.

[0023] Once the HIV virion has opened an access portal through the T-Helper cell's outer plasma membrane, the HIV virion inserts two positive strand RNA molecules and the associated enzymes it carries into the T-Helper cell. Each RNA strand is approximately 9500 nucleotides in length. Inserted along with the RNA strands are the enzymes reverse transcriptase, protease and integrase. Once the virus's genome gains access to the interior of the T-Helper cell, in the cytoplasm the pair of RNA molecules are transformed to deoxyribonucleic acid by the reverse transcriptase enzyme. Following modification of the virus's genome to DNA, the virus's genetic information migrates to the host cell's nucleus. In the nucleus, with the assistance of the integrase protein, the HIV's DNA becomes inserted into the T-Helper cell's native nuclear DNA. When the timing is appropriate, the now integrated viral DNA is decoded by the host cell's polymerase molecules and the virus's genetic information commands certain cell functions to carry out the replication process to construct copies of the human immunodeficiency virus.

[0024] The outer layer of the HIV virion is comprised of a portion of the T-Helper cell's outer cell membrane. In the final stage of the replication process, as a copy of the HIV virion, carrying the HIV genome, buds through the host cell's cell membrane the outer protein shell acquires as its exterior envelope, a wrapping of lipid bilayer from the host cell's cell membrane. In the case of HIV, since the surface of the pathogen is covered by an envelope comprised of lipid bilayer taken from the host T-Helper cells, this feature allows the HIV virion the capacity to elude the two immune systems, since the detectors comprising the innate immune system and the adaptable immune system may find it difficult to distinguish between the surface of an infectious HIV virion and the surface characteristics of a noninfected T-Helper cell.

[0025] The Hepatitis C virus (HCV) is a positive sense RNA virus, meaning a type of RNA that is capable of bypassing the need for involving the host cell's nucleus by having its RNA genome function as messenger RNA. Hepatitis C infects liver cells. The Hepatitis C viral genome becomes divided once it gains access to the interior of a liver host cell. Portions of the subdivisions of the Hepatitis C genome directly interact with ribosomes to produce proteins necessary to construct copies of the virus.

[0026] HCV belongs to the Flaviviridae family and is the only member of the Hepacivirus genus. There are considered to be at least 100 different strains of Hepatitis C virus based on genome sequencing variability.

[0027] HCV is comprised of an outer lipoprotein envelope and an internal nucleocapsid. The genetic payload is carried within the nucleocapsid. In its natural state, present on the surface of the outer envelope of the Hepatitis C virus are probes that detect receptors present on the surface of liver cells. The glycoprotein E1 probe and the glycoprotein E2 probe have been identified to be affixed to the surface of HCV. The E2 probe binds with high affinity to the large external loop of a CD81 cell-surface receptor. CD81 is found on the surface of many cell types including liver cells. Once the E2 probe has engaged the CD81 cell-surface receptor, cofactors on the surface of HCV's exterior envelope engage either or both the low density lipoprotein receptor (LDLR) or the scavenger receptor class B type I (SR-BI) present on the liver cell in order to effect the mechanism to facilitate HCV breaching the cell membrane and inserting its RNA genome payload through the plasma cell membrane of the liver cell into the liver cell. Upon successful engagement of the HCV surface probes with a liver cell's cell-surface receptors, HCV inserts the single strand of RNA and other payload elements it carries into the liver cell targeted to be a host cell. The HCV RNA genome then interacts with enzymes and ribosomes inside the liver cell in a translational process to produce the proteins required to construct copies of the protein components of HCV. The HCV genome undergoes a method of transcription to replicate copies of the virus's RNA genome. Inside the host, pieces of the HCV virus are assembled together and ultimately loaded with a copy of the HCV genome. Replicas of the original HCV then escape the host cell and migrate the environment in search of additional host liver cells to infect and continue the replication process.

[0028] The HCV's naturally occurring genetic payload consists of a single molecule of linear positive sense, single stranded RNA approximately 9600 nucleotides in length. By means of a translational process a polyprotein of approximately 3000 amino acids is generated. This polyprotein is cleaved post translation by host and viral proteases into individual viral proteins which include: the structural proteins of C, E1, E2, the nonstructural proteins NS1, NS2, NS3, NS4A, NS4B, NS5A, NS5B, p7 and ARFP/F protein. Hepatitis C virus's proteins direct the host liver cell to construction copies of the Hepatitis C virus. A membrane associated replicase complex consisting of the virus's nonstructural proteins NS3 and NS5B facilitate the replication of the viral genome. The membrane of the endoplasmic reticulum appears to be the site of protein maturation and viral assembly. Once copies of the Hepatitis C Virus are generated, they exit the host cell and each copy of HCV migrates in search of another appropriate liver cell that will act as a host to continue the replication process.

[0029] Hepatitis C virus life-cycle demonstrates that copies of a virus virion can be generated by inserting RNA into a host cell that functions as messenger RNA in the host cell. The Hepatitis C viral RNA genome functions as messenger RNA, acting as the template in conjunction with the biologic machinery of a host cell to produce the components that comprise copies of the Hepatitis C virion and the Hepatitis C viral RNA provides the biologic instructions to assemble the components into complete copies of the Hepatitis C virions. The Hepatitis C virus life-cycle clearly demonstrates that viral virions can be manufactured by a host cell without involving the nucleus of the cell.

[0030] Deciphering the existence, replication and behavior of viruses provides clear examples of several fundamental concepts, which include: (1) Viruses target specific cells in the body by means of identifying and engaging such target cells utilizing the probes projecting outward from the virus's exterior shell to make contact with cell-surface receptors located on the surface of their host cells, and (2) Viruses are capable of carrying a variety of different types of payloads including DNA, RNA and a variety of proteins.

[0031] Current gene therapy approach to attempting to deliver a payload to cells in the body use modified forms of existing viruses to act as transport devices to deliver genetic information. This approach is severely limited by restricting the virus virion to the target only cells the viral vector naturally seeks out and infects. Current gene therapy approach is further limited by using the pre-existing size of naturally occurring viruses, rather than being able to modify the size of the structure to be able to tailor the volumetric carrying capacity of the payload portion of the modified virus. Further, gene therapy is restricted to utilizing naturally occurring viruses to deliver only genetic information; it has not previously been appreciated by those skilled in the art that virus-like transport devices might deliver to a variety of specific cell types a wide variety of differing payloads.

[0032] Ribonucleic acids are inherent to a cell and RNAs are used by some viruses to act as the virus's genome to generate copies of the virus. RNAs inherent to a cell are referred to as 'cellular RNAs' and include protein coding RNAs and non-coding RNAs (ncRNA). Protein coding RNAs, generally referred to as messenger RNAs, code for proteins and undergo translation to produce protein molecules. Non-coding RNA represent a variety of functional RNA molecules that do not undergo translation to produce a protein. Non-coding RNAs are highly abundant and functionally important for the cell. Non-coding RNAs have also referred by such terms as non-protein-coding RNAs (npcRNA) or non-messenger RNA (nmRNA) or small non-messenger RNA (snmRNA) or functional RNAs (fRNA). The non-coding RNAs include: transfer RNAs (tRNA), ribosomal RNAs (rRNA), small nuclear RNAs (snRNA), small nucleolar RNAs (snoRNA), signal recognition particle RNA (SRP RNA), antisense RNA (aRNA), micro RNA (miRNA), small interfering RNA (siRNA), Y RNA, telomerase RNA. RNA found in naturally occurring viruses are referred to as 'viral RNA'.

[0033] Transfer RNAs (tRNA), are RNAs that carries amino acids and deliver them to a ribosome. Ribosomal RNAs (rRNA), are RNAs that couple with ribosomal proteins and participate in translation of mRNA to produce protein molecules. Small nuclear RNAs (snRNA) are RNAs involved in splicing and other nuclear functions. Small nucleolar RNAs (snoRNA) are RNAs involved in nucleotide modification. Signal recognition particle RNA (SRP RNA) are RNAs are involved in membrane integration. Antisense RNA (aRNA) are RNAs involved in transcription attenuation, mRNA degradation, mRNA stabilization, and translation blockage. Micro RNA (miRNA) are RNAs involved in gene regulation and have been implicated in a wide range of cell functions including cell growth, apoptosis, neuronal plasticity, insulin secretion. Small interfering RNA (siRNA) are RNAs involved in gene regulation, often interfering with the expression of a single gene. Y RNA are RNAs involved in RNA processing and DNA replication. Telomerase RNA are RNAs involved in telomere synthesis. The primary purpose of 'viral

RNA' is to make copies of the virus that carries of a genome RNA.

[0034] Messenger RNA molecules are comprised of three regions (or segments). These three regions include: (1) a 5' untranslatable region, (2) a coding region and (3) a 3' untranslatable region. The 5' untranslatable region acts as the initiation point for a ribosome to attach to the mRNA. The 'coding region' acts as the template from which a protein is constructed. An 'untranslatable region' represents a segment of a messenger RNA molecule that does not code for a protein and is not used to yield a protein and therefore 'translation' does not occur in such a region. The 3' untranslatable region is associated with the degradation of the usefulness of the mRNA. Different mRNAs have different service life expectancies. The half-life of the naturally occurring mRNA that acts as the template responsible for the production of the protein 'glucokinase' is two hours. The half-life of the naturally occurring mRNA that acts as the template to produce the protein 'alcohol dehydrogenase' is ten hours. The half-life of the naturally occurring mRNA that acts as the template to produce the protein 'glucuronidase' is thirty hours. By modifying the nucleotides that comprise the 3' untranslatable unit of an mRNA, the service half-life of the mRNA may be altered to be lengthened or shortened depending upon the need for the quantity of protein and timeframe over which the mRNA is required to produce the protein coded in the protein template of the mRNA's coding region.

[0035] RNA found in naturally occurring viruses are referred to as 'viral RNA'. The primary function of 'viral RNA' is dedicated to making copies of the virus that carries the RNA genome. Cellular RNAs are inherent to a cell and do not include 'viral RNAs'. Modifications to messenger RNA molecules occur naturally due to errors that occur in the DNA and errors that occurring during the transcription phase and maturation phase of generating messenger RNA. Modifications to ribonucleic acid molecules may occur purposely to produce a medical therapeutic response.

[0036] Modified ribonucleic acid molecules are naturally occurring cellular ribonucleic acid molecules that have purposely undergone modification to the nucleotide sequence to enhance the performance of the naturally occurring cellular ribonucleic acid molecule. Naturally occurring cellular ribonucleic acid molecules can purposely have their nucleotide sequence modified in the 3'untranslatable region, the coding region or the 5' untranslatable region or modification may be made in any combination of the three regions to enhance the performance of the modified ribonucleic acid molecule above and beyond that of the naturally occurring ribonucleic acid molecule. Naturally occurring cellular ribonucleic acid molecules that purposely have a quantity of their nucleotides altered to produce a medical benefit are termed 'modified ribonucleic acids', versus naturally occurring cellular ribonucleic acid molecules that undergo mutation due to an error that occurs in production of the molecule would be termed 'mutant ribonucleic acids'.

[0037] Research has demonstrated that natural proteins can be altered to produce medically beneficial effects. The parathyroid hormone (PTH) is one example. Intact PTH is produced by cells in the parathyroid glands. There are four parathyroid glands present in the neck, generally in the vicinity of the thyroid gland. The term 'para-' means 'next to', so early anatomists identified the four glands 'parathyroid glands' because they were generally found 'next to' the thyroid gland in the neck. Parathyroid hormone is released in response to the cells of the parathyroid gland sensing a decline in the level of serum calcium. Parathyroid hormone, in its natural state, acts to stimulate osteoclast cells present in bone to release calcium from bone, thereby acting as a mechanism to return the serum calcium level to the normal range whenever the serum calcium drops below the normal range. On the other hand, it has been quite well demonstrated that if (1) the amino acid chain of the parathyroid hormone is shortened and (2) the shorter parathyroid hormone molecule is pulsed, by injecting it into the body once a day, the action of this modified parathyroid hormone molecule is opposite of the intact parathyroid hormone. One such form of a shorter length parathyroid hormone molecule is termed 'teriparatide'. Teriparatide (1-34) has the identical sequence from 1 to the 34th N-terminal amino acid of the 84-amino acid endogenous human parathyroid hormone. The skeletal effects of the modified protein molecule act on bone cells to preferentially cause osteoblastic activity over osteoclastic activity, which results in storage of calcium into bone, rather than a release of calcium from bone if the teriparatide is administered once a day. Teriparatide has been a recognized and widely used treatment of osteoporosis since at least as far back as the year 2000.

[0038] Purposely modifying the 'coding region' of a messenger RNA modifies the protein the messenger RNA produces when ribosomes attach to and translate such a modified messenger RNA. As demonstrated by the case of modifying the naturally occurring parathyroid hormone by administering a molecule that is comprised of fewer amino acids than the original PTH molecule, modifying proteins the messenger RNAs produce may provide health care providers with an entirely new and widely spanning armamentarium of medically beneficial therapies.

[0039] The 5' untranslatable region of a messenger RNA molecule is used to identify the messenger RNA and utilized as a point of attachment by ribosomes to the messenger RNA molecule. Modifying the 5' untranslatable region of a messenger RNA by altering the nucleotide sequence in the 5' untranslatable region may make it easier to identify a modified messenger ribonucleic acid molecules in a fashion that the modified messenger ribonucleic acid molecules can be more easily and readily engaged by ribosomes. Altering the nucleotide sequence of the 5' untranslatable region of a modified messenger ribonucleic acid molecule to create a unique identifier, facilitates ribosomes to preferentially engage the modified messenger ribonucleic acid molecule to preferentially produce the protein for which the modified messenger ribonucleic acid molecule is acting as a template.

[0040] Modifying the nucleotide sequence of messenger ribonucleic acid molecules in the 3' untranslatable region extends or shortens the service life of said modified messenger ribonucleic acid molecules, compared to naturally occurring messenger ribonucleic acid molecules. Service life refers to the quantity of time a messenger RNA molecule, present in the cytoplasm, will be able to undergo translation before it is degraded by cellular enzymes. By modifying the nucleotide sequence of a messenger RNA molecule to extend its service life, this allows additional time for ribosomes to decode the information present on the modified messenger ribonucleic acid molecules. Modifying the naturally occurring messenger ribonucleic acid molecule in the 3' untranslatable region in a fashion to cause the molecule to resist degradation by cellular enzymes without compromising the functionality of said modified messenger ribonucleic acid molecules increases production of proteins by ribosomes which results in an enhanced medically therapeutic treatment.

[0041] A dramatic, not previously recognized by those expert in the art is the need to develop a transport vehicle that can be fashioned to seek out specific types of cells and deliver to these cells cellular ribonucleic acid molecules to treat medical conditions related to a protein deficiency. By providing cellular RNAs to these specific target cells a wide variety of cellular functions can be enhanced including gene expression, protein production, telomere synthesis. The exterior envelope of a transport should be constructed so as not to alert the immune system to its presence to prevent rejection of these vehicles. Transport vehicles should be capable of being configured to target any specific type of cell and engage and deliver their payload only to that specific type of cell. To this point, no such device or process has been conceived.

BRIEF SUMMARY OF THE INVENTION

[0042] This medical method for utilization of configurable microscopic medical payload delivery devices to deliver ribonucleic acid molecules to specific cell types facilitates a dramatic new approach to managing a wide variety of medical conditions. By selecting the type of probes that will effectively engage cell-surface receptors on target cells and fixing these probes on the surface of the configurable microscopic medical payload delivery devices, specific types of cells can be targeted. By utilizing configurable microscopic medical payload delivery devices to deliver cellular ribonucleic acid molecules to specific cell types, medical conditions including protein deficient states, genetic deficiencies, conditions related to over expression of genes previously incapable of being treated, are now treatable utilizing this new and unique approach.

DETAILED DESCRIPTION

[0043] The future of medical treatment includes the aggressive, widespread utilization of configurable microscopic medical payload delivery devices (CMMPDD) to deliver a wide variety of ribonucleic acid molecules directly to targeted cell types in the body.

[0044] This patent introduces the concepts: (1) configurable microscopic medical payload delivery devices can carry ribonucleic acid molecules inherent to the cell as the payload, and (2) glycoprotein probes present on the exterior of the configurable microscopic medical payload delivery devices include specific glycoprotein probes or protein structure probes affixed to the exterior, these glycoprotein probes or protein structure probes intended to seek out and engage cell-surface receptors attached to the exterior of whichever cell the configurable microscopic medical payload delivery devices is intended to deliver its payload of cellular RNAs to in order to produce a predetermined medically beneficial effect.

[0045] For purposes of this text, the use of the terms 'specific target cell type', 'target cell', 'specific cell type', 'specific cell', 'specific type of cell' are equivalent and interchangeable; the configuration of cell-surface receptors that a specific cell type has located on and protruding from its outer cell membrane determines the cell type.

[0046] For purposes of this text an 'external envelope' refers to the outermost covering of a virus or a virus-like transport device or a configurable microscopic medical payload delivery device. The external envelope may be comprised of a lipid layer, a lipid bilayer, the combination of a lipid layer affixed to a protein matrix or the combination of a lipid bilayer affixed to a protein matrix. A protein matrix is equivalent to a protein shell and may be referred to as a protein matrix shell. The terms protein matrix, protein shell, protein matrix shell are equivalent to the term capsid, where the term capsid is meant to represent 'a protein coat or shell of a virus particle, surrounding the nucleic acid or nucleoprotein core'. For purposes of this text, the term 'particle' is equivalent to the term 'virion'; further the term 'virus particle' is equivalent to 'viral virion'.

[0047] For purposes of this text an 'internal shell' refers to a protein matrix shell nested inside the external envelope. Multiple inner shells may exist, with those of smaller diameter concentrically nested inside those of a larger diameter. The innermost protein matrix shell is termed the nucleocapsid. The proteins that comprise the nucleocapsid are termed capsid proteins. In the cavity created by the nucleocapsid, referred to as the center or core of the nucleocapsid, is where the payload of ribonucleic acid molecules is carried.

[0048] For purposes of this text 'external probes' are molecular structures that are utilized to locate and engage cell-surface receptors on biologically active cells. External probes are generally comprised of a portion which is anchored or fixed in the external envelope and a second portion that extends out and away from the external envelope. The portion of the external probe that extends out and away from the external envelope is intended to make contact and engage a specific cell-surface receptor located on a biologically active cell. External probes may be comprised solely of a protein structure or an external probe may be a glycoprotein molecule.

[0049] For purposes of this text 'glycoprotein molecule' refers to a molecule comprised of a carbohydrate region and a protein region. Glycoprotein molecules that act as probes are generally anchored or fixed to a lipid layer utilizing the carbohydrate portion of the molecule as an anchor. The protein portion of the glycoprotein molecule which extends outward and away from the exterior envelope the glycoprotein has been affixed such that the protein region may function as a probe to locate and attach to the cell-surface receptor it was created to engage.

[0050] The concept of configurable microscopic medical payload delivery devices is modeled after naturally existing viruses. Configurable microscopic medical payload delivery devices in general are spherical in shape; though other shapes may be used as function might warrant the use of a particular shape. The spherical configurable microscopic medical payload delivery devices are comprised of an exterior envelope and one or more nested inner protein shells. A quantity of exterior protein structure probes and/or glycoprotein probes are anchored in the exterior envelope and a portion extends out and away from the exterior envelope. Nesting of protein shells refers to progressively smaller diameter shells fitting snugly inside protein shells of a larger diameter. Inside the innermost protein shell, referred to as the nucleocapsid, is a cavity referred to as the core of the device. The core of the device is the space where the medically therapeutic payload the device carries is located. The payload of the device is comprised of ribonucleic acid molecules.

[0051] Configurable microscopic medical payload delivery devices (CMMPDD) target specific types of cells in the body. Configurable microscopic medical payload delivery devices engage specific types of cells by the configuration of probes affixed to the exterior envelope of the CMMPDD. By fixing specific probes to the exterior envelope of the CMMPDD, these probes intended to engage and attach only to specific cell-surface receptors located on certain cell types in the body, the CMMPDD will deliver its payload to only those cell types that express compatible and engagable specific cell-surface receptors. In a similar fashion where the exterior probes of a naturally occurring virus engage specific cell-surface receptors present on the surface of the virus's host cell and only the designated host cell, the CMMPDD's exterior probes are configured to engage cell-surface receptors on a specific type of target cell and only those cells. In this manner, the payload of cellular RNAs carried by CMMPDD will be delivered only to specific types of cells in the body. The configuration of the exterior probes on the surface of a CMMPDD varies as needed so as to effect the CMMPDD delivery of specific cellular RNA payloads to specific cell types as needed to effect a particular predetermined medical treatment.

[0052] The size of the configurable microscopic medical payload delivery devices is dependent upon the diameter of the inner protein matrix shells and this is dictated by the volume size of the payload the CMMPDD is required to carry and deliver to a target cell. The diameter of each inner protein matrix shell is governed by the number of protein molecules utilized to construct the protein matrix shell at the time the protein matrix shell is generated. Increasing the number of proteins that comprise a protein matrix shell increases the diameter of the protein matrix shell. When applicable, as dictated by the capacity the CMMPDD is to be utilized to function as, an external lipid envelope wraps around and covers the outermost protein matrix shell. The larger the volume of the core of the CMMPDD, the greater the physical size of the payload the CMMPDD is able to carry. The size of the configurable microscopic medical payload delivery device is to be generally the size of cell (approximately 10^{-4} m in diameter) or less, generally detectable by a light microscope or, as needed, an electron microscope. The size of the CMMPDD is not to be too large such that it would generate a burden to the body by damaging organ tissues through clogging blood vessels or the glomeruli in the kidneys. The dimensions of each type of CMMPDD are to be tailored to the mission of the CMMPDD, which takes into account factors such as the type of target cell, the size of the payload that is to be delivered to the target cells and the length of time the CMMPDD may have to engage the target cell.

[0053] The payload of the configurable microscopic medical payload delivery devices include cellular RNAs, which include protein coding RNAs and non-coding RNAs. Protein coding RNAs include messenger RNAs. The non-coding RNAs include: transfer RNAs (tRNA), ribosomal RNAs (rRNA), small nuclear RNAs (snRNA), small nucleolar RNAs (snoRNA), signal recognition particle RNA (SRP RNA), antisense RNA (aRNA), micro RNA (miRNA), small interfering RNA (siRNA), Y RNA, telomerase RNA.

[0054] Being enveloped in an external lipid layer, configurable microscopic medical payload delivery devices possess the advantage of having their exterior appear similar to the plasma membrane that acts as an outside covering for the cells that comprise the body. By appearing similar to existing plasma membranes, the CMMPDDs appear similar to naturally occurring structures found in the body. CMMPDD are afforded the capability to avoid detection by a body's immune system because the exterior of the CMMPDD mimics the cells comprising the body and the surveillance elements of the immune system find it difficult to discern between the CMMPDD and naturally occurring cells comprising the body.

[0055] To carry out the process of manufacturing a configurable microscopic medical payload delivery device, a primitive cell such as a stem cell is selected. The reason for utilizing primitive cells such as stems cells as the host cell, is that the CMMPDD acquires its outer envelope from the host cell and the more primitive the host cell, the fewer in number the identifying protein markers are present on the surface of the CMMPDD. The fewer the identifying surface proteins present on the outer envelope of the CMMPDD, the less likely a body's immune system will identify the CMMPDD as an intruder and therefore less likely the body's immune system will react to the presence of the CMMPDD and reject the CMMPDD by attacking and neutralizing the CMMPDD.

[0056] Stem cells used as host cells to manufacture quantities of CMMPDD product are selected per histocompatibility markers present on their surface. Certain histocompatibility markers present on the surface of the final CMMPDD product will be less likely to cause a reaction in a specific patient based on the genetic profile of the patient's histocompatibility markers. A similar histocompatibility match is done when donor organs are selected to be given to recipients to avoid rejection of the donor organ by the recipient's immune system.

[0057] The selected stem cells used to manufacture configurable microscopic medical payload delivery devices goes through several steps of maturation before it is capable of generating therapeutic CMMPDD product. RNA inserted into the host stem cell code for the general physical outer structures of the CMMPDD. RNA inserted into the host generate surface probes that target the cell-surface receptors on specific target cell types. RNA is inserted into the host that is used to generate the payload of ribonucleic acid molecules. Similar to how copies of a naturally occurring virus, such as the Hepatitis C virus or HIV, are produced, assembled and released from a host cell, copies of the CMMPDD are produced, assembled and released from a stem cell functioning as a de facto host cell. Once released from the host cell, the copies of the CMMPDD are collected, then pooled together to produce a therapeutic dose that results in a medically beneficial effect.

[0058] The stem cells used as host cells are suspended in a broth of nutrients and are kept at an optimum temperature to govern the rate of production of the CMMPDD product. Similar to the natural production of the Hepatitis C virus, the configurable microscopic medical payload delivery devices 'production genome' is introduced into the host stem cells. The configurable microscopic medical payload delivery devices production genome carries genetic instructions to cause the host cells to manufacture the configurable microscopic medical payload delivery devices' outer protein wall, the inner protein matrixes, the surface probes the configurable microscopic medical payload delivery device is to have affixed to its outer envelope, the ribonucleic acid molecules the configurable microscopic medical payload delivery devices are to carry, and the instructions to assemble the various pieces into the final form of the configurable microscopic medical payload delivery devices along with the instructions to activate the budding process. The resultant configurable microscopic medical payload delivery devices are collected from the nutrient broth surrounding the host cells and placed together into doses to be used as a treatment for a protein deficiency state.

[0059] The 'production genome' are an array of RNAs, which include messenger RNAs that are directly translated by the host cell's ribosomes. The production genome dictates the characteristics of the final version of the CMMPDD that buds from the host stem cell and is released and is to be utilized as a medical treatment. The production genome is specifically tailored to code for the surface probes that will seek and engage a specific type of target cell. The production genome also carries the instructions to code for the production of the type of ribonucleic acid molecules to be delivered to the specific type of target cell. The 'production genome' varies depending upon the configuration of the CMMPDD and the specific type of ribonucleic acid molecules the CMMPDD will transport to effect a specific predetermined medical treatment in a specific type of cell.

[0060] The configurable microscopic medical payload delivery device transporting ribonucleic acid molecules represents a very versatile medical treatment delivery device. CMMPDD is used to deliver a number of different ribonucleic acid molecules to a wide variety of cells in the body.

[0061] The construction of a naturally occurring virus can be likened to the act of following a programmed script to produce a specific result. It is known that the genetic code that a virus carries dictates the production of copies of the virus. It is known that specific segments of the viral genetic code represent instructions that dictate the construction of different parts of the virus so that copies of the virus can be made inside the host cell. It is well documented that there exist different subtypes of most viruses, based off of mutations that have occurred to the viral genome over time; these mutations to the viral genome producing variants in the construction of the virus. Configurable microscopic medical payload delivery devices which carry RNA are constructed much like a naturally occurring virus virion would be constructed in a host cell. Altering the production RNA alters the configuration of the external probes or alters the configuration of the size of the inner shells or alters the type of RNA the CMMPDD will carry or alters any combination of the three.

[0062] As an example of this method, to treat diabetes mellitus the following production process is followed in the lab: (1) Human stem cells are selected. (2) Into the selected stem cells is placed the RNA production genome constructed, in this case, specifically as a means to treat diabetes mellitus. The RNA production genome contains genetic instructions to cause the host stem cells to manufacture the CMMPDDs' outer protein wall, the inner protein matrix, surface probes to include a quantity of glycoprotein probes that engage the GPR40 cell-surface receptor present on the surface of Beta cells located in the Islets of Langerhans in the pancreas, and the messenger RNA payload to facilitate the production of the insulin molecule; and the biologic instructions to assemble the components into the final form of the CMMPDD and the biologic instructions to activate the budding process. (3) Upon insertion of the RNA production genome into the host stem cells, host stem cells' protein production cellular machinery responds by simultaneously translating the different segments of the RNA production genome to produce the proteins that comprise the exterior protein wall, the inner protein matrix molecules, the surface probes, the mRNA payload to produce insulin and decode the instructions to assemble the components into the CMMPDDs. (4) Upon assembly, the CMMPDDs bud through the cell membrane of the host stem cell. (5) At the time of the budding process, the CMMPDDs acquire an outside envelope over the outer protein shell, this outer envelope comprised of a portion of the plasma membrane from the host stem cell the CMMPDD exits. (6) The resultant CMMPDDs are collected from the nutrient broth surrounding the host stem cells. (7) The CMMPDD product is washed in a sterile solution to remove unwanted elements of the nutrient broth. (8) The configurable microscopic medical payload delivery devices are removed from the sterile solution wash and suspended in a sterile hypoallergenic liquid medium. (9) The CMMPDD are separated into individual quantities to facilitate storage and delivery to physicians and patients. (10) The CMMPDD product carried in the sterile hypoallergenic liquid medium is administered to a diabetic patient per injection in a dose that is tailored to receiving patient's requirement to produce sufficient amount of insulin to control the blood sugar. (11) Upon being injected into the body, the CMMPDD product migrates to the Beta cells located in the Islets of Langerhans by means of the blood stream. (12) Upon the CMMPDD product reaching the Beta cells, the probes on the surface of the CMMPDDs engage the cell-surface receptors located on the Beta cells and inserts the RNA payload, including mRNA, into the Beta cells. The mRNA payload is translated by the cell's ribosomes to produce insulin molecules. The increase in insulin production by Beta cells successfully treats diabetes mellitus.

[0063] In a similar fashion, configurable microscopic medical payload delivery devices can be fashioned to deliver a payload of a specific type of ribonucleic acid molecule to any type of cell in the body. Different cell types express different cell-surface markers on the exterior of their plasma membrane. The differing configurations of cell-surface markers on differing types of cells distinguish one cell type from another cell type. By configuring the exterior probes that extend from the surface of the configurable microscopic medical payload delivery device to seek out and engage specific cell-surface receptors present on a specific cell type, payloads of any messenger ribonucleic acid molecule or any non-coding ribonucleic acid molecule can be delivered to specific cells in the body.

Conclusions, Ramification, and Scope

[0064] Accordingly, the reader will see that the configurable microscopic medical payload delivery device to deliver cellular ribonucleic acid molecules to specific targeted cell types provides advantages over existing art by (1) being a delivery device that seeks out specific types of cells, (2) by being a delivery device that is versatile enough to deliver a variety of cellular ribonucleic acid molecules to accomplish various medical treatments and (3) by being a delivery device constructed with a surface envelope that will avoid detection by the innate immune system and the adaptable immune system so as not to activate the immune system to its presence; for these reasons this represents a new and unique medical delivery device that has never before been recognized nor appreciated by those skilled in the art.

[0065] Although the description above contains specificities, these should not be construed as limiting the scope of the invention but as merely providing illustrations of some of the presently preferred embodiments of the invention.

[0066] Thus the scope of the invention should be determined by the appended claims and their legal equivalents, rather than by the examples given.

CLAIMS: Reserved.

No. 4: ADAPTABLE MODIFIED VIRUS VECTOR TO DE-
LIVER MODIFIED MESSENGER RIBONUCLEIC ACID AS A
MEDICAL TREATMENT DEVICE TO MANAGE DIABETES
MELLITUS AND OTHER PROTEIN DEFICIENT DISEASES

INDIVIDUALS REQUESTING PATENT: Dr. Lane B. Scheiber
II, MD and Dr. Lane B. Scheiber, ScD

©2009 Lane B. Scheiber II and Lane B. Scheiber. A portion
of the disclosure of this patent document contains material
which is subject to copyright protection. The copyright owners
have no objection to the facsimile reproduction by anyone of
the patent document or the patent disclosure, as it appears
in the Patent and Trademark Office patent file or records, but
otherwise reserves all copyright rights whatsoever.

ABSTRACT

Diabetes mellitus is a disease of elevated blood glucose, often
directly related to a deficiency in insulin production or insulin
receptor production. The innovative strategy of treatment
described here utilizes modified viruses and virus-like vehicles
to act as a transport mechanism to deliver modified messenger
RNA molecules to target cells in the body. Delivering to the
Beta cells in the body the modified messenger RNA needed to
construction of insulin or insulin receptors will lead to enhanced
production of biologically active insulin or insulin receptors
by Beta cells as necessary, which will lead to correcting
deficiencies in insulin or insulin receptors the result of which
will help properly regulate blood glucose levels throughout the
body utilizing innate regulatory mechanisms.

BACKGROUND OF THE INVENTION

Field of the Invention

This invention relates to any medical device intended to correct
a protein deficiency in the body by increasing the intracellular

production of the deficient protein by utilizing a modified virus to insert one or more modified messenger ribonucleic acid molecules into one or more cells of the body.

Description of Background Art

[0001] For purposes of this text there are several general definitions. A 'ribose' is a five carbon or pentose sugar ($C_5H_{10}O_5$) present in the structural components of ribonucleic acid, riboflavin, and other nucleotides and nucleosides. A 'deoxyribose' is a deoxypentose ($C_5H_{10}O_4$) found in deoxyribonucleic acid. A 'nucleoside' is a compound of a sugar usually ribose or deoxyribose with a nitrogenous base by way of an N-glycosyl link. A 'nucleotide' is a single unit of a nucleic acid, composed of a five carbon sugar (either a ribose or a deoxyribose), a nitrogenous base and a phosphate group. There are two families of 'nitrogenous bases', which include: pyrimidine and purine. A 'pyrimidine' is a six member ring made up of carbon and nitrogen atoms, the members of the pyrimidine family include cytosine (C), thymine (T) and uracil (U). A 'purine' is a five-member ring fused to a pyrimidine type ring; the members of the purine family include adenine (A) and guanine (G). A 'nucleic acid' is a polynucleotide which is a biologic molecule such as ribonucleic acid or deoxyribonucleic acid that allow organisms to reproduce. A 'ribonucleic acid' (RNA) is a linear polymer of nucleotides formed by repeated riboses linked by phosphodiester bonds between the 3-hydroxyl group of one and the 5-hydroxyl group of the next; RNAs are a single strand macromolecule comprised of a sequence of nucleotides, these nucleotides generally referred to by their nitrogenous bases, which include: adenine, cytosine, guanine or uracil. RNAs are subset into different types which include messenger RNA (mRNA), transport RNA (tRNA), and ribosomal RNA (rRNA). Messenger RNAs act as templates to produce proteins. A ribosome is a complex comprised of RNAs and proteins and is responsible for the correct positioning of mRNA and charged tRNA to facilitate the proper alignment and bonding of amino acids into a strand to produce a protein. A 'charged' tRNA is a tRNA that is carrying an amino acid. Ribosomal RNA (rRNA) represents a subset of RNAs that form part of the physical structure of a ribosome.

[0002] Diabetes mellitus represents an important health issue that affects a significant portion of the world population. In the United States, about 16 million people suffer from diabetes mellitus. Every year, about 650,000 additional people are diagnosed with this disease. Diabetes mellitus is the seventh leading cause of all deaths.

[0003] Diabetes mellitus represents a state of hyperglycemia, a serum blood sugar that is higher than what is considered the normal range for humans. Glucose, a six-carbon molecule, is a form of sugar. Glucose is absorbed by the cells of the body and converted to energy by the processes of glycolysis, the Krebs cycle and phosporylation. Insulin, a protein, facilitates the transfer of glucose from the blood into cells. Normal range for blood glucose in humans is generally defined as a fasting blood plasma glucose level of between 70 to 110 mg/dl. For descriptive purposes, the term 'plasma' refers to the fluid portion of blood.

[0004] Diabetes mellitus is classified as Type One and Type Two. Type One diabetes mellitus is insulin dependent, which refers to the condition where there is a lack of sufficient insulin circulating in the blood stream and insulin must be provided to the body in order to properly regulate the blood glucose level. When insulin is required to regulate the blood glucose level in the body, this condition is often referred to as insulin dependent diabetes mellitus (IDDM). Type Two diabetes mellitus is noninsulin dependent, often referred to as noninsulin dependent diabetes mellitus (NIDDM), meaning the blood glucose level can be managed without insulin, and instead by means of diet, exercise or intervention with oral medications. Type Two diabetes mellitus is considered a progressive disease, the underlying pathogenic mechanisms including pancreatic Beta cell (also often designated as β-Cell) dysfunction and insulin resistance.

[0005] The pancreas serves as an endocrine gland and an exocrine gland. Functioning as an endocrine gland the pancreas produces and secretes hormones including insulin and glucagon. Insulin acts to reduce levels of glucose circulating in the blood. Beta cells secrete insulin into the blood when a higher than normal level of glucose is detected in the serum. For purposes of this description the terms 'blood', 'blood stream' and 'serum' refer to the same substance. Glucagon acts to stimulate an increase in glucose circulating in the blood. Beta cells in the pancreas secrete glucagon when a low level of glucose is detected in the serum.

[0006] Glucose enters the body and then the blood stream as a result of the digestion of food. The Beta cells of the Islets of Langerhans continuously sense the level of glucose in the blood and respond to elevated levels of blood glucose by secreting insulin into the blood. Beta cells produce the protein 'insulin' in their endoplasmic reticulum and store the insulin in vacuoles until it is needed. When Beta cells detect an increase in the glucose level in the blood, Beta cells release insulin into the blood from the described storage vacuoles.

[0007] Insulin is a protein. An insulin protein consists of two chains of amino acids, an alpha chain and a beta chain, linked by two disulfide (S-S) bridges. One chain, the alpha chain consists of 21 amino acids. The second chain the beta chain consists of 30 amino acids.

[0008] Insulin interacts with the cells of the body by means of a cell-surface receptor termed the 'insulin receptor' located on the exterior of a cell's 'outer membrane', otherwise known as the 'plasma membrane'. Insulin interacts with muscle and liver cells by means of the insulin receptor to rapidly remove excess blood sugar when the glucose level in the blood is higher than the upper limit of the normal physiologic range. Recognized functions of insulin include stimulating cells to take up glucose from the blood and convert it to glycogen to facilitate the cells in the body to utilize glucose to generate biochemically usable energy, and to stimulate fat cells to take up glucose and synthesize fat.

[0009] Diabetes Mellitus may be the result of one or more factors. Causes of diabetes mellitus may include: (1) mutation of the insulin gene itself causing miscoding, which results in the production of ineffective insulin molecules; (2) mutations to genes that code for the 'transcription factors' needed for transcription of the insulin gene in the deoxyribonucleic acid (DNA) to create messenger ribonucleic acid (mRNA) molecules, which facilitate the manufacture of the insulin molecule; (3) mutations of the gene encoding for the insulin receptor, which produces inactive or an insufficient number of insulin receptors; (4) mutation to the gene encoding for glucokinase, the enzyme that phosphorylates glucose in the first step of glycolysis; (5) mutations to the genes encoding portions of the potassium channels in the plasma membrane of the Beta cells, preventing proper closure of the channel, thus blocking insulin release; (6) mutations to mitochondrial genes that as a result, decreases the energy available to be used facilitate the release of insulin, therefore reducing insulin secretion; (7) failure of glucose transporters to properly permit the facilitated diffusion of glucose from plasma into the cells of the body.

[0010] A 'eukaryote' refers to a nucleated cell. Eukaryotes comprise nearly all animal and plant cells. A human eukaryote or nucleated cell is comprised of an exterior lipid bilayer plasma membrane, cytoplasm, a nucleus, and organelles. The exterior plasma membrane defines the perimeter of the cell, regulates the flow of nutrients, water and regulating molecules in and out of the cell, and has embedded into its structure receptors that the cell uses to detect properties of the environment surrounding the cell membrane. The cytoplasm acts as a filling medium inside the boundaries of the plasma cell membrane and is comprised mainly of water and nutrients such as amino acids, oxygen, and glucose. The nucleus, organelles, and ribosomes are suspended in the cytoplasm. The nucleus contains the majority of the cell's genetic information in the form of double stranded deoxyribonucleic acid (DNA). Organelles generally carry out specialized functions for the cell and include such structures as the mitochondria, the endoplasmic reticulum, storage vacuoles, lysosomes and Golgi complex (sometimes referred to as a Golgi apparatus). Floating in the cytoplasm, but also located in the endoplasmic reticulum and mitochondria are ribosomes. Ribosomes are complex macromolecule structures comprised of ribosomal ribonucleic acid (rRNA) and several strands of proteins that combine and couple to a messenger ribonucleic acid (mRNA) molecule. The rRNA and the ribosomal proteins congregate to form a macromolecule structure that surrounds a mRNA molecule. Ribosomes decode genetic information in a mRNA molecule and manufacture proteins to the specifications of the instruction code physically present in the mRNA molecule. More than one ribosome may be attached to a single mRNA at a time.

[0011] The majority of the deoxyribonucleic acid (DNA) comprises the chromosomes, double stranded helical structures located in the nucleus of the cell. DNA in a circular form, can also be found in the mitochondria, the powerhouse of the cell, an organelle that assists in converting glucose into usable energy molecules. DNA represents the genetic information a cell needs to manufacture the materials it requires to sustain life and to replicate. Genetic information is stored in the DNA by arrangements of four nucleotides referred to as: adenine, thymine, guanine and cytosine. DNA represents instruction coding, that in the process known as transcription, the DNA's genetic information is decoded by transcription protein complexes referred to as polymerases (or polymerase complex), to produce ribonucleic acid (RNA). RNA is a single strand of genetic information comprised of coded arrangements of four nucleotides: adenine, uracil, guanine and cytosine. In a RNA, 'uracil' takes the place of 'thymine', thymine being present in the DNA. Several different types of RNAs have been identified, which include messenger RNAs (mRNA), transport RNAs (tRNA) and ribosomal RNAs (rRNA).

[0012] Proteins are comprised of a series of amino acids bonded together in a linear strand, sometimes referred to as a chain; a protein may be further modified to be a structure comprised of one or more similar or differing strands of amino acids bonded together. Insulin is a protein structure comprised of two strands of amino acids, one strand comprised of 21 amino acids long and the second strand comprised of 30 amino acids, the two strands attached by two disulfide bridges. There are an estimated 30,000 different proteins the cells of the human body may manufacture. The human body is comprised of a wide variety of cells, many with specialized functions requiring unique combinations of proteins and protein structures such as glycoproteins (a protein combined with a carbohydrate) to accomplish the required task or tasks a specialized cell is designed to perform. Forms of glycoproteins are known to be utilized as cell-surface receptors. Messenger RNAs (mRNA) are created by transcription of DNA, they generally migrate to other locations inside the cell, and are utilized by ribosomes as protein manufacturing templates. A ribosome is a protein complex that manufactures proteins by deciphering the instruction code located in a mRNA molecule. When a specific protein is needed, pieces of the ribosome complex, which include rRNA molecules and ribosomal proteins, bind around the strand of a mRNA that carries the specific instruction code that will generate the required protein. The ribosome traverses the mRNA strand and deciphers the genetic information coded into the sequence of nucleotides that comprise the mRNA molecule to produce a protein molecule and this process is referred to as translation.

[0013] A ribosome is complex macromolecule comprised of ribosomal RNA (rRNA) molecules and ribosomal proteins. Ribosomal RNAs and ribosomal proteins are often designated with a number measured in Svedberg (S) units which represents the sediment coefficient. The sediment coefficient is influenced by both molecular weight of the molecule and surface area of the molecule. In humans there are generally recognized at this time two mitochondrial rRNAs identified as 12S rRNA and 16S rRNA, and there are generally recognized four rRNAs that reside in the cytoplasm of a cell identified as 5S rRNA, 5.8S rRNA, 18S rRNA and 28S rRNA. There may be other rRNAs, as of yet unidentified, that reside in some of the other structures in the cell that engage in manufacturing of macromolecules, such as the smooth endoplasmic reticulum, the rough endoplasmic reticulum and the Golgi complex.

[0014] In eukaryotes, in the cytoplasm, the ribosome complex is referred to as an 80S ribosome. Generally two ribosomal proteins comprise a ribosome complex. This 80S ribosome is comprised of one 'dome-shape' 60S ribosomal protein and one 'cap-shaped' 40S ribosomal protein.

[0015] In the forms of life referred to as vertebrates (Humans are classified as a form of vertebrate), of the four rRNAs that reside in the cytoplasm of a eukaryote cell, the 18S rRNA is found in and helps comprise the physical structure of the 40S protein subunit of the ribosome complex and the 5S rRNA, 5.8S rRNA, and 28S rRNA molecules are found in and help comprise the physical structure of the 60S protein subunit of the ribosome complex.

[0016] The rRNA molecules are thought to provide at least three different functions for the ribosome complex. The rRNA molecules are thought to: (1) assist with identification of the messenger RNA to be translated, (2) act as an enzyme to facilitate the production of the protein molecule being translated from the mRNA molecule undergoing translation, (3) possibly cause folding at certain locations in the three dimensional structure of the protein being generated as the ribosome complex decodes the mRNA molecule.

[0017] Ribosomal RNAs (rRNA) are generated by polymerase molecule deciphering the instruction code present in the DNA. The rRNAs generally migrate to locations where mRNAs are to be utilized as templates. The rRNA molecules connect to their respective ribosome proteins and this macromolecule complex, referred to as a ribosome or ribosome complex, surrounds the beginning segment of a mRNA molecule. Utilizing inherent coding, the rRNA molecules direct the ribosome pieces to build the ribosome complex around a particular strand of mRNA or particular type of mRNA. The inherent coding the rRNA molecules harbor is a sequence of nucleotides which represent a unique name, unique base-four number or unique combination of a name and base-four number that corresponds to a particular mRNA or particular type of mRNA. In this manner, rRNA acts to control which mRNA molecule will undergo translation to produce proteins, rather than a ribosome complex randomly engaging any mRNA template that happens to be available. With the DNA producing rRNA molecules that cause a ribosome to attach to a particular mRNA molecule or particular type of mRNA molecule, the DNA is able to exert control over the manufacturing capacity of the cell and produce proteins as needed, rather than producing proteins in a random fashion. Producing proteins as needed by the cell, rather than in a random fashion, conserves valuable resources and conserves energy inside the cell.

[0018] RNAs are generally degraded by enzymes known as ribonucleases or RNAases. Ribonucleases act to inactive the RNA molecules. Different RNAs have different half-lives.

[0019] Transport RNAs (tRNA) are constructed in the nucleus or in the mitochondria, and are coded for one of the 20 amino acids the cells of the human body use to construct proteins. Once a tRNA is created by transcription of the DNA, the tRNA seeks out the type of amino acid it has been coded for and attaches to that specific amino acid. A tRNA molecule is considered to be 'charged' when it is carrying an amino acid. The charged tRNA delivers the amino acid it carries to a ribosome that is waiting for the specific amino acid the tRNA is carrying. Proteins are manufactured by the ribosomes binding together sequences of amino acids. The order by which the amino acids are bonded together is dictated by the way the sequencing of the nucleotides comprising the mRNA is constructed and how the ribosome interprets the information encoded in the string of nucleotides present in the mRNA strand.

[0020] Messenger RNA molecules are divided into three regions. The three regions include (1) the 5' untranslatable region, (2) the coding region, and (3) the 3' untranslatable region. An 'untranslatable region' represents a segment of a messenger RNA molecule that does not code for a protein and is not used to yield a protein and therefore 'translation' does not occur in such a region. The 'coding region' is the portion of the mRNA that is decoded by the ribosomes by the process known as translation to produce a particular protein molecule. A sequence of three nucleotides present in the coding region of a mRNA molecule represents a unit of information referred to as a codon. Codons code for all of the 20 amino acids used to construct protein molecules and also for START and STOP commands. In the process known as translation, the ribosome decodes the codons present in the coding region in the mRNA, initiating the protein manufacturing process at a START codon, then interfacing with charged tRNAs carrying the amino acids that match the sequence of codons in the mRNA as the ribosome traverses the length of the coding region of the mRNA molecule. The ribosome functions as a protein factory by taking amino acids delivered by charged tRNAs and binding the amino acids together in the order dictated by the sequence of codon instructions coded into the mRNA template as directed by the manner of the nucleic acid arrangement in the mRNA molecule.

Protein synthesis ceases when a ribosome encounters a STOP code. The protein molecule is then released by the ribosome. Ribosomes do not decode the nucleotide sequences to produce proteins in a mRNA's 5' untranslatable region or a mRNA's 3' untranslatable region.

[0021] The insulin molecule is a protein produced by Beta cells located in the pancreas. The 'insulin messenger RNA' is created in a Beta cell by a polymerase complex transcribing the insulin gene from nuclear DNA in the nucleus of the cell. The native messenger RNA (mRNA) for insulin then travels to the endoplasmic reticulum, where numerous ribosomes, comprised of rRNA and ribosomal proteins, engage these mRNA molecules. Many ribosomes may be attached to a single strand of mRNA simultaneously, each generating an identical copy of the protein as dictated by the information encoded in the mRNA. Insulin is produced by ribosomes translating the information in a mRNA molecule coded for the insulin protein, which produce strands of amino acids that are coded for an immature form of the biologically active insulin molecule referred to as 'pro-insulin'. Once the pro-insulin molecule is generated it then undergoes modification by several enzymes including prohormone convertase one (PC1), prohormone convertase two (PC2) and carboxypeptidase E, which results in the production of a biologically active insulin molecule. Once the biologically active insulin protein is generated it is stored in a vacuole in the Beta cell to await being released into the blood stream.

[0022] Insulin receptors, which appear on the surface of cells, offer binding sites for insulin circulating in the blood. When insulin binds to an insulin receptor, the biologic response inside the cell causes glucose to enter the cell and undergo processing in the cytoplasm. Processed glucose molecules then enter the mitochondria. The mitochondria further process the modified glucose molecules to produce usable energy in the form of adenosine triphosphate molecules (ATP). Thirty-eight ATP molecules may be generated from one molecule of glucose during the process of aerobic respiration. ATP molecules are utilized as an energy source by biologic processes throughout the cell.

[0023] The current medical therapeutic approach to the management of diabetes mellitus has produced limited results. Patients with diabetes generally struggle with an inadequate production of insulin, or an ineffective release of biologically active insulin molecules, or a release of an insufficient number of biologically active insulin molecules, or an insufficient production of cell-surface receptors, or a production of ineffective cell-surface receptors, or a production of ineffective insulin molecules that are unable to interact properly with insulin receptors to produce the required biologic effect. Type One diabetes requires administration of exogenous insulin. The traditional approach to Type Two diabetes has generally first been to adjust the diet to limit the caloric intake the individual consumes. Exercise is used as an initial approach to both Type One and Type Two diabetes as a means of up-regulating the utilization of fats and sugar so as to reduce the amount of circulating plasma glucose. When diet and exercise are inadequate in properly managing Type Two diabetes, oral medications are often introduced. The action of sulfonylureas, a commonly prescribed class of oral medication, is to stimulate the Beta cells to produce additional insulin receptors and enhance the insulin receptors' response to insulin. Biguanides, another form of oral treatment, inhibit gluconeogenesis, the production of glucose in the liver, thereby attempting to reduce plasma glucose levels. Thiazolidinediones (TZDs) lower blood sugar levels by activating peroxisome proliferator-activated receptor gamma (PPAR-γ), a transcription factor, which when activated regulates the activity of various target genes, particularly ones involved in glucose and lipid metabolism. If diet, exercise and oral medications do not produce a satisfactory control of the level of blood glucose in a diabetic patient, exogenous insulin is injected into the body in an effort to normalize the amount of glucose present in the serum. Insulin, a protein, has not successfully been made available as an oral medication to date due to the fact that proteins in general become degraded when they encounter the acid environment present in the stomach.

[0024] Despite strict monitoring of blood glucose and potentially multiple doses of insulin injected throughout the day, many patients with diabetes mellitus still experience devastating adverse effects from elevated blood glucose levels. Microvascular damage and elevated tissue sugar levels contribute to such complications as renal failure, retinopathy involving the eyes, neuropathy, and accelerated heart disease despite aggressive efforts to maintain the blood sugar within the physiologic normal range using exogenous insulin by itself or a combination of exogenous insulin and one or more oral medications. Diabetes remains the number one cause of renal failure in the United States. Especially in diabetic patients that are dependent upon administering exogenous insulin into their body, though dosing of the insulin may be four or more times a day and even though this may produce adequate control of the blood glucose level to prevent the clinical symptoms of hyperglycemia; this does not unerringly supplement the body's natural capacity to monitor the blood sugar level minute to minute, twenty-four hours a day, and deliver an immediate response to a rise in blood glucose by the release of insulin from Beta cells as required. The deleterious effects of diabetes may still evolve despite strict and persistent control of the glucose level in the blood stream.

[0025] The current treatment of diabetes may be augmented by the unique approach to utilizing modified viruses as vehicles to transport exogenous modified messenger ribonucleic acid (mRNA) molecules to participate with ribosomes to manufacture pro-insulin, insulin, the enzymes utilized to modify proinsulin to the biologically active insulin molecule and insulin receptors. By delivering mRNA coded to facilitate the manufacture of pro-insulin, insulin, the enzymes utilized to modify proinsulin to the biologically active insulin molecule and/or insulin receptors, the Beta cells in the pancreas would be stimulated to generate additional biologically active insulin.

[0026] Viruses are obligate parasites. Viruses simply represent a carrier of genetic material and by themselves viruses are unable to replicate or carry out any form of biologic function outside their host cell. Viruses are generally comprised of one or more nested shells constructed of one or more layers of protein or lipid material, a genetic payload that represents the instruction code necessary to replicate the virus, and protein enzymes to help facilitate the genetic payload in the function of replicating copies of the virus once the genetic payload has been delivered to a host cell. Located on the outer shell or envelope of a virus are probes. The function of a virus's probes is to locate and engage a host cell's receptors. The virus's surface probes are designed to detect, make contact with and functionally engage one or more receptors located on the exterior of a cell type that will offer the virus the proper environment in which to construct copies of itself. A host cell provides the virus the proper biochemical machinery for the virus to successfully replicate itself.

[0027] Protected by an outer protein coat or lipid envelope, viruses carry a genetic payload in the form of deoxyribonucleic acid (DNA) or ribonucleic acid (RNA). Once a virus's exterior probes locate and functionally engage the surface receptor or receptors on a host cell, the virus inserts its genetic payload into the interior of the host cell. In the event a virus is carrying a DNA payload, the virus's DNA travels to the host cell's nucleus and is known to become inserted into the host cell's own native DNA. In the case where a virus is carrying its genetic payload as RNA, the virus inserts the RNA payload into the host cell and may also insert one or more enzymes to facilitate the RNA being utilized properly to replicate copies of the virus. Once inside the host cell, some species of virus facilitate use of their RNA by having the RNA converted to DNA. Once the viral RNA has been converted to DNA, the virus's DNA travels to the host cell's nucleus and is known to become inserted into the host cell's native DNA. Once a virus's genetic material has been inserted into the host cell's native DNA, the virus's genetic material takes command of certain cell functions and redirects the resources of the host cell to generate copies of the virus. Other forms of RNA viruses bypass the need to use the nuclear DNA and simply utilize portions of the viral genome to act as messenger RNA (mRNA). RNA viruses that bypass the host cell's DNA, cause the cell to in general generate copies of the necessary parts of the virus directly from the virus's RNA genome.

[0028] The Hepatitis C virus (HCV) is a positive sense RNA virus, meaning HCV's genome is a type of RNA that is capable of bypassing the need for involving the host cell's nucleus by having its RNA genome function as messenger RNA. The Hepatitis C virus infects liver cells. The Hepatitis C viral genome becomes divided once it gains access to the interior of a liver host cell. Portions of the subdivisions of the Hepatitis C viral genome directly interact with ribosomes to produce proteins necessary to construct copies of the virus.

[0029] HCV belongs to the Flaviviridae family and is the only member of the Hepacivirus genus. There are considered to be at least 100 different strains of Hepatitis C virus based on genome sequencing variability.

[0030] HCV is comprised of an outer lipoprotein envelope and an internal nucleocapsid. The genetic payload is carried within the nucleocapsid. In its natural state, present on the surface of the outer envelope of the Hepatitis C virus are probes that detect receptors present on the surface of liver cells. The glycoprotein E1 probe and the glycoprotein E2 probe have been identified to be affixed to the surface of HCV. The E2 probe binds with high affinity to the large external loop of a CD81 cell-surface receptor. CD81 is found on the surface of many cell types including liver cells. Once the E2 probe has engaged the CD81 cell-surface receptor, cofactors on the surface of HCV's exterior envelope engage either or both the low density lipoprotein receptor (LDLR) or the scavenger receptor class B type I (SR-BI) present on the liver cell in order to effect the mechanism to facilitate HCV breaching the cell membrane and inserting its viral RNA genome payload through the plasma cell membrane of the liver cell, thus delivering the HCV RNA genome into the liver cell. Upon successful engagement of the HCV surface probes with a liver cell's cell-surface receptors, HCV inserts the single strand of RNA and other payload elements it carries into the liver cell targeted to be a host cell. The HCV RNA genome then interacts with enzymes and ribosomes inside the liver cell in a translational process to produce the proteins required to construct copies of the protein components of HCV. The HCV genome undergoes a method of transcription to replicate copies of the virus's RNA genome. Inside the host, pieces of the HCV virus are assembled together and ultimately loaded with a copy of the HCV genome. Replicas of the original HCV then escape the host cell and migrate the environment in search of additional host liver cells to infect and continue the replication process.

[0031] HCV's naturally occurring genetic payload consists of a single molecule of linear positive sense, single stranded RNA approximately 9600 nucleotides in length. By means of a translational process a polyprotein of approximately 3000 amino acids is generated. This polyprotein is cleaved post translation by host and viral proteases into individual viral proteins which include: the structural proteins of C, E1, E2, the nonstructural proteins NS1, NS2, NS3, NS4A, NS4B, NS5A, NS5B, p7 and ARFP/F protein. Hepatitis C virus's proteins direct the host liver cell to construction copies of the Hepatitis C virus. A membrane associated replicase complex consisting of the virus's nonstructural proteins NS3 and NS5B facilitate the replication of the viral genome. The membrane of the endoplasmic reticulum appears to be the site of protein maturation and viral assembly. Once copies of the Hepatitis C Virus are generated, they exit the host cell and each copy of HCV migrates in search of another appropriate liver cell that will act as a host to continue the replication process.

[0032] A modified Hepatitis C virus offers a naturally occurring vehicle mechanism to transport and insert medically therapeutic modified messenger ribonucleic acid (mRNA) molecules into specific targeted cells of the human body. The surface probes present on the Hepatitis C virus's outer protein coat can be modified to seek out specific receptors on specific target cells. Once the modified Hepatitis C virus's probes properly engage the cell-surface receptors on a target cell, the modified Hepatitis C virus would insert into the target cell one or more medically therapeutic modified messenger ribonucleic acid (mRNA) molecules for the purpose of having the target cell generate proteins to achieve a medically therapeutic response.

[0033] Current state of gene therapy generally refers to efforts directed toward inserting an exogenous subunit of DNA into a vehicle such as a naturally occurring virus. The vehicle is intended to insert the exogenous subunit of DNA into a cell the virus naturally targets. The exogenous DNA subunit then migrates to the target cell's nucleus. The exogenous DNA subunit then inserts into the native DNA of the cell. This represents a permanent alteration of the cell's nuclear DNA. The nuclear transcription proteins then read the exogenous DNA subunit's nucleotide coding to produce the intended cellular response. The approach described hereunder involves RNA versus DNA. DNA is comprised of the nucleotides adenine, thymine, guanine and cytosine. RNA is composed of the nucleotides: adenine, uracil, guanine and cytosine. DNA codes for the manufacture of RNAs, which are composed of nucleotides. RNAs facilitate the manufacture of proteins, which are composed of amino acids. The virus chosen as the transport vehicle, Hepatitis C virus, is a RNA virus versus a virus that naturally carries a DNA genome.

[0034] Beta cells located in the Islets of Langerhans in the pancreas are thought to have at least one unique identifying surface receptor. The exterior receptor GPR40 appears specific to Beta cells located in the Islets of Langerhans in the pancreas. A virus equipped with a surface probe designed to engage the GPR40 Beta cell receptor, could travel the blood stream of the body until it locates a GPR40 receptor on a Beta cell, engage the receptor with its surface probe, and then insert the genetic payload it carries into the Beta cell. A genetic payload of one or more modified mRNAs could be used to enhance proper protein production by cells deficient in a particular protein. Hormones are proteins that circulate the body and stimulate biologic activity specific to the hormone's role. In the case of a deficiency of a hormone, production of a deficient hormone could be enhanced by inserting one or more modified mRNAs into specific target cells in the body to stimulate production of the required hormone. In the case of diabetes mellitus, utilizing a modified Hepatitis C virus as a vehicle, modified mRNA molecules could be inserted into Beta cells, to assist the Beta cells are with generating an adequate insulin production and adequate release of insulin into the blood to meet the body's needs.

[0035] Viruses are constructed in a number of ways and shapes. The shape of a virus may be rod or filament like, icosahedral, or complex structures combining filament and polygonal shapes. Viruses may have an outer protein coat or an outer envelope comprised of lipids. Icosahedral viruses with an outer lipid envelope appear spherical in shape. An outer envelope is often comprised of two lipid layers often termed a lipid bilayer. Spherical viruses may be in the form of being comprised of an outer envelope and one inner shell or an outer envelope and two inner shells. In the case of a spherical virus with an outer envelope and one inner shell, the inner shell is often referred to as a nucleocapsid shell comprised of capsid proteins. In the case of a spherical virus being comprised of an outer envelope and two inner shells, the outer most inner viral shell may be referred to as comprised of matrix proteins, the innermost of the two shells being referred to as a nucleocapsid shell being comprised of capsid proteins. The inner protein shell is nested inside the outer protein shell.

[0036] An alternative means to treat diabetes might include the use of a quantity of virus-like transport vehicles. The virus-like transport vehicles would be spherical in shape. The virus-like transport vehicles would be comprised of a lipid bilayer envelope and one or more inner nested protein shells, depending upon the size of the payload. Nesting of protein shells refers to progressively smaller diameter shells fitting snugly inside protein shells of a larger diameter. The virus-like transport vehicles would be similar in construction to viruses, and such virus-like transport vehicles would carry a payload consisting of ribosomal RNA molecules. The size of the virus-like transport vehicle would depend upon the payload the virus-like transport vehicle would be required to carry. Embedded in the virus-like transport vehicle's outer lipid bilayer surface would be a quantity of probes that are intended to target cell-surface receptors on specific cells. The virus-like transport vehicle would be introduced into a patient's blood stream or tissues so that the virus-like transport vehicle could deliver the therapeutic genetic payload that it carries to Beta cells in the pancreas. When one or more probes on the surface of the virus-like transport vehicle engage one or more cell-surface receptors on a Beta cell located in the pancreas, the virus-like transport vehicle will insert its therapeutic payload of ribosomal RNA into the Beta cell to enhance the Beta cell's biologic function of producing insulin and/or insulin receptors.

[0037] The action of altering the type of probe or probes present on the surface of the modified virus, the modified Hepatitis C virus, or the virus-like transport vehicle would change the target the modified virus or virus-like transport vehicle would seek out. By changing the probe on the surface of the modified virus, the modified Hepatitis C virus, or the virus-like transport vehicle the payload carried by the modified virus, the modified Hepatitis C virus, or the virus-like transport vehicle could be delivered to any cell that carried on its surface a cell-surface receptor that would engage the probes the modified virus, the modified Hepatitis C virus, or the virus-like transport vehicle was carrying on its surface. In this fashion, specific payloads could be delivered to specific cells throughout the body.

[0038] The utilization of modified messenger ribonucleic acid (mRNA) molecules does not alter the cell's DNA. Modified mRNAs degrade and become unusable after a period of time. Use of RNA as a therapeutic modality offers a therapeutic opportunity that could have a reversible or an attenuable effect when required. Using modified mRNA to produce proteins bypasses the action of decoding the DNA and errors or deficiencies that might occur during the process of transcription. By employing a medically therapeutic virus to carry modified mRNAs to cells, deficiencies of any of the approximately 30,000 proteins that comprise the tissues that exist in the body and on the surface of the body can be successfully treated or averted.

[0039] Messenger RNA molecules are comprised of three regions (or segments). These three regions include: (1) a 5' untranslatable region, (2) a coding region and (3) a 3' untranslatable region. The 5' untranslatable region acts as the initiation point for a ribosome to attach to the mRNA. The 'coding region' acts as the template from which a protein is constructed. An 'untranslatable region' represents a segment of a messenger RNA molecule that does not code for a protein and is not used to yield a protein and therefore 'translation' does not occur in such a region. The 3' untranslatable region is associated with the degradation of the usefulness of the mRNA. Different mRNAs have different service life expectancies. The half-life of the naturally occurring mRNA that acts as the template responsible for the production of the protein 'glucokinase' is two hours. The half-life of the naturally occurring mRNA that acts as the template to produce the protein 'alcohol dehydrogenase' is ten hours. The half-life of the naturally occurring mRNA that acts as the template to produce the protein 'glucuronidase' is thirty hours. By modifying the nucleotides that comprise the 3' untranslatable unit of an mRNA, the service half-life of the mRNA may be altered to be lengthened or shortened depending upon the need for the quantity of protein and timeframe over which the mRNA is required to produce the protein coded in the protein template of the mRNA's coding region.

[0040] Research has demonstrated that natural proteins can be altered to produce medically beneficial effects. The parathyroid hormone (PTH) is one example. Intact PTH is produced by cells in the parathyroid glands. There are four parathyroid glands present in the neck, generally in the vicinity of the thyroid gland. The term 'para-' means 'next to', so early anatomists identified the four glands 'parathyroid glands' because they were generally found 'next to' the thyroid gland in the neck. Parathyroid hormone is released in response to the cells of the parathyroid gland sensing a decline in the level of serum calcium. Parathyroid hormone, in its natural state, acts to stimulate osteoclast cells present in bone to release calcium from bone, thereby acting as a mechanism to return the serum calcium level to the normal range whenever the serum calcium drops below the normal range. On the other hand, it has been quite well demonstrated that if (1) the amino acid chain of the parathyroid hormone is shortened and (2) the shorter parathyroid hormone molecule is pulsed, by injecting it into the body once a day, the action of this modified parathyroid hormone molecule is opposite of the intact parathyroid hormone. One such form of a shorter length parathyroid hormone molecule is termed 'teriparatide'. Teriparatide (1-34) has the identical sequence from 1 to the 34th N-terminal amino acid of the 84-amino acid endogenous human parathyroid hormone. The skeletal effects of the modified protein molecule act on bone cells to preferentially cause osteoblastic activity over osteoclastic activity, which results in storage of calcium into bone, rather than a release of calcium from bone if the teriparatide is administered once a day. Teriparatide has been a recognized and widely used treatment of osteoporosis since at least as far back as the year 2000.

[0041] Modifying the 'coding region' of a messenger RNA will modify the protein the messenger RNA will produce when the ribosomes decode such a modified messenger RNA. As demonstrated by the case of modifying the naturally occurring parathyroid hormone by administering a molecule that is comprised of fewer amino acids than the original PTH molecule, modifying proteins the messenger RNAs produce may provide health care providers with an entirely new and widely spanning armamentarium of medically beneficial therapies.

[0042] The 5' untranslatable region of a messenger RNA molecule is used to identify the messenger RNA and utilized as a point of attachment by ribosomes to the messenger RNA molecule. Modifying the 5' untranslatable region by altering the nucleotide sequence in the 5' untranslatable region may make it easier to identify a modified messenger ribonucleic acid molecules in a fashion that the modified ribonucleic acid molecules can be engaged by ribosomes. Altering the nucleotide sequence of the 5' untranslatable region of a modified messenger ribonucleic acid molecule to create a unique identifier would facilitate ribosomes to preferentially engage the modified messenger ribonucleic acid molecule to preferentially produce the protein for which the modified messenger ribonucleic acid molecule is acting as a template.

BRIEF SUMMARY OF THE INVENTION

[0043] A modified virus is used as a transport medium to carry a payload of one or more modified messenger ribonucleic acid molecules. The modified virus is intended to make contact with a target Beta cell located in the Islets of Langerhans in the pancreas by means of the modified virus's exterior probes including one or more probes meant to engage GPR40 exterior cell-surface receptors on a Beta cell. Once the virus's exterior probes engage a target Beta cell's receptors, the modified virus inserts into the target cell one or more modified messenger ribonucleiç acid molecules it is carrying. A virus-like transport vehicle may be used in the place of a modified virus. Messenger RNA molecules act as a template for protein production. Ribosomes engage messenger RNA molecules to generate proteins. Medical disease states such as diabetes mellitus that are the result of a deficiency of one or more proteins can be successfully treated by utilizing viruses to insert the proper modified messenger RNA into specific cells to enhance the production of proteins that are identified as being deficient, thus correcting the deficiency. The deficiency of insulin production is a prime example of a medical condition that is capable of being corrected by utilizing a modified virus to transport modified messenger RNA molecules to assist ribosomes with the production of the pro-insulin molecule, the insulin molecule, the insulin receptor molecule, prohormone convertase one (PC1), prohormone convertase two (PC2), and/or carboxypeptidase E for the purpose of enhancing the Beta cells' production of the insulin molecule and/or the insulin receptor.

DETAILED DESCRIPTION

[0044] Diabetes mellitus is a medical condition often recognized when an individual's fasting blood glucose level is persistently higher than the generally accepted normal range of 60-110 mg/dl. An elevated blood glucose level may occur as the result of a lack of sufficient insulin; a lack of sufficient biologically effective insulin; a deficiency of the number of insulin receptors available to interact with insulin; a deficiency in the number of biologically active insulin receptors available to properly interact with insulin; insufficient release of insulin into the blood stream.

[0045] Insulin, a protein, is generated in Beta cells located in the Islets of Langerhans in the pancreas. Insulin is produced by decoding DNA through a process called transcription. Initially, transcription of the DNA produces a messenger ribonucleic acid (mRNA) molecule coded for the pro-insulin molecule. This mRNA coded for the 'pro-insulin' molecule, is then decoded by one or more ribosomes through a process called translation to produce a chain of amino acids that is referred to as the 'pro-insulin' molecule. The 'pro-insulin' molecule is modified by enzymes to produce the biologically active 'insulin' protein. Insulin molecules are stored in vacuoles in the Beta cells of the pancreas. Insulin is released from storage vacuoles in response to a rise in the level of glucose in the blood. Other proteins are manufactured in a similar fashion as pro-insulin and insulin.

[0046] Errors in the DNA or errors that occur in the process that generates the messenger RNA or a deficiency in the number of messenger RNA or a deficiency in the number of biologically active messenger RNA results in a deficiency of, or errors in the 'pro-insulin' molecule. Deficiencies in the biologically active enzymes intended to modify the 'pro-insulin' molecule to produce the biologically active insulin protein may result in deficiencies in adequate insulin production.

[0047] Correcting deficiencies or errors associated with the production of the protein insulin would correct diabetes mellitus, when diabetes mellitus is related to an insufficient quantity of biologically active insulin. Correcting deficiencies or errors associated with the production of insulin receptors would correct diabetes mellitus, when diabetes mellitus is related to an insufficient quantity of biologically active insulin receptors.

[0048] Naturally occurring messenger ribonucleic acids (mRNA) act as templates from which proteins are manufactured inside a cell. Modified messenger ribonucleic acid (mRNA) molecules would act similarly as templates from which proteins would be manufactured inside a cell. Ribosomal ribonucleic acids (rRNA) congregate with ribosomal proteins to produce a complex referred to as ribosome. Ribosomes would attach to a modified mRNA and then in conjunction with charged tRNAs, linear amino acid strings would be constructed to form proteins.

[0049] The Hepatitis C virus (HCV) is comprised of an outer lipid bilayer envelope and an internal nucleocapsid. The virus's genetic payload is carried within the nucleocapsid. The HCV's naturally occurring genetic payload consists of a single molecule of linear positive sense, single stranded RNA approximately 9600 nucleotides in length, which includes: the structural proteins of C, E1, E2, the nonstructural proteins NS1, NS2, NS3, NS4A, NS4B, NS5A, NS5B, p7 and ARFP/F protein. Present on the surface of the outer envelope of the Hepatitis C virus are probes that detect receptors present on the surface of liver cells. The glycoproteins E1 and E2 have been identified to be affixed to the surface of HCV. Portions of the Hepatitis C virus genome, when separated into individual pieces, behave like messenger RNA. Naturally occurring HCV is constructed with surface probes fashioned to recognize a receptor on the surface of a liver cell. Once the naturally occurring HCV's surface probe E2 engages a liver cell's CD81 receptor, and cofactors on the surface of HCV's exterior envelope engage the low density lipoprotein receptor (LDLR) or the scavenger receptor class B type I (SR-BI) on the liver cell, HCV then has the opportunity to insert its RNA genetic payload into the engaged target liver cell.

[0050] Replicating viruses and constructing viruses to carry DNA payloads is a form of manufacturing technology that has already been well established and is in use facilitating gene therapy. Replicating viruses and designing these viruses to carry one or more modified messenger ribonucleic acid molecules as the genetic payload would incorporate similar techniques as already proven useful in current gene therapy technologies.

[0051] To carry out the process to manufacture a modified medically therapeutic Hepatitis C virus, messenger RNA would be inserted into the host that would code for the general physical outer structures of the Hepatitis C virus. Messenger RNA would be inserted into the host that would generate surface probes that would target the surface receptors on Beta cells. Messenger RNA would be inserted into the host that would generate copies of the therapeutic modified messenger RNA that would take the place of the Hepatitis C virus's innate genome. Therapeutic modified mRNA that would act as the modified HCV's genome would encode for proteins that would include the pro-insulin molecule, the insulin molecule, the insulin receptor, the enzyme prohormone convertase one, the enzyme prohormone convertase two, the enzyme carboxypeptidase E. Similar to how copies of a naturally occurring Hepatitis C virus are produced, assembled and released from a host cell, copies of the modified medically therapeutic Hepatitis C virus would be produced, assembled and released from a host cell. The copies of the modified medically therapeutic Hepatitis C virus would be collected and utilized as a medical treatment.

[0052] To treat the various different forms of diabetes mellitus various combinations of messenger RNA molecules would be inserted into the host, and the host would produce copies of modified Hepatitis C virus that target Beta cells and carry a genetic payload consisting of modified messenger RNA molecules that would consist of one or more copies of a modified messenger RNA that codes for the insulin molecule, the insulin receptor, the enzyme prohormone convertase one, the enzyme prohormone convertase two, the enzyme carboxypeptidase E, and/or the insulin receptor. Depending upon the physical size of the modified messenger RNAs and the available space inside the modified Hepatitis C virus more than one type of modified messenger RNA may be packaged into a single modified Hepatitis C virus, which may produce more than one therapeutic action in a cell.

[0053] The modified Hepatitis C virus would be incapable of replication on its own due to the fact that the messenger RNA that a naturally occurring Hepatitis C virus would normally carry would not be present in the modified form of the Hepatitis C virus.

[0054] To treat diabetes, a quantity of modified Hepatitis C virus would be introduced into a patient's blood stream or tissues so that the modified virus could deliver the therapeutic genetic payload that it carries to Beta cells in the pancreas. When the probes on the surface of the modified Hepatitis C virus engage a cell-surface receptor or receptors on a Beta cell, the modified Hepatitis C virus will insert its therapeutic payload of modified messenger RNA molecules into the Beta cell to enhance the Beta cell's biologic function of producing insulin and/or insulin receptors.

[0055] An alternative means to treat diabetes might include the use of a quantity of virus-like transport vehicles. The virus-like transport vehicles would be comprised of a bilayer lipid envelope and a nucleocapsid inner shell, similar to the construction of a virus, and such virus-like transport vehicles would carry a payload consisting of modified messenger RNA molecules. Embedded in the virus-like transport vehicle's outer lipid bilayer surface envelope would be a quantity of probes that target cell-surface receptors on specific cells. The virus-like would be introduced into a patient's blood stream or tissues so that the virus-like transport vehicle could deliver the therapeutic genetic payload that it carries to Beta cells in the pancreas. When the probes on the surface of the virus-like transport vehicle engage a cell-surface receptor or receptors on a Beta cell located in the pancreas, the virus-like transport vehicle will insert its therapeutic payload of modified mRNA into the Beta cell to enhance the Beta cell's biologic function of producing insulin and/or insulin receptors.

[0056] RNAs are generally degraded by enzymes known as ribonucleases or RNAases. Ribonucleases act to inactive the

RNA molecules. Different RNAs are known to have different half-lives.

[0057] Messenger RNA molecules are comprised of three regions (or segments). These three regions include a (1) 5' untranslatable region, (2) a coding region and (3) a 3' untranslatable region. The '5' untranslatable region' acts as the initiation point for a ribosome to attach to the mRNA. The 'coding region' acts as the template from which a protein is constructed. An 'untranslatable region' represents a segment of a messenger RNA molecule that does not code for a protein and is not used to yield a protein and therefore 'translation' does not occur in such a region. The 3' untranslatable region is associated with the degradation of the usefulness of the mRNA. Different mRNAs have different service life expectancies. The half-life of the naturally occurring mRNA that acts as the template responsible for the production of the protein 'glucokinase' is two hours. The half-life of the naturally occurring mRNA that produces the protein 'alcohol dehydrogenase' is ten hours. The half-life of the naturally occurring mRNA that produces the protein 'glucuronidase' is thirty hours. By modifying the nucleotides that comprise the 3' untranslatable unit of an mRNA the service half life of the mRNA may be altered to be lengthened or shortened depending upon the need for the quantity of protein and timeframe over which the mRNA is required to produce the protein coded in the mRNA's protein coding region.

[0058] Modifying the 'coding region' of a messenger RNA will modify the protein the messenger RNA will produce when the ribosomes decode such a modified messenger RNA. As demonstrated by the case of modifying the naturally occurring parathyroid hormone by administering a molecule that is comprised of fewer amino acids than the original PTH molecule, modifying proteins the messenger RNAs produce will provide health care providers with an entirely new and widely spanning armamentarium of medically beneficial therapies.

[0059] The action of altering the type of probe or probes present on the surface of the modified virus, the modified Hepatitis C virus, or the virus-like transport vehicle would change the target the modified virus or virus-like transport vehicle would seek. By changing the probes on the surface of the modified virus, the modified Hepatitis C virus, or the virus-like transport vehicle the payload carried by the modified virus, the modified Hepatitis C virus, or the virus-like transport vehicle could be delivered to any cell that carried on its surface a cell-surface receptor that would engage the probes the modified virus, the modified Hepatitis C virus, or the virus-like transport vehicle was carrying on its surface. In this fashion, specific payloads could be delivered to specific cells throughout the body.

[0060] By providing Beta cells with the above-mentioned modified messenger RNAs, the capacity of Beta cells to carrying out the biologic processes of producing insulin and recognizing and responding to blood glucose levels is enhanced, which results in an efficient means to control the glucose levels in the blood stream on a constant and persistent basis utilizing innate regulatory mechanisms and thus diabetes mellitus can be effectively treated and the harmful effects of this disease can be averted.

[0061] By providing any target cell with medically therapeutic modified messenger RNAs to enhance a cell's capacity to produce one or more proteins, any protein deficiency can be effectively treated and the harmful effects of the protein deficiency can be averted.

CLAIMS: Reserved.

No. 5: ADAPTABLE MODIFIED VIRUS VECTOR TO DE-
LIVER RIBOSOMAL RIBONUCLEIC ACID AS A MEDICAL
TREATMENT DEVICE TO MANAGE DIABETES MELLITUS
AND OTHER PROTEIN DEFICIENT DISEASES

INDIVIDUALS REQUESTING PATENT: Dr. Lane B. Scheiber
II, MD and Dr. Lane B. Scheiber, ScD

©2009 Lane B. Scheiber II and Lane B. Scheiber. A portion
of the disclosure of this patent document contains material
which is subject to copyright protection. The copyright owners
have no objection to the facsimile reproduction by anyone of
the patent document or the patent disclosure, as it appears
in the Patent and Trademark Office patent file or records, but
otherwise reserves all copyright rights whatsoever.

ABSTRACT

Diabetes mellitus is a disease of elevated blood glucose, often
directly related to a deficiency in insulin production or insulin
receptor production. The innovative strategy of treatment
described here utilizes modified viruses and virus-like vehicles
to act as a transport mechanism to deliver ribosomal RNA
molecules to target cells in the body. Delivering to the Beta cells
in the body the ribosomal RNA needed to assist ribosomes
with the construction of insulin or insulin receptors will lead
to enhanced production of biologically active insulin or insulin
receptors by Beta cells as necessary, which will lead to correcting
deficiencies in insulin or insulin receptors, the result of which
will help properly regulate blood glucose levels throughout the
body utilizing innate cellular regulatory mechanisms.

BACKGROUND OF THE INVENTION

Field of the Invention

This invention relates to any medical device intended to correct
a protein deficiency in the body by increasing the intracellular

production of the deficient protein by utilizing a modified virus to insert one or more ribosomal ribonucleic acid molecules into one or more cells of the body.

Description of Background Art

[0001] For purposes of this text there are several general definitions. A 'ribose' is a five carbon or pentose sugar ($C_5H_{10}O_5$) present in the structural components of ribonucleic acid, riboflavin, and other nucleotides and nucleosides. A 'deoxyribose' is a deoxypentose ($C_5H_{10}O_4$) found in deoxyribonucleic acid. A 'nucleoside' is a compound of a sugar usually ribose or deoxyribose with a nitrogenous base by way of an N-glycosyl link. A 'nucleotide' is a single unit of a nucleic acid, composed of a five carbon sugar (either a ribose or a deoxyribose), a nitrogenous base and a phosphate group. There are two families of 'nitrogenous bases', which include pyrimidine and purine. A 'pyrimidine' is a six member ring made up of carbon and nitrogen atoms, the members of the pyrimidine family include: cytosine (C), thymine (T) and uracil (U). A 'purine' is a five-member ring fused to a pyrimidine type ring; the members of the purine family include: adenine (A) and guanine (G). A 'nucleic acid' is a polynucleotide which is a biologic molecule such as ribonucleic acid or deoxyribonucleic acid that allow organisms to reproduce. A 'ribonucleic acid' (RNA) is a linear polymer of nucleotides formed by repeated riboses linked by phosphodiester bonds between the 3-hydroxyl group of one and the 5-hydroxyl group of the next; RNAs are a single strand macromolecule comprised of a sequence of nucleotides, these nucleotides generally referred to by their nitrogenous bases, which include: adenine, cytosine, guanine or uracil. RNAs are subset into different types which include messenger RNA (mRNA), transport RNA (tRNA), and ribosomal RNA (rRNA). Messenger RNAs act as templates to produce proteins. A ribosome is a complex comprised of RNAs and proteins and is responsible for the correct positioning of mRNA and charged tRNA to facilitate the proper alignment and bonding of amino acids into a strand to produce a protein. A 'charged' tRNA is a tRNA that is carrying an amino acid. Ribosomal RNA (rRNA) represents a subset of RNAs that form part of the physical structure of a ribosome.

[0002] Diabetes mellitus represents an important health issue that affects a significant portion of the world population. In the United States, about 16 million people suffer from diabetes mellitus. Every year, about 650,000 additional people are diagnosed with this disease. Diabetes mellitus is the seventh leading cause of all deaths.

[0003] Diabetes mellitus represents a state of hyperglycemia, a serum blood sugar that is higher than what is considered the normal range for humans. Glucose, a six-carbon molecule, is a form of sugar. Glucose is absorbed by the cells of the body and converted to energy by the processes of glycolysis, the Krebs cycle and phosporylation. Insulin, a protein, facilitates the transfer of glucose from the blood into cells. Normal range for blood glucose in humans is generally defined as a fasting blood plasma glucose level of between 70 to 110 mg/dl. For descriptive purposes, the term 'plasma' refers to the fluid portion of blood.

[0004] Diabetes mellitus is classified as Type One and Type Two. Type One diabetes mellitus is insulin dependent, which refers to the condition where there is a lack of sufficient insulin circulating in the blood stream and insulin must be provided to the body in order to properly regulate the blood glucose level. When insulin is required to regulate the blood glucose level in the body, this condition is often referred to as insulin dependent diabetes mellitus (IDDM). Type Two diabetes mellitus is noninsulin dependent, often referred to as noninsulin dependent diabetes mellitus (NIDDM), meaning the blood glucose level can be managed without insulin, and instead by means of diet, exercise or intervention with oral medications. Type Two diabetes mellitus is considered a progressive disease, the underlying pathogenic mechanisms including pancreatic Beta cell (also often designated as β-Cell) dysfunction and insulin resistance.

[0005] The pancreas serves as an endocrine gland and an exocrine gland. Functioning as an endocrine gland the pancreas produces and secretes hormones including insulin and glucagon. Insulin acts to reduce levels of glucose circulating in the blood. Beta cells secrete insulin into the blood when a higher than normal level of glucose is detected in the serum. For purposes of this description the terms 'blood', 'blood stream' and 'serum' refer to the same substance. Glucagon acts to stimulate an increase in glucose circulating in the blood. Beta cells in the pancreas secrete glucagon when a low level of glucose is detected in the serum.

[0006] Glucose enters the body and then the blood stream as a result of the digestion of food. The Beta cells of the Islets of Langerhans continuously sense the level of glucose in the blood and respond to elevated levels of blood glucose by secreting insulin into the blood. Beta cells produce the protein 'insulin' in their endoplasmic reticulum and store the insulin in vacuoles until it is needed. When Beta cells detect an increase in the glucose level in the blood, Beta cells release insulin into the blood from the described storage vacuoles.

[0007] Insulin is a protein. An insulin protein consists of two chains of amino acids, an alpha chain and a beta chain, linked by two disulfide (S-S) bridges. One chain, the alpha chain consists of 21 amino acids. The second chain, the beta chain consists of 30 amino acids.

[0008] Insulin interacts with the cells of the body by means of a cell-surface receptor termed the 'insulin receptor' located on the exterior of a cell's 'outer membrane', otherwise known as the 'plasma membrane'. Insulin interacts with muscle and liver cells by means of the insulin receptor to rapidly remove excess blood sugar when the glucose level in the blood is higher than the upper limit of the normal physiologic range. Recognized functions of insulin include stimulating cells to take up glucose from the blood and convert it to glycogen to facilitate the cells in the body to utilize glucose to generate biochemically usable energy, and to stimulate fat cells to take up glucose and synthesize fat.

[0009] Diabetes Mellitus may be the result of one or more factors. Causes of diabetes mellitus may include: (1) mutation of the insulin gene itself causing miscoding, which results in the production of ineffective insulin molecules; (2) mutations to genes that code for the 'transcription factors' needed for transcription of the insulin gene in the deoxyribonucleic acid (DNA) to create messenger ribonucleic acid (mRNA) molecules, which facilitate the manufacture of the insulin molecule; (3) mutations of the gene encoding for the insulin receptor, which produces inactive or an insufficient number of insulin receptors; (4) mutation to the gene encoding for glucokinase, the enzyme that phosphorylates glucose in the first step of glycolysis; (5) mutations to the genes encoding portions of the potassium channels in the plasma membrane of the Beta cells, preventing proper closure of the channel, thus blocking insulin release; (6) mutations to mitochondrial genes that as a result, decreases the energy available to be used facilitate the release of insulin, therefore reducing insulin secretion; (7) failure of glucose transporters to properly permit the facilitated diffusion of glucose from plasma into the cells of the body.

[0010] The term 'eukaryote' refers to a nucleated cell. Eukaryotes comprise nearly all animal and plant cells. A human eukaryote or nucleated cell is comprised of an exterior lipid bilayer plasma membrane, cytoplasm, a nucleus, and organelles. The exterior plasma membrane defines the perimeter of the cell, regulates the flow of nutrients, water and regulating molecules in and out of the cell, and has embedded into its structure receptors that the cell uses to detect properties of the environment surrounding the cell membrane. The cytoplasm acts as a filling medium inside the boundaries of the plasma cell membrane and is comprised mainly of water and nutrients such as amino acids, oxygen, and glucose. The nucleus, organelles, and ribosomes are suspended in the cytoplasm. The nucleus contains the majority of the cell's genetic information in the form of double stranded deoxyribonucleic acid (DNA). Organelles generally carry out specialized functions for the cell and include such structures as the mitochondria, the endoplasmic reticulum, storage vacuoles, lysosomes and Golgi complex (sometimes referred to as the Golgi apparatus). Floating in the cytoplasm, but also located in the endoplasmic reticulum and mitochondria are ribosomes. Ribosomes are complex macromolecule structures comprised of ribosomal ribonucleic acid (rRNA) molecules and ribosomal proteins that combine and couple to a messenger ribonucleic acid (mRNA) molecule. The rRNAs and the ribosomal proteins congregate to form a macromolecule structure that surrounds a mRNA molecule. Ribosomes decode genetic information in a mRNA molecule and manufacture proteins to the specifications of the instruction code physically present in the mRNA molecule. More than one ribosome may be attached to a single mRNA at a time.

[0011] The majority of the deoxyribonucleic acid (DNA) comprises the chromosomes, double stranded helical structures located in the nucleus of the cell. DNA in a circular form, can also be found in the mitochondria, the powerhouse of the cell, an organelle that assists in converting glucose into usable energy molecules. DNA represents the genetic information a cell needs to manufacture the materials it requires to sustain life and to replicate. Genetic information is stored in the DNA by arrangements of four nucleotides referred to as: adenine, thymine, guanine and cytosine. DNA represents instruction coding, that in the process known as transcription, the DNA's genetic information is decoded by transcription protein complexes referred to as polymerases (or polymerase complex), to produce ribonucleic acid (RNA). RNA is a single strand of genetic information comprised of coded arrangements of four nucleotides: adenine, uracil, guanine and cytosine. In a RNA, 'uracil' takes the place of 'thymine', thymine being present in the DNA. Several different types of RNAs have been identified, which include messenger RNAs (mRNA), transport RNAs (tRNA) and ribosomal RNAs (rRNA).

[0012] Proteins are comprised of a series of amino acids bonded together in a linear strand, sometimes referred to as a chain; a protein may be further modified to be a structure comprised of one or more similar or differing strands of amino acids bonded together. Insulin is a protein structure comprised of two strands of amino acids, one strand comprised of 21 amino acids long and the second strand comprised of 30 amino acids, the two strands attached by two disulfide bridges. There are an estimated 30,000 different proteins the cells of the human body may manufacture. The human body is comprised of a wide variety of cells, many with specialized functions requiring unique combinations of proteins and protein structures such as glycoproteins (a protein combined with a carbohydrate) to accomplish the required task or tasks a specialized cell is designed to perform. Forms of glycoproteins are known to be utilized as cell-surface receptors. Messenger RNAs (mRNA) are created by transcription of DNA; they generally migrate to other locations inside the cell and are utilized by ribosomes as protein manufacturing templates. A ribosome is a protein macromolecule complex that manufactures proteins by deciphering the instruction code located in a mRNA molecule. When a specific protein is needed, pieces of the ribosome complex, which include rRNA molecules and ribosomal proteins, bind around the strand of a mRNA that carries the specific instruction code that will generate the required protein. The ribosome traverses the mRNA strand and deciphers the genetic information coded into the sequence of nucleotides that comprise the mRNA molecule to produce a protein molecule and this process is referred to as translation.

[0013] A ribosome is complex macromolecule comprised of ribosomal RNA (rRNA) molecules and ribosomal proteins. Ribosomal RNAs and ribosomal proteins are often designated with a number measured in Svedberg (S) units, which represents the sediment coefficient. The sediment coefficient is influenced by both molecular weight of the molecule and surface area of the molecule. In humans there are generally recognized at this time two mitochondrial rRNAs identified as 12S rRNA and 16S rRNA, and there are generally recognized four rRNAs that reside in the cytoplasm of a cell identified as 5S rRNA, 5.8S rRNA, 18S rRNA and 28S rRNA. There may be other rRNAs, as of yet unidentified, that reside in some of the other structures in the cell that engage in manufacturing of macromolecules, such as the smooth endoplasmic reticulum, the rough endoplasmic reticulum and the Golgi complex.

[0014] In eukaryotes, in the cytoplasm, the ribosome complex is referred to as an 80S ribosome. Generally two ribosomal proteins comprise a ribosome complex. This 80S ribosome is comprised of one 'dome-shape' 60S ribosomal protein and one 'cap-shaped' 40S ribosomal protein.

[0015] In the forms of life referred to as vertebrates (Humans are classified as a form of vertebrate), of the four rRNAs that reside in the cytoplasm of a eukaryote cell, the 18S rRNA is found in and helps comprise the physical structure of the 40S protein subunit of the ribosome complex and the 5S rRNA, 5.8S rRNA, and 28S rRNA molecules are found in and help comprise the physical structure of the 60S protein subunit of the ribosome complex.

[0016] The rRNA molecules are thought provide at least three different functions for the ribosome complex. The rRNA molecules are thought to: (1) assist with identification of the messenger RNA to be translated, (2) act as an enzyme to facilitate the production of the protein molecule being translated from the mRNA molecule undergoing translation, (3) possibly

344

cause folding at certain locations in the three dimensional structure of the protein being generated as the ribosome complex decodes the mRNA molecule.

[0017] Ribosomal RNAs (rRNA) are generated by polymerase molecules deciphering the instruction code present in the DNA. The rRNAs generally migrate to locations where mRNAs are to be utilized as templates. The rRNA molecules connect to their respective ribosome proteins and this macromolecule complex, referred to as a ribosome or ribosome complex, surrounds the beginning segment of a mRNA molecule. Utilizing inherent coding, the rRNA molecules direct the ribosome pieces to build the ribosome complex around a particular strand of mRNA or particular type of mRNA. The 'inherent coding' the rRNA molecules harbor is a sequence of nucleotides which represent a unique 'name', unique 'base-four number' or unique 'combination of a name and base-four number' that corresponds to a particular mRNA or particular type of mRNA. In this manner, rRNAs act to control which mRNA molecule will undergo translation to produce proteins, rather than a ribosome complex randomly engaging any mRNA template that happens to be available. With the DNA producing rRNA molecules that cause a ribosome to attach to a particular mRNA molecule or particular type of mRNA molecule, the DNA is able to exert control over the manufacturing capacity of the cell and produce proteins as needed, rather than producing proteins in a random fashion. Producing proteins as needed by the cell, rather than in a random fashion, conserves valuable resources and conserves energy inside the cell.

[0018] RNAs are generally degraded by enzymes known as ribonucleases or RNAases. Ribonucleases act to inactive the RNA molecules. Different RNAs have different half-lives. The nucleotide sequencing of the rRNA molecule could be altered from that of the naturally occurring molecule to lengthen or shorten the service half-life of the native rRNA. Lengthening the service life of rRNA molecules such that the rRNAs could combine with ribosomal proteins to participate in ribosomes over a longer than the naturally occurring period of time would be especially useful in diabetic patients to facilitate a greater production of insulin molecules in the Beta cells.

[0019] The rate of degradation of rRNA molecules by ribonucleases could be varied by changing the nucleotide sequence of the rRNA molecule or by altering the folding characteristics of the rRNA molecule or by altering both the nucleotide sequence and the folding characteristics of the rRNA molecule. By making changes to the nucleotide sequence and/or the folding characteristics of the rRNA molecules the rate of degradation of the rRNA molecules by ribonucleases could be caused to vary in length of time from seconds to minutes to hours to days to weeks to months to years.

[0020] Transport RNAs (tRNA) are constructed in the nucleus or in the mitochondria, and are coded for one of the 20 amino acids the cells of the human body use to construct proteins. Once a tRNA is created by transcription of the DNA, the tRNA seeks out the type of amino acid it has been coded for and attaches to that specific amino acid. A tRNA molecule is considered to be 'charged' when it is carrying an amino acid. The charged tRNA delivers the amino acid it carries to a ribosome that is waiting for the specific amino acid the tRNA is carrying. Proteins are manufactured by the ribosomes binding together sequences of amino acids. The order by which the amino acids are bonded together is dictated by the way the sequencing of the nucleotides comprising the mRNA is constructed and how the ribosome interprets the information encoded in the string of nucleotides present in the mRNA strand.

[0021] Messenger RNA molecules are divided into three regions (or segments). The three regions include: (1) the 5' untranslatable region, (2) the coding region, and (3) the 3' untranslatable region. The '5' untranslatable region' acts as the initiation point for a ribosome to attach to the mRNA. The 'coding region' acts as the template from which a protein is constructed. The '3' untranslatable region' is associated with the degradation of the usefulness of the mRNA. An 'untranslatable region' represents a segment of a messenger RNA molecule that does not code for a protein and is not used to yield a protein and therefore 'translation' does not occur in such a region. Different mRNAs have different service life expectancies. The half-life of the mRNA that acts as the template that is responsible for the production of the protein 'glucokinase' is two hours. The half-life of the mRNA that produces the protein 'alcohol dehydrogenase' is ten hours. The half-life of the mRNA that produces the protein 'glucuronidase' is thirty hours. By modifying the nucleotides that comprise the 3' untranslatable unit of an mRNA the service half-life of the mRNA may be altered to be lengthened or shortened.

[0022] The coding region is the portion of the mRNA that is decoded by the ribosomes to produce a particular protein molecule by the process known as translation. A sequence of three nucleotides present in the coding region of a mRNA molecule represents a unit of information referred to as a codon. Codons code for all of the 20 amino acids used to construct protein molecules and also for START and STOP commands. In the process known as translation, the ribosome decodes the codons present in the coding region of the mRNA, initiating the protein manufacturing process at a START codon, then interfacing with tRNAs carrying the amino acids that match the sequence of codons in the mRNA as the ribosome traverses the length of the coding region of the mRNA molecule. The ribosome functions as a protein factory by taking amino acids delivered by charged tRNAs and binding the amino acids together in the order dictated by the sequence of codon instructions coded into the mRNA template as directed by the manner of the nucleic acid arrangement in the mRNA molecule. Protein synthesis ceases when a ribosome encounters a STOP code. The protein molecule is then released by the ribosome. Ribosomes do not decode the nucleotide sequences to produce proteins in a mRNA's 5' untranslatable region or a mRNA's 3' untranslatable region.

[0023] The insulin molecule is a protein produced by Beta cells located in the pancreas. The 'insulin messenger RNA' is created in a Beta cell by a polymerase complex transcribing the insulin gene from nuclear DNA in the nucleus of the cell. The native messenger RNA (mRNA) for insulin then travels to the endoplasmic reticulum, where numerous ribosomes, comprised of rRNA and ribosomal proteins, engage these mRNA molecules. Many ribosomes may be attached to a single strand of mRNA simultaneously, each generating an identical copy of the protein as dictated by the information encoded in the mRNA. Insulin is produced by ribosomes translating the information in a mRNA molecule coded for the insulin protein, which produce strands of amino acids that are coded for an immature form of the biologically active insulin molecule referred to as 'pro-insulin'. Once the pro-insulin molecule is generated it then undergoes modification by several enzymes including prohormone convertase one (PC1), prohormone convertase two (PC2) and carboxypeptidase E, which results in the production of a biologically active insulin molecule. Once the biologically active insulin protein is generated it is stored in a vacuole in the Beta cell to await being released into the blood stream.

[0024] Insulin receptors, which appear on the surface of cells, offer binding sites for insulin circulating in the blood. When insulin binds to an insulin receptor, the biologic response inside the cell causes glucose to enter the cell and undergo processing in the cytoplasm. Processed glucose molecules then enter the mitochondria. The mitochondria further process the modified glucose molecules to produce usable energy in the form of adenosine triphosphate molecules (ATP). Thirty-eight ATP molecules may be generated from one molecule of glucose during the process of aerobic respiration. ATP molecules are utilized as an energy source by biologic processes throughout the cell.

[0025] The current medical therapeutic approach to the management of diabetes mellitus has produced limited results. Patients with diabetes generally struggle with an inadequate production of insulin, or an ineffective release of biologically active insulin molecules, or a release of an insufficient number of biologically active insulin molecules, or an insufficient production of cell-surface receptors, or a production of ineffective cell-surface receptors, or a production of ineffective insulin molecules that are unable to interact properly with insulin receptors to produce the required biologic effect. Type One diabetes requires administration of exogenous insulin. The traditional approach to Type Two diabetes has generally first been to adjust the diet to limit the caloric intake the individual consumes. Exercise is used as an initial approach to both Type One and Type Two diabetes as a means of up-regulating the utilization of fats and sugar so as to reduce the amount of circulating plasma glucose. When diet and exercise are inadequate in properly managing Type Two diabetes, oral medications are often introduced. The action of sulfonylureas, a commonly prescribed class of oral medication, is to stimulate the Beta cells to produce additional insulin receptors and enhance the insulin receptors' response to insulin. Biguanides, another form of oral treatment, inhibit gluconeogenesis, the production of glucose in the liver, thereby attempting to reduce plasma glucose levels. Thiazolidinediones (TZDs) lower blood sugar levels by activating peroxisome proliferator-activated receptor gamma (PPAR-γ), a transcription factor, which when activated regulates the activity of various target genes, particularly ones involved in glucose and lipid metabolism. If diet, exercise and oral medications do not produce a satisfactory control of the level of blood glucose in a diabetic patient, exogenous insulin is injected into the body in an effort to normalize the amount of glucose present in the serum. Insulin, a protein, has not successfully been made available as an oral medication to date due to the fact that proteins in general become degraded when they encounter the acid environment present in the stomach.

[0026] Despite strict monitoring of blood glucose and potentially multiple doses of insulin injected throughout the day, many patients with diabetes mellitus still experience devastating adverse effects from elevated blood glucose levels. Microvascular damage and elevated tissue sugar levels contribute to such complications as renal failure, retinopathy involving the eyes, neuropathy, and accelerated heart disease despite aggressive efforts to maintain the blood sugar within the physiologic normal range using exogenous insulin by itself or a combination of exogenous insulin and one or more oral medications. Diabetes remains the number one cause of renal failure in the United States. Especially in diabetic patients that are dependent upon administering exogenous insulin into their body, though dosing of the insulin may be four or more times a day and even though this may produce adequate control of the blood glucose level to prevent the clinical symptoms of hyperglycemia; this does not unerringly supplement the body's natural capacity to monitor the blood sugar level minute to minute, twenty-four hours a day, and deliver an immediate response to a rise in blood glucose by the release of insulin from Beta cells as required. The deleterious effects of diabetes may still evolve despite strict and persistent control of the glucose level in the blood stream.

[0027] The current treatment of diabetes may be augmented by the unique approach to utilizing modified viruses as vehicles to transport ribosomal ribonucleic acid (rRNA) molecules to facilitate the assembly of ribosomes that will attach to messenger ribonucleic acid (mRNA) molecules coded to facilitate the manufacture of pro-insulin and insulin and the enzymes utilized to modify proinsulin to the biologically active insulin molecule, and messenger ribonucleic acids (mRNA) coded to manufacture insulin receptors.

[0028] Viruses are obligate parasites. Viruses simply represent a carrier of genetic material and by themselves viruses are unable to replicate or carry out any form of biologic function outside their host cell. Viruses are generally comprised of one or more nested shells constructed of one or more layers of protein or lipid material, a genetic payload that represents the instruction code necessary to replicate the virus, and protein enzymes to help facilitate the genetic payload in the function of replicating copies of the virus once the genetic payload has been delivered to a host cell. Located on the outer shell or envelope of a virus are probes. The function of a virus's probes is to locate and engage a host cell's receptors. The virus's surface probes are designed to detect, make contact with and functionally engage one or more receptors located on the exterior of a cell type that will offer the virus the proper environment in which to construct copies of itself. A host cell provides the virus the proper biochemical machinery for the virus to successfully replicate itself.

0029] Protected by an outer protein coat or lipid envelope, viruses carry a genetic payload in the form of deoxyribonucleic acid (DNA) or ribonucleic acid (RNA). Once a virus's exterior probes locate and functionally engage the surface receptor or receptors on a host cell, the virus inserts its genetic payload into the interior of the host cell. In the event a virus is carrying a DNA payload, the virus's DNA travels to the host cell's nucleus and is known to become inserted into the host cell's own native DNA. In the case where a virus is carrying its genetic payload as RNA, the virus inserts the RNA payload into the host cell and may also insert one or more enzymes to facilitate the RNA being utilized properly to replicate copies of the virus. Once inside the host cell, some species of virus facilitate use of their RNA by having the RNA converted to DNA. Once the viral RNA has been converted to DNA, the virus's DNA travels to the host cell's nucleus and is known to become inserted into the host cell's native DNA. Once a virus's genetic material has been inserted into the host cell's native DNA, the virus's genetic material takes command of certain cell functions and redirects the resources of the host cell to generate copies of the virus. Other forms of RNA viruses bypass the need to use the nuclear DNA and simply utilize portions of the viral genome to act as messenger RNA (mRNA). RNA viruses that bypass the host cell's DNA, cause the cell to in general generate copies of the necessary parts of the virus directly from the virus's RNA genome.

[0030] The Hepatitis C virus (HCV) is a positive sense RNA virus, meaning HCV's genome is a type of RNA that is capable of bypassing the need for involving the host cell's nucleus by having its RNA genome function as messenger RNA. The Hepatitis C virus infects liver cells. The Hepatitis C viral genome becomes divided once it gains access to the interior of a liver host cell. Portions of the subdivisions of the Hepatitis C viral genome directly interact with ribosomes to produce proteins necessary to construct copies of the virus.

[0031] HCV belongs to the Flaviviridae family and is the only member of the Hepacivirus genus. There are considered to be at least 100 different strains of Hepatitis C virus based on genome sequencing variability.

[0032] HCV is comprised of an outer lipoprotein envelope and an internal nucleocapsid. The genetic payload is carried within the nucleocapsid. In its natural state, present on the surface of the outer envelope of the Hepatitis C virus are probes that detect receptors present on the surface of liver cells. The glycoprotein E1 probe and the glycoprotein E2 probe have been identified to be affixed to the surface of HCV. The E2 probe binds with high affinity to the large external loop of a CD81 cell-surface receptor. CD81 is found on the surface of many cell types including liver cells. Once the E2 probe has engaged the CD81 cell-surface receptor, cofactors on the surface of HCV's exterior envelope engage either or both the low density lipoprotein receptor (LDLR) or the scavenger receptor class B type I (SR-

BI) present on the liver cell in order to effect the mechanism to facilitate HCV breaching the cell membrane and inserting its viral RNA genome payload through the plasma cell membrane of the liver cell, thus delivering the HCV RNA genome into the liver cell. Upon successful engagement of the HCV surface probes with a liver cell's cell-surface receptors, HCV inserts the single strand of RNA and other payload elements it carries into the liver cell targeted to be a host cell. The HCV RNA genome then interacts with enzymes and ribosomes inside the liver cell in a translational process to produce the proteins required to construct copies of the protein components of HCV. The HCV genome undergoes a method of transcription to replicate copies of the virus's RNA genome. Inside the host, pieces of the HCV virus are assembled together and ultimately loaded with a copy of the HCV genome. Replicas of the original HCV then escape the host cell and migrate the environment in search of additional host liver cells to infect and continue the replication process.

[0033] HCV's naturally occurring genetic payload consists of a single molecule of linear positive sense, single stranded RNA approximately 9600 nucleotides in length. By means of a translational process a polyprotein of approximately 3000 amino acids is generated. This polyprotein is cleaved post translation by host and viral proteases into individual viral proteins which include: the structural proteins of C, E1, E2, the nonstructural proteins NS1, NS2, NS3, NS4A, NS4B, NS5A, NS5B, p7 and ARFP/F protein. Hepatitis C virus's proteins direct the host liver cell to construction copies of the Hepatitis C virus. A membrane associated replicase complex consisting of the virus's nonstructural proteins NS3 and NS5B facilitate the replication of the viral genome. The membrane of the endoplasmic reticulum appears to be the site of protein maturation and viral assembly. Once copies of the Hepatitis C Virus are generated, they exit the host cell and each copy of HCV migrates in search of another appropriate liver cell that will act as a host to continue the replication process.

[0034] A modified Hepatitis C virus offers a naturally occurring vehicle mechanism to transport and insert medically therapeutic ribosomal ribonucleic acid (rRNA) molecules into specific targeted cells of the human body. The surface probes present on the Hepatitis C virus's outer protein coat can be modified to seek out specific receptors on specific target cells. Once the modified Hepatitis C virus's probes properly engage the cell-surface receptors on a target cell, the modified Hepatitis C virus would insert into the target cell one or more medically therapeutic ribosomal ribonucleic acid (rRNA) molecules for the purpose of having the target cell generate proteins to achieve a medically therapeutic response.

[0035] Current state of gene therapy generally refers to efforts directed toward inserting an exogenous subunit of DNA into a vehicle such as a naturally occurring virus. The vehicle is intended to insert the exogenous subunit of DNA into a cell the virus naturally targets. The exogenous DNA subunit then migrates to the target cell's nucleus. The exogenous DNA subunit then inserts into the native DNA of the cell. This represents a permanent alteration of the cell's nuclear DNA. The nuclear transcription proteins then read the exogenous DNA subunit's nucleotide coding to produce the intended cellular response. The approach described hereunder involves RNA versus DNA. DNA is comprised of the nucleotides adenine, thymine, guanine and cytosine. RNA is composed of the nucleotides: adenine, uracil, guanine and cytosine. DNA codes for the manufacture of RNAs, which are composed of nucleotides. RNAs facilitate the manufacture of proteins, which are composed of amino acids. The virus chosen as the transport vehicle, Hepatitis C virus, is a RNA virus versus a virus that naturally carries a DNA genome.

[0036] Beta cells located in the Islets of Langerhans in the pancreas are thought to have at least one unique identifying surface receptor. The exterior receptor GPR40 appears specific to Beta cells located in the Islets of Langerhans in the pancreas.

A virus equipped with a surface probe designed to engage the GPR40 Beta cell receptor, could travel the blood stream of the body until it locates a GPR40 receptor on a Beta cell, engage the receptor with its surface probe, and then insert the genetic payload it carries into the Beta cell. A genetic payload of one or more ribosomal RNAs could be used to enhance proper protein production by cells deficient in a particular protein. Hormones are proteins that circulate the body and stimulate biologic activity specific to the hormone's role. In the case of a deficiency of a hormone, production of a deficient hormone could be enhanced by inserting one or more ribosomal RNAs into specific target cells in the body to stimulate production of the required hormone. In the case of diabetes mellitus, utilizing a modified Hepatitis C virus as a vehicle, ribosomal RNA molecules could be inserted into Beta cells, to assist the individual's Beta cells are with generating an adequate insulin production and adequate release of insulin into the blood to meet the body's needs.

[0037] Viruses are constructed in a number of ways and shapes. The shape of a virus may be rod or filament like, icosahedral, or complex structures combining filament and polygonal shapes. Viruses may have an outer protein coat or an outer envelope comprised of lipids. Icosahedral viruses with an outer lipid envelope appear spherical in shape. An outer envelope is often comprised of two lipid layers often termed a lipid bilayer. Spherical viruses may be in the form of being comprised of an outer envelope and one inner shell or an outer envelope and two inner shells. In the case of a spherical virus with an outer envelope and one inner shell, the inner shell is often referred to as a nucleocapsid shell comprised of capsid proteins. In the case of a spherical virus being comprised of an outer envelope and two inner shells, the outer most inner viral shell may be referred to as comprised of matrix proteins, the innermost of the two shells being referred to as a nucleocapsid shell being comprised of capsid proteins. The inner protein shell is nested inside the outer protein shell.

[0038] An alternative means to treat diabetes might include the use of a quantity of virus-like transport vehicles. The virus-like transport vehicles would be spherical in shape. The virus-like transport vehicles would be comprised of a lipid bilayer envelope and one or more inner nested protein shells, depending upon the size of the payload. Nesting of protein shells refers to progressively smaller diameter shells fitting snugly inside protein shells of a larger diameter. The virus-like transport vehicles would be similar in construction to viruses, and such virus-like transport vehicles would carry a payload consisting of ribosomal RNA molecules. The size of the virus-like transport vehicle would depend upon the payload the virus-like transport vehicle would be required to carry. Embedded in the virus-like transport vehicle's outer lipid bilayer surface would be a quantity of probes that are intended to target cell-surface receptors on specific cells. The virus-like transport vehicle would be introduced into a patient's blood stream or tissues so that the virus-like transport vehicle could deliver the therapeutic genetic payload that it carries to Beta cells in the pancreas. When one or more probes on the surface of the virus-like transport vehicle engage one or more cell-surface receptors on a Beta cell located in the pancreas, the virus-like transport vehicle will insert its therapeutic payload of ribosomal RNA into the Beta cell to enhance the Beta cell's biologic function of producing insulin and/or insulin receptors.

[0039] The action of altering the type of probe or probes present on the surface of the modified virus, the modified Hepatitis C virus, or the virus-like transport vehicle would change the target the modified virus or virus-like transport vehicle would seek out. By changing the probe on the surface of the modified virus, the modified Hepatitis C virus, or the virus-like transport vehicle, the payload carried by the modified virus, the modified Hepatitis C virus, or the virus-like transport vehicle could be delivered to any cell that carried on its surface a cell-surface receptor that would engage the probes the modified virus, the modified Hepatitis C virus, or the virus-like transport vehicle was carrying on its surface. In this fashion, specific payloads could be delivered to specific cells throughout the body.

[0040] The utilization of ribosomal RNA molecules does not alter the cell's DNA. Ribosomal RNAs degrade and become unusable after a period of time. Use of RNA as a therapeutic modality offers a therapeutic opportunity that could have a reversible or an attenuable effect when required. Ribosomal RNA assisting in decoding messenger RNA bypasses the action of decoding the DNA and errors or deficiencies that might occur during the process of transcription that occurs in the nucleus of the cell. By employing a medically therapeutic virus to carry ribosomal RNA to cells, deficiencies of any of the approximately 30,000 proteins that comprise the tissues that exist in the body and on the surface of the body can be successfully treated or averted.

BRIEF SUMMARY OF THE INVENTION

[0041] A modified virus is used as a transport medium to carry a payload of one or more ribosomal ribonucleic acid molecules. The modified virus is intended to make contact with a target Beta cell located in the Islets of Langerhans in the pancreas by means of the modified virus's exterior probes including one or more probes meant to engage GPR40 exterior cell-surface receptors on a Beta cell. Once the virus's exterior probes engage a target Beta cell's receptors, the modified virus inserts into the target cell one or more ribonucleic acid molecules it is carrying. A virus-like transport vehicle may be used in the place of a modified virus. The exogenous ribosomal RNA molecules connect to ribosome proteins and the resultant complex, referred to as a ribosome, surrounds the beginning segment of a mRNA molecule. Utilizing its own inherent coding, exogenous rRNA molecules direct the ribosome pieces to build the ribosome complex around a mRNA. Medical disease states such as diabetes mellitus that are the result of a deficiency of one or more proteins can be successfully treated by utilizing viruses to insert the proper ribosomal RNA into specific cells to enhance the production of proteins that are identified as being deficient, thus correcting the deficiency. The deficiency of insulin production is a prime example of a medical condition that is capable of being corrected by utilizing a modified virus to transport ribosomal RNA molecules to assist ribosomes with reading native messenger RNA molecules coded for the pro-insulin molecule, the insulin molecule, the insulin receptor molecule, prohormone convertase one (PC1), prohormone convertase two (PC2), and/or carboxypeptidase E, delivering such ribosomal RNA molecules to Beta cells for the purpose of enhancing the Beta cells' production of the insulin molecule and/or the insulin receptor.

DETAILED DESCRIPTION

[0042] Diabetes mellitus is a medical condition often recognized when an individual's fasting blood glucose level is persistently higher than the generally accepted normal range of 60-110 mg/dl. An elevated blood glucose level may occur as the result of a lack of sufficient insulin; a lack of sufficient biologically effective insulin; a deficiency of the number of insulin receptors available to interact with insulin; a deficiency in the number of biologically active insulin receptors available to properly interact with insulin; insufficient release of insulin into the blood stream.

[0043] Insulin, a protein, is generated in Beta cells located in the Islets of Langerhans in the pancreas. Insulin is produced by decoding DNA through a process called transcription. Initially, transcription of the DNA produces a messenger ribonucleic acid (mRNA) molecule coded for the pro-insulin molecule. This mRNA coded for the 'pro-insulin' molecule, is then decoded by one or more ribosomes through a process called translation to produce a chain of amino acids that is referred to as the 'pro-insulin' molecule. The 'pro-insulin' molecule is modified by enzymes to produce the biologically active 'insulin' protein. Insulin molecules are stored in vacuoles in the Beta cells of the pancreas. Insulin is released from storage vacuoles in response to a rise in the level of glucose in the blood. Other proteins are manufactured in a similar fashion as pro-insulin and insulin.

[0044] Errors in the DNA or errors that occur in the process that generates the messenger RNA or a deficiency in the number of messenger RNA or a deficiency in the number of biologically active messenger RNA results in a deficiency of, or errors in the 'pro-insulin' molecule. Deficiencies in the biologically active enzymes intended to modify the 'pro-insulin' molecule to produce the biologically active insulin protein may result in deficiencies in adequate insulin production.

[0045] Correcting deficiencies or errors associated with the production of the protein insulin would correct diabetes mellitus, when diabetes mellitus is related to an insufficient quantity of biologically active insulin. Correcting deficiencies or errors associated with the production of insulin receptors would correct diabetes mellitus, when diabetes mellitus is related to an insufficient quantity of biologically active insulin receptors.

[0046] Messenger ribonucleic acids (mRNA) act as templates from which proteins are manufactured inside a cell. Ribosomal ribonucleic acids (rRNA) congregate with ribosomal proteins to produce a complex referred to as ribosome. Ribosomes attach to a mRNA and then in conjunction with charged tRNAs amino acid strings are constructed to form proteins.

[0047] The Hepatitis C virus (HCV) is comprised of an outer lipid bilayer envelope and an internal nucleocapsid. The virus's genetic payload is carried within the nucleocapsid. The HCV's naturally occurring genetic payload consists of a single molecule of linear positive sense, single stranded RNA approximately 9600 nucleotides in length, which includes: the structural proteins of C, E1, E2, the nonstructural proteins NS1, NS2, NS3, NS4A, NS4B, NS5A, NS5B, p7 and ARFP/F protein.

Present on the surface of the outer envelope of the Hepatitis C virus are probes that detect receptors present on the surface of liver cells. The glycoproteins E1 and E2 have been identified to be affixed to the surface of HCV. Portions of the Hepatitis C virus genome, when separated into individual pieces, behave like messenger RNA. Naturally occurring HCV is constructed with surface probes fashioned to recognize a receptor on the surface of a liver cell. Once the naturally occurring HCV's surface probe E2 engages a liver cell's CD81 receptor, and cofactors on the surface of HCV's exterior envelope engage the low density lipoprotein receptor (LDLR) or the scavenger receptor class B type I (SR-BI) on the liver cell, HCV then has the opportunity to insert its RNA genetic payload into the engaged target liver cell.

[0048] Replicating viruses and constructing viruses to carry DNA payloads is a form of manufacturing technology that has already been well established and is in use facilitating gene therapy. Replicating viruses and designing these viruses to carry ribosomal ribonucleic acid molecules as the genetic payload would incorporate similar techniques as already proven useful and are being used in current gene therapy technologies.

[0049] To carry out the process to manufacture a modified medically therapeutic Hepatitis C virus, messenger RNA would be inserted into the host that would code for the general physical outer structures of the Hepatitis C virus. Messenger RNA would be inserted into the host that would generate surface probes that would target the surface receptors on Beta cells. Messenger RNA would be inserted into the host that would generate copies of the ribosomal RNA that would provide a therapeutic action that would take the place of the Hepatitis C virus's innate genome. Similar to how copies of a naturally occurring Hepatitis C virus is produced, assembled and released from a host cell, copies of the modified medically therapeutic Hepatitis C virus carrying medically therapeutic ribosomal RNA would be produced, assembled and released from a host cell.

[0050] To treat the various different forms of diabetes mellitus various combinations of ribosomal RNA may be inserted into the host, and the host would produce copies of modified Hepatitis C virus that target Beta cells and carry a genetic payload consisting of ribosomal RNA molecules that would consist of one or more copies of ribosomal RNAs that interact with ribosomes that attach and decode messenger RNA that code for the insulin molecule, the insulin receptor, the enzyme prohormone convertase one, the enzyme prohormone convertase two, the enzyme carboxypeptidase E. Depending upon the physical size of the ribosomal RNA and the available space inside the modified Hepatitis C virus, more than one type of ribosomal RNA may be packaged into a single modified Hepatitis C virus.

[0051] The modified Hepatitis C virus would be incapable of replication on its own due to the fact that the messenger RNA that a naturally occurring Hepatitis C virus would normally carry would not be present in the modified form of the Hepatitis C virus.

[0052] To treat diabetes, a quantity of modified Hepatitis C virus would be introduced into a patient's blood stream or tissues so that the modified virus could deliver the therapeutic ribosomal RNA payload that it carries to Beta cells in the pancreas. When the probes on the surface of the modified Hepatitis C virus engage a cell-surface receptor or receptors on a Beta cell, the modified Hepatitis C virus will insert its therapeutic payload of ribosomal RNA molecules into the Beta cell to enhance the Beta cell's biologic function of producing insulin and/or insulin receptors.

[0053] An additional means to treat diabetes might include the use of a quantity of virus-like transport vehicles. The virus-like transport vehicles would be comprised of a bilayer lipid envelope and a nucleocapsid inner shell, similar to the construction of a virus, and such virus-like transport vehicles would carry a payload consisting of ribosomal RNA molecules. Embedded in the virus-like transport vehicle's outer lipid bilayer surface envelope would be a quantity of probes that target cell-surface receptors on specific cells. The virus-like transport vehicle would be introduced into a patient's blood stream or tissues so that the virus-like transport vehicle could deliver the therapeutic genetic payload that it carries to Beta cells in the pancreas. When the probes on the surface of the virus-like transport vehicle engage a cell-surface receptor or receptors on a Beta cell located in the pancreas, the virus-like transport vehicle will insert its therapeutic payload of ribosomal RNA into the Beta cell to enhance the Beta cell's biologic function of producing insulin and/or insulin receptors. The ribosomal ribonucleic acid molecules carried as a payload in the virus-like transport vehicle would consist of a quantity of 5S ribosomal ribonucleic acid molecules, a quantity of 5.8S ribosomal ribonucleic acid molecules, a quantity of 12S ribosomal ribonucleic acid molecules, a quantity of 16S ribosomal ribonucleic acid molecules, a quantity of 18S ribosomal ribonucleic acid molecules, and/or a quantity of 28S ribosomal ribonucleic acid molecules. The quantity of each variety of ribosomal acid molecule determined by the need to decode messenger RNA molecules.

[0054] RNAs are generally degraded by enzymes known as ribonucleases or RNAases. Ribonucleases act to inactive the RNA molecules. Different RNAs are known to have different half-lives. The nucleotide sequencing of the rRNA molecule could be altered from that of the natural occurring molecule to lengthen or shorten the service half-life of the native rRNA. Depending upon the application, the rate of degradation of rRNA molecules by ribonucleases could be varied. By changing the nucleotide sequence of the rRNA molecule or by altering the folding characteristics of the rRNA molecule or by altering both the nucleotide sequence and the folding characteristics of the rRNA molecule the rate of degradation of the rRNA molecules by ribonucleases could be caused to vary in length of time from seconds to minutes to hours to days to weeks to months to years. The rate of degradation of the rRNA molecules could be tailored to the treatment objectives of the rRNA molecule. Lengthening the service life of rRNA molecules such that the rRNAs could combine with ribosomal proteins to participate in ribosomes over a longer than the naturally occurring period of time would be especially useful in diabetic patients to facilitate a greater production of insulin molecules in the Beta cells and to increase the interval that would be required between treatments.

[0055] The action of altering the type of probe or probes present on the surface of the modified virus, the modified Hepatitis C virus, or the virus-like transport vehicle would change the target the modified virus or virus-like transport vehicle would seek. By changing the probes on the surface of the modified virus, the modified Hepatitis C virus, or the virus-like transport vehicle the payload carried by the modified virus, the modified Hepatitis C virus, or the virus-like transport vehicle could be delivered to any cell that carried on its surface a cell-surface receptor that would engage the probes the modified virus, the modified Hepatitis C virus, or the virus-like transport vehicle was carrying on its surface. In this fashion, specific payloads could be delivered to specific cells throughout the body.

[0056] By providing Beta cells with the above-mentioned ribosomal RNAs the capacity of Beta cells to carrying out the biologic processes of producing insulin and recognizing and responding to blood glucose levels is enhanced, which results in an efficient means to control the glucose levels in the blood stream on a constant and persistent basis utilizing innate regulatory mechanisms and thus diabetes mellitus can be effectively treated and the harmful effects of this disease can be averted.

[0057] By providing any target cell with medically therapeutic ribosomal RNAs to enhance a cell's capacity to produce one or more proteins, any protein deficiency can be effectively treated and the harmful effects of the protein deficiency can be averted.

CLAIMS: Reserved.

No. 6: ADAPTABLE MODIFIED VIRUS VECTOR TO DELIV-
ER RIBOSOMAL RIBONUCLEIC ACID COMBINED WITH
MESSENGER RIBONUCLEIC ACID AS A MEDICAL TREAT-
MENT DEVICE TO MANAGE DIABETES MELLITUS AND
OTHER PROTEIN DEFICIENT DISEASES

INDIVIDUALS REQUESTING PATENT: Dr. Lane B. Scheiber
II, MD and Dr. Lane B. Scheiber, ScD

©2009 Lane B. Scheiber II and Lane B. Scheiber. A portion
of the disclosure of this patent document contains material
which is subject to copyright protection. The copyright owners
have no objection to the facsimile reproduction by anyone of
the patent document or the patent disclosure, as it appears
in the Patent and Trademark Office patent file or records, but
otherwise reserves all copyright rights whatsoever.

ABSTRACT

Diabetes mellitus is a disease of elevated blood glucose, often
directly related to a deficiency in insulin production or insulin
receptor production. The innovative strategy of treatment
described here utilizes modified viruses and virus-like vehicles
to act as a transport mechanism to deliver ribosomal RNA
molecules along with messenger RNA molecules to target
cells in the body. Delivering to the Beta cells in the body the
ribosomal RNA needed to assist ribosomes with the construction
of insulin or insulin receptors along with messenger RNA will
lead to enhanced production of biologically active insulin or
insulin receptors by Beta cells as necessary, which will lead
to correcting deficiencies in insulin or insulin receptors the
result of which will help properly regulate blood glucose levels
throughout the body utilizing innate regulatory mechanisms.

BACKGROUND OF THE INVENTION

Field of the Invention

This invention relates to any medical device intended to correct a protein deficiency in the body by increasing the intracellular production of the deficient protein by utilizing a modified virus to insert one or more ribosomal ribonucleic acid molecules along with one or more messenger ribonucleic acid molecules into one or more cells of the body.

Description of Background Art

[0001] For purposes of this text there are several general definitions. A 'ribose' is a five carbon or pentose sugar ($C_5H_{10}O_5$) present in the structural components of ribonucleic acid, riboflavin, and other nucleotides and nucleosides. A 'deoxyribose' is a deoxypentose ($C_5H_{10}O_4$) found in deoxyribonucleic acid. A 'nucleoside' is a compound of a sugar usually ribose or deoxyribose with a nitrogenous base by way of an N-glycosyl link. A 'nucleotide' is a single unit of a nucleic acid, composed of a five carbon sugar (either a ribose or a deoxyribose), a nitrogenous base and a phosphate group. There are two families of 'nitrogenous bases', which include: pyrimidine and purine. A 'pyrimidine' is a six member ring made up of carbon and nitrogen atoms; the members of the pyrimidine family include: cytosine (C), thymine (T) and uracil (U). A 'purine' is a five-member ring fused to a pyrimidine type ring; the members of the purine family include: adenine (A) and guanine (G). A 'nucleic acid' is a polynucleotide which is a biologic molecule such as ribonucleic acid or deoxyribonucleic acid that allow organisms to reproduce. A 'ribonucleic acid' (RNA) is a linear polymer of nucleotides formed by repeated riboses linked by phosphodiester bonds between the 3-hydroxyl group of one and the 5-hydroxyl group of the next; RNAs are a single strand macromolecule comprised of a sequence of nucleotides, these nucleotides generally referred to by their nitrogenous bases, which include: adenine, cytosine, guanine or uracil. RNAs are subset into different types which include messenger RNA (mRNA), transport RNA (tRNA), and ribosomal RNA (rRNA). Messenger RNAs act as templates to produce proteins. A ribosome is a complex comprised of rRNAs and proteins and is responsible for the correct positioning of mRNA and charged tRNA to facilitate the proper alignment and bonding of amino acids into a strand to produce a protein. A 'charged' tRNA is a tRNA that is carrying an amino acid. Ribosomal RNA (rRNA) represents a subset of RNAs that form part of the physical structure of a ribosome.

[0002] Diabetes mellitus represents an important health issue that affects a significant portion of the world population. In the United States, about 16 million people suffer from diabetes mellitus. Every year, about 650,000 additional people are diagnosed with this disease. Diabetes mellitus is the seventh leading cause of all deaths.

[0003] Diabetes mellitus represents a state of hyperglycemia, a serum blood sugar that is higher than what is considered the normal range for humans. Glucose, a six-carbon molecule, is a form of sugar. Glucose is absorbed by the cells of the body and converted to energy by the processes of glycolysis, the Krebs cycle and phosporylation. Insulin, a protein, facilitates the transfer of glucose from the blood into cells. Normal range for blood glucose in humans is generally defined as a fasting blood plasma glucose level of between 70 to 110 mg/dl. For descriptive purposes, the term 'plasma' refers to the fluid portion of blood.

[0004] Diabetes mellitus is classified as Type One and Type Two. Type One diabetes mellitus is insulin dependent, which refers to the condition where there is a lack of sufficient insulin circulating in the blood stream and insulin must be provided to the body in order to properly regulate the blood glucose level. When insulin is required to regulate the blood glucose level in the body, this condition is often referred to as insulin dependent diabetes mellitus (IDDM). Type Two diabetes mellitus is noninsulin dependent, often referred to as noninsulin dependent diabetes mellitus (NIDDM), meaning the blood glucose level can be managed without insulin, and instead by means of diet, exercise or intervention with oral medications. Type Two diabetes mellitus is considered a progressive disease, the underlying pathogenic mechanisms including pancreatic Beta cell (also often designated as β-Cell) dysfunction and insulin resistance.

[0005] The pancreas serves as an endocrine gland and an exocrine gland. Functioning as an endocrine gland the pancreas produces and secretes hormones including insulin and glucagon. Insulin acts to reduce levels of glucose circulating in the blood. Beta cells secrete insulin into the blood when a higher than normal level of glucose is detected in the serum. For purposes of this description the terms 'blood', 'blood stream' and 'serum' refer to the same substance. Glucagon acts to stimulate an increase in glucose circulating in the blood. Beta cells in the pancreas secrete glucagon when a low level of glucose is detected in the serum.

[0006] Glucose enters the body and then the blood stream as a result of the digestion of food. The Beta cells of the Islets of Langerhans continuously sense the level of glucose in the blood and respond to elevated levels of blood glucose by secreting insulin into the blood. Beta cells produce the protein 'insulin' in their endoplasmic reticulum and store the insulin in vacuoles until it is needed. When Beta cells detect an increase in the glucose level in the blood, Beta cells release insulin into the blood from the described storage vacuoles.

[0007] Insulin is a protein. An insulin protein consists of two chains of amino acids, an alpha chain and a beta chain, linked by two disulfide (S-S) bridges. One chain, the alpha chain consists of 21 amino acids. The second chain the beta chain consists of 30 amino acids.

[0008] Insulin interacts with the cells of the body by means of a cell-surface receptor termed the 'insulin receptor' located on the exterior of a cell's 'outer membrane', otherwise known as the 'plasma membrane'. Insulin interacts with muscle and liver cells by means of the insulin receptor to rapidly remove excess blood sugar when the glucose level in the blood is higher than the upper limit of the normal physiologic range. Recognized functions of insulin include stimulating cells to take up glucose from the blood and convert it to glycogen to facilitate the cells in the body to utilize glucose to generate biochemically usable energy, and to stimulate fat cells to take up glucose and synthesize fat.

[0009] Diabetes Mellitus may be the result of one or more factors. Causes of diabetes mellitus may include: (1) mutation of the insulin gene itself causing miscoding, which results in the production of ineffective insulin molecules; (2) mutations to genes that code for the 'transcription factors' needed for transcription of the insulin gene in the deoxyribonucleic acid (DNA) to create messenger ribonucleic acid (mRNA) molecules, which facilitate the manufacture of the insulin molecule; (3) mutations of the gene encoding for the insulin receptor, which produces inactive or an insufficient number of insulin receptors; (4) mutation to the gene encoding for glucokinase, the enzyme that phosphorylates glucose in the first step of glycolysis; (5) mutations to the genes encoding portions of the potassium channels in the plasma membrane of the Beta cells, preventing proper closure of the channel, thus blocking insulin release; (6) mutations to mitochondrial genes that as a result, decreases the energy available to be used facilitate the release of insulin, therefore reducing insulin secretion; (7) failure of glucose transporters to properly permit the facilitated diffusion of glucose from plasma into the cells of the body.

[0010] A 'eukaryote' refers to a nucleated cell. Eukaryotes comprise nearly all animal and plant cells. A human eukaryote or nucleated cell is comprised of an exterior lipid bilayer plasma membrane, cytoplasm, a nucleus, and organelles. The exterior plasma membrane defines the perimeter of the cell, regulates the flow of nutrients, water and regulating molecules in and out of the cell, and has embedded into its structure receptors that the cell uses to detect properties of the environment surrounding the cell membrane. The cytoplasm acts as a filling medium inside the boundaries of the plasma cell membrane and is comprised mainly of water and nutrients such as amino acids, oxygen, and glucose. The nucleus, organelles, and ribosomes are suspended in the cytoplasm. The nucleus contains the majority of the cell's genetic information in the form of double stranded deoxyribonucleic acid (DNA). Organelles generally carry out specialized functions for the cell and include such structures as the mitochondria, the endoplasmic reticulum, storage vacuoles, lysosomes and Golgi complex (sometimes referred to as a Golgi apparatus). Floating in the cytoplasm, but also located in the endoplasmic reticulum and mitochondria are ribosomes. Ribosomes are complex macromolecule structures comprised of ribosomal ribonucleic acid (rRNA) molecules and ribosomal proteins that combine and couple to a messenger ribonucleic acid (mRNA) molecule. The rRNAs and the ribosomal proteins congregate to form a macromolecule structure that surrounds a mRNA molecule. Ribosomes decode genetic information in a mRNA molecule and manufacture proteins to the specifications of the instruction code physically present in the mRNA molecule. More than one ribosome may be attached to a single mRNA at a time.

[0011] The majority of the deoxyribonucleic acid (DNA) comprises the chromosomes, double stranded helical structures located in the nucleus of the cell. DNA in a circular form, can also be found in the mitochondria, the powerhouse of the cell, an organelle that assists in converting glucose into usable energy molecules. DNA represents the genetic information a cell needs to manufacture the materials it requires to sustain life and to replicate. Genetic information is stored in the DNA by arrangements of four nucleotides referred to as: adenine, thymine, guanine and cytosine. DNA represents instruction coding, that in the process known as transcription, the DNA's genetic information is decoded by transcription protein complexes referred to as polymerases (or polymerase complex), to produce ribonucleic acid (RNA). RNA is a single strand of genetic information comprised of coded arrangements of four nucleotides: adenine, uracil, guanine and cytosine. In a RNA, 'uracil' takes the place of 'thymine', thymine being present in the DNA. Several different types of RNAs have been identified, which include messenger RNAs (mRNA), transport RNAs (tRNA) and ribosomal RNAs (rRNA).

[0012] Proteins are comprised of a series of amino acids bonded together in a linear strand, sometimes referred to as a chain; a protein may be further modified to be a structure comprised of one or more similar or differing strands of amino acids bonded together. Insulin is a protein structure comprised of two strands of amino acids; one strand comprised of 21 amino acids long and the second strand comprised of 30 amino acids, the two strands attached by two disulfide bridges. There are an estimated 30,000 different proteins the cells of the human body may manufacture. The human body is comprised of a wide variety of cells, many with specialized functions requiring unique combinations of proteins and protein structures such as glycoproteins (a protein combined with a carbohydrate) to accomplish the required task or tasks a specialized cell is designed to perform. Forms of glycoproteins are known to be utilized as cell-surface receptors. Messenger RNAs (mRNA) are created by transcription of DNA, they generally migrate to other locations inside the cell and are utilized by ribosomes as protein manufacturing templates. A ribosome is a protein complex that manufactures proteins by deciphering the instruction code located in a mRNA molecule. When a specific protein is needed, pieces of the ribosome complex, which include rRNA molecules and ribosomal proteins, bind around the strand of a mRNA that carries the specific instruction code that will generate the required protein. The ribosome traverses the mRNA strand and deciphers the genetic information coded into the sequence of nucleotides that comprise the mRNA molecule to produce a protein molecule and this process is referred to as translation.

[0013] A ribosome is complex macromolecule comprised of ribosomal RNA (rRNA) molecules and ribosomal proteins. Ribosomal RNAs and ribosomal proteins are often designated with a number measured in Svedberg (S) units, which represents the sediment coefficient. The sediment coefficient is influenced by both molecular weight of the molecule and surface area of the molecule. In humans there are generally recognized at this time two mitochondrial rRNAs identified as 12S rRNA and 16S rRNA, and there are generally recognized four rRNAs that reside in the cytoplasm of a cell identified as 5S rRNA, 5.8S rRNA, 18S rRNA and 28S rRNA. There may be other rRNAs, as of yet unidentified, that reside in some of the other structures in the cell that engage in manufacturing of macromolecules, such as the smooth endoplasmic reticulum, the rough endoplasmic reticulum and the Golgi complex.

[0014] In eukaryotes, in the cytoplasm, the ribosome complex is referred to as an 80S ribosome. Generally two ribosomal proteins comprise a ribosome complex. This 80S ribosome is comprised of one 'dome-shape' 60S ribosomal protein and one 'cap-shaped' 40S ribosomal protein.

[0015] In the forms of life referred to as vertebrates (Humans are classified as a form of vertebrate), of the four rRNAs that reside in the cytoplasm of a eukaryote cell, the 18S rRNA is found in and helps comprise the physical structure of the 40S protein subunit of the ribosome complex and the 5S rRNA, 5.8S rRNA, and 28S rRNA molecules are found in and help comprise the physical structure of the 60S protein subunit of the ribosome complex.

[0016] The rRNA molecules are thought to provide at least three different functions for the ribosome complex. The rRNA molecules are thought to: (1) assist with identification of the messenger RNA to be translated, (2) act as an enzyme to facilitate the production of the protein molecule being translated from the mRNA molecule undergoing translation, (3) possibly cause folding at certain locations in the three dimensional structure of the protein being generated as the ribosome complex decodes the mRNA molecule.

[0017] Ribosomal RNAs (rRNA) are generated by polymerase molecules deciphering the instruction code present in the DNA. The rRNAs generally migrate to locations where mRNAs are to be utilized as templates. The rRNA molecules connect to their respective ribosome proteins and this macromolecule complex, referred to as a ribosome or ribosome complex, surrounds the beginning segment of a mRNA molecule. Utilizing inherent coding, the rRNA molecules direct the ribosome pieces to build the ribosome complex around a particular strand of mRNA or particular type of mRNA. Given there are four unique types of nucleotides that make up the physical linear strand of any RNA molecule, these four unique types of nucleotides may in some circumstances represent a base-four numbering system. As an analogy, at the core of the current digital computer technology, binary coding or base-two coding, which is comprised of 'ones' and 'zeros', is utilized in certain formats to code for names and numbers. The inherent coding the rRNA molecules harbor is a sequence of nucleotides which represent a unique 'name' (coded in the base-four numbering system), unique 'base-four number' or unique 'combination of a name and base-four number' that corresponds to a particular mRNA or particular type of mRNA. In this manner, rRNAs act to control which mRNA molecule will undergo translation to produce proteins, rather than a ribosome complex randomly engaging any mRNA template that happens to be available. With the DNA producing rRNA molecules that cause a ribosome to attach to a particular mRNA molecule or particular type of mRNA molecule, the DNA is able to exert control over the manufacturing capacity of the cell and produce proteins as needed, rather than producing proteins in a random fashion. Producing proteins as needed by the cell, rather than in a random fashion, conserves valuable resources and conserves energy inside the cell.

[0018] RNAs are generally degraded by enzymes known as ribonucleases or RNAases. Ribonucleases act to split RNA molecules, which tends to inactive the RNA molecules; preventing RNA molecules from performing their duties. Different RNAs have different half-lives. A 'service life' refers to the amount of time an RNA molecule may participate in the biologic functions it was originally created to participate in within a cell. A 'half-life' or 'service half-life' is the amount of time it takes for half of a given amount of RNA molecules to degrade to a form to which the RNA molecules are unable to participate in the biologic processes they were created to participate in within a cell. The 'life' or 'service life' or 'time span of participation in biologic processes' of biologic macromolecules is generally measured and reported in the science community in terms of the macromolecule's half-life. The nucleotide sequencing of the rRNA molecule could be altered from that of the naturally occurring molecule to lengthen or shorten the service half-life of the native rRNA. Lengthening the service life of rRNA molecules such that the rRNAs could combine with ribosomal proteins to participate in ribosomes over a longer than the naturally occurring period of time would be especially useful in diabetic patients to facilitate a greater production of insulin molecules in the Beta cells.

[0019] The rate of degradation of rRNA molecules by ribonucleases could be varied by changing the nucleotide sequence of the rRNA molecule or by altering the folding characteristics of the rRNA molecule or by altering both the nucleotide sequence and the folding characteristics of the rRNA molecule. By making changes to the nucleotide sequence and/ or the folding characteristics of the rRNA molecules the rate of degradation of the rRNA molecules by ribonucleases could be caused to vary in length of time from seconds to minutes to hours to days to weeks to months to years.

[0020] Transport RNAs (tRNA) are constructed in the nucleus or in the mitochondria, and are coded for one of the 20 amino acids the cells of the human body use to construct proteins. Once a tRNA is created by transcription of the DNA, the tRNA seeks out the type of amino acid it has been coded for and attaches to that specific amino acid. A tRNA molecule is considered to be 'charged' when it is carrying an amino acid. The charged tRNA delivers the amino acid it carries to a ribosome that is waiting for the specific amino acid the tRNA is carrying. Proteins are manufactured by the ribosomes binding together sequences of amino acids. The order by which the amino acids are bonded together is dictated by the way the sequencing of the nucleotides comprising the mRNA is constructed and how the ribosome interprets the information encoded in the string of nucleotides present in the mRNA strand.

[0021] Messenger RNA molecules are divided into three regions. The three regions include the (1) 5' untranslatable region, (2) the coding region, and (3) the 3' untranslatable region. An 'untranslatable region' represents a segment of a messenger RNA molecule that does not code for a protein and is not used to yield a protein and therefore 'translation' does not occur in such a region. The 'coding region' is the portion of the mRNA that is decoded by the ribosomes by the process known as translation to produce a particular protein molecule. A sequence of three nucleotides present in the coding region of a mRNA molecule represents a unit of information referred to as a codon. Codons code for all of the 20 amino acids used to construct protein molecules and also for START and STOP commands. In the process known as translation, the ribosome decodes the codons present in the coding region in the mRNA, initiating the protein manufacturing process at a START codon, then interfacing with charged tRNAs carrying the amino acids that match the sequence of codons in the mRNA as the ribosome traverses the length of the coding region of the mRNA molecule. The ribosome functions as a protein factory by taking amino acids delivered by tRNAs and binding the amino acids together in the order dictated by the sequence of codon instructions coded into the mRNA template as directed by the manner of the nucleic acid arrangement in the mRNA molecule. Protein synthesis ceases when a ribosome encounters a STOP code. The protein molecule is then released by the ribosome. Ribosomes do not decode the nucleotide sequences to produce proteins in a mRNA's 5' untranslatable region or a mRNA's 3' untranslatable region.

[0022] The insulin molecule is a protein produced by Beta cells located in the pancreas. The 'insulin messenger RNA' is created in a Beta cell by a polymerase complex transcribing the insulin gene from nuclear DNA in the nucleus of the cell. The native messenger RNA (mRNA) for insulin then travels to the endoplasmic reticulum, where numerous ribosomes, comprised of rRNA and ribosomal proteins, engage these mRNA molecules. Many ribosomes may be attached to a single strand of mRNA simultaneously, each generating an identical copy of the protein as dictated by the information encoded in the mRNA. Insulin is produced by ribosomes translating the information in a mRNA molecule coded for the insulin protein, which produce strands of amino acids that are coded for an immature form of the biologically active insulin molecule referred to as 'pro-insulin'. Once the pro-insulin molecule is generated it then undergoes modification by several enzymes including prohormone convertase one (PC1), prohormone convertase two (PC2) and carboxypeptidase E, which results in the production of a biologically active insulin molecule. Once the biologically active insulin protein is generated it is stored in a vacuole in the Beta cell to await being released into the blood stream.

[0023] Insulin receptors, which appear on the surface of cells, offer binding sites for insulin circulating in the blood. When insulin binds to an insulin receptor, the biologic response inside the cell causes glucose to enter the cell and undergo processing in the cytoplasm. Processed glucose molecules then enter the mitochondria. The mitochondria further process the modified glucose molecules to produce usable energy in the form of adenosine triphosphate molecules (ATP). Thirty-eight ATP molecules may be generated from one molecule of glucose during the process of aerobic respiration. ATP molecules are utilized as an energy source by biologic processes throughout the cell.

[0024] The current medical therapeutic approach to the management of diabetes mellitus has produced limited results. Patients with diabetes generally struggle with an inadequate production of insulin, or an ineffective release of biologically active insulin molecules, or a release of an insufficient number of biologically active insulin molecules, or an insufficient production of cell-surface receptors, or a production of ineffective cell-surface receptors, or a production of ineffective insulin molecules that are unable to interact properly with insulin receptors to produce the required biologic effect. Type One diabetes requires administration of exogenous insulin. The traditional approach to Type Two diabetes has generally first been to adjust the diet to limit the caloric intake the individual consumes. Exercise is used as an initial approach to both Type One and Type Two diabetes as a means of up-regulating the utilization of fats and sugar so as to reduce the amount of circulating plasma glucose. When diet and exercise are inadequate in properly managing Type Two diabetes, oral medications are often introduced. The action of sulfonylureas, a commonly prescribed class of oral medication, is to stimulate the Beta cells to produce additional insulin receptors and enhance the insulin receptors' response to insulin. Biguanides, another form of oral treatment, inhibit gluconeogenesis, the production of glucose in the liver, thereby attempting to reduce plasma glucose levels. Thiazolidinediones (TZDs) lower blood sugar levels by activating peroxisome proliferator-activated receptor gamma (PPAR-γ), a transcription factor, which when activated regulates the activity of various target genes, particularly ones involved in glucose and lipid metabolism. If diet, exercise and oral medications do not produce a satisfactory control of the level of blood glucose in a diabetic patient, exogenous insulin is injected into the body in an effort to normalize the amount of glucose present in the serum. Insulin, a protein, has not successfully been made available as an oral medication to date due to the fact that proteins in general become degraded when they encounter the acid environment present in the stomach.

[0025] Despite strict monitoring of blood glucose and potentially multiple doses of insulin injected throughout the day, many patients with diabetes mellitus still experience devastating adverse effects from elevated blood glucose levels. Microvascular damage and elevated tissue sugar levels contribute to such complications as renal failure, retinopathy involving the eyes, neuropathy, and accelerated heart disease despite aggressive efforts to maintain the blood sugar within the physiologic normal range using exogenous insulin by itself or a combination of exogenous insulin and one or more oral medications. Diabetes remains the number one cause of renal failure in the United States. Especially in diabetic patients that are dependent upon administering exogenous insulin into their body, though dosing of the insulin may be four or more times a day and even though this may produce adequate control of the blood glucose level to prevent the clinical symptoms of hyperglycemia; this does not unerringly supplement the body's natural capacity to monitor the blood sugar level minute to minute, twenty-four hours a day, and deliver an immediate response to a rise in blood glucose by the release of insulin from Beta cells as required. The deleterious effects of diabetes may still evolve despite strict and persistent control of the glucose level in the blood stream.

[0026] The current treatment of diabetes may be augmented by the unique approach to utilizing modified viruses as vehicles to transport ribosomal ribonucleic acid (rRNA) molecules along with exogenous messenger ribonucleic acid (mRNA) into cells in order to increase the production of biologically active insulin. By utilizing modified viruses to transport rRNA to facilitate assembly of ribosomes that are intended to attach to exogenous messenger ribonucleic acid molecules delivered into the cell by the modified virus or to attach to native messenger ribonucleic acid (mRNA) molecules already present in the cell would offer a new treatment option for patients with diabetes. By delivering both rRNA along with mRNA coded to facilitate the manufacture of pro-insulin, insulin, the enzymes utilized to modify proinsulin to the biologically active insulin molecule and/ or insulin receptors, the Beta cells in the pancreas would be stimulated to generate additional insulin. The above-mentioned concept would be analogous to providing cells with both the 'elements of the decoder' and the 'template' needed to construct copies of one or more proteins that a cell is lacking.

[0027] Viruses are obligate parasites. Viruses simply represent a carrier of genetic material and by themselves viruses are unable to replicate or carry out any form of biologic function outside their host cell. Viruses are generally comprised of one or more nested shells constructed of one or more layers of protein or lipid material, a genetic payload that represents the instruction code necessary to replicate the virus, and protein enzymes to help facilitate the genetic payload in the function of replicating copies of the virus once the genetic payload has been delivered to a host cell. Located on the outer shell or envelope of a virus are probes. The function of a virus's probes is to locate and engage a host cell's receptors. The virus's surface probes are designed to detect, make contact with and functionally engage one or more receptors located on the exterior of a cell type that will offer the virus the proper environment in which to construct copies of itself. A host cell provides the virus the proper biochemical machinery for the virus to successfully replicate itself.

[0028] Protected by an outer protein coat or lipid envelope, viruses carry a genetic payload in the form of deoxyribonucleic acid (DNA) or ribonucleic acid (RNA). Once a virus's exterior probes locate and functionally engage the surface receptor or receptors on a host cell, the virus inserts its genetic payload into the interior of the host cell. In the event a virus is carrying a DNA payload, the virus's DNA travels to the host cell's nucleus and is known to become inserted into the host cell's own native DNA. In the case where a virus is carrying its genetic payload as RNA, the virus inserts the RNA payload into the host cell and may also insert one or more enzymes to facilitate the RNA being utilized properly to replicate copies of the virus. Once inside the host cell, some species of virus facilitate use of their RNA by having the RNA converted to DNA. Once the viral RNA has been converted to DNA, the virus's DNA travels to the host cell's nucleus and is known to become inserted into the host cell's native DNA. Once a virus's genetic material has been inserted into the host cell's native DNA, the virus's genetic material takes command of certain cell functions and redirects the resources of the host cell to generate copies of the virus. Other forms of RNA viruses bypass the need to use the nuclear DNA and simply utilize portions of the viral genome to act as messenger RNA (mRNA). RNA viruses that bypass the host cell's DNA, cause the cell to in general generate copies of the necessary parts of the virus directly from the virus's RNA genome.

[0029] The Hepatitis C virus (HCV) is a positive sense RNA virus, meaning HCV's genome is a type of RNA that is capable of bypassing the need for involving the host cell's nucleus by having its RNA genome function as messenger RNA. The Hepatitis C virus infects liver cells. The Hepatitis C viral genome becomes divided once it gains access to the interior of a liver host cell. Portions of the subdivisions of the Hepatitis C viral genome directly interact with ribosomes to produce proteins necessary to construct copies of the virus.

[0030] HCV belongs to the Flaviviridae family and is the only member of the Hepacivirus genus. There are considered to be at least 100 different strains of Hepatitis C virus based on genome sequencing variability.

[0031] HCV is comprised of an outer lipoprotein envelope and an internal nucleocapsid. The genetic payload is carried within the nucleocapsid. In its natural state, present on the surface of the outer envelope of the Hepatitis C virus are probes that detect receptors present on the surface of liver cells. The glycoprotein E1 probe and the glycoprotein E2 probe have been identified to be affixed to the surface of HCV. The E2 probe binds with high affinity to the large external loop of a CD81 cell-surface receptor. CD81 is found on the surface of many cell types including liver cells. Once the E2 probe has engaged the CD81 cell-surface receptor, cofactors on the surface of HCV's exterior envelope engage either or both the low density lipoprotein receptor (LDLR) or the scavenger receptor class B type I (SR-BI) present on the liver cell in order to effect the mechanism to facilitate HCV breaching the cell membrane and inserting its viral RNA genome payload through the plasma cell membrane of the liver cell, thus delivering the HCV RNA genome into the liver cell. Upon successful engagement of the HCV surface probes with a liver cell's cell-surface receptors, HCV inserts the single strand of RNA and other payload elements it carries into the liver cell targeted to be a host cell. The HCV RNA genome then interacts with enzymes and ribosomes inside the liver cell in a translational process to produce the proteins required to construct copies of the protein components of HCV. The HCV genome undergoes a method of transcription to replicate copies of the virus's RNA genome. Inside the host, pieces of the HCV virus are assembled together and ultimately loaded with a copy of the HCV genome. Replicas of the original HCV then escape the host cell and migrate the environment in search of additional host liver cells to infect and continue the replication process.

[0032] HCV's naturally occurring genetic payload consists of a single molecule of linear positive sense, single stranded

RNA approximately 9600 nucleotides in length. By means of a translational process a polyprotein of approximately 3000 amino acids is generated. This polyprotein is cleaved post translation by host and viral proteases into individual viral proteins which include: the structural proteins of C, E1, E2, the nonstructural proteins NS1, NS2, NS3, NS4A, NS4B, NS5A, NS5B, p7 and ARFP/F protein. Hepatitis C virus's proteins direct the host liver cell to construction copies of the Hepatitis C virus. A membrane associated replicase complex consisting of the virus's nonstructural proteins NS3 and NS5B facilitate the replication of the viral genome. The membrane of the endoplasmic reticulum appears to be the site of protein maturation and viral assembly. Once copies of the Hepatitis C Virus are generated, they exit the host cell and each copy of HCV migrates in search of another appropriate liver cell that will act as a host to continue the replication process.

[0033] A modified Hepatitis C virus offers a naturally occurring vehicle mechanism to transport and insert medically therapeutic ribosomal ribonucleic acid (rRNA) molecules along with one or more messenger ribonucleic acid (mRNA) molecules into specific targeted cells of the human body. The surface probes present on the Hepatitis C virus's outer protein coat can be modified to seek out specific receptors on specific target cells. Once the modified Hepatitis C virus's probes properly engage the cell-surface receptors on a target cell, the modified Hepatitis C virus would insert into the target cell one or more medically therapeutic ribosomal ribonucleic acid (rRNA) molecules along with one or more messenger ribonucleic acid (mRNA) molecules for the purpose of having the target cell generate proteins to achieve a medically therapeutic response.

[0034] Current state of gene therapy generally refers to efforts directed toward inserting an exogenous subunit of DNA into a vehicle such as a naturally occurring virus. The vehicle is intended to insert the exogenous subunit of DNA into a cell the virus naturally targets. The exogenous DNA subunit then migrates to the target cell's nucleus. The exogenous DNA subunit then inserts into the native DNA of the cell. This represents a permanent alteration of the cell's nuclear DNA. The nuclear transcription proteins then read the exogenous DNA subunit's nucleotide coding to produce the intended cellular response. The approach described hereunder involves RNA versus DNA. DNA is comprised of the nucleotides: adenine, thymine, guanine and cytosine. RNA is composed of the nucleotides: adenine, uracil, guanine and cytosine. DNA codes for the manufacture of RNAs, which are composed of nucleotides. RNAs facilitate the manufacture of proteins, which are composed of amino acids. The virus chosen as the transport vehicle, Hepatitis C virus, is a RNA virus versus a virus that naturally carries a DNA genome.

[0035] Beta cells located in the Islets of Langerhans in the pancreas are thought to have at least one unique identifying surface receptor. The exterior receptor GPR40 appears specific to Beta cells located in the Islets of Langerhans in the pancreas. A virus equipped with a surface probe designed to engage the GPR40 Beta cell receptor, could travel the blood stream of the body until it locates a GPR40 receptor on a Beta cell, engage the receptor with its surface probe, and then insert the genetic payload it carries into the Beta cell. A genetic payload of one or more ribosomal RNAs along with one or more messenger RNAs could be used to enhance proper protein production by cells deficient in a particular protein. Hormones are proteins that circulate the body and stimulate biologic activity specific to the hormone's role. In the case of a deficiency of a hormone, production of a deficient hormone could be enhanced by inserting one or more ribosomal RNAs along with one or more messenger RNAs into specific target cells in the body to stimulate production of the required hormone. In the case of diabetes mellitus, utilizing a modified Hepatitis C virus as a vehicle, ribosomal RNA molecules along with messenger RNA molecules could be inserted into Beta cells, to assist the Beta cells are with generating an adequate insulin production and adequate release of insulin into the blood to meet the body's needs.

[0036] Viruses are constructed in a number of ways and shapes. The shape of a virus may be rod or filament like, icosahedral, or complex structures combining filament and polygonal shapes. Viruses may have an outer protein coat or an outer envelope comprised of lipids. Icosahedral viruses with an outer lipid envelope appear spherical in shape. An outer envelope is often comprised of two lipid layers often termed a lipid bilayer. Spherical viruses may be in the form of being comprised of an outer envelope and one inner shell or an outer envelope and two inner shells. In the case of a spherical virus with an outer envelope and one inner shell, the inner shell is often referred to as a nucleocapsid shell comprised of capsid proteins. In the case of a spherical virus being comprised of an outer envelope and two inner shells, the outer most inner viral shell may be referred to as comprised of matrix proteins, the innermost of the two shells being referred to as a nucleocapsid shell being comprised of capsid proteins. The inner protein shell is nested inside the outer protein shell.

[0037] An alternative means to treat diabetes might include the use of a quantity of virus-like transport vehicles. The virus-like transport vehicles would in general be spherical in shape; though other shapes may be used as function might warrant the use of a particular shape. The spherical virus-like transport vehicles would be comprised of a lipid bilayer envelope and one or more inner nested protein shells, depending upon the size of the payload. Nesting of protein shells refers to progressively smaller diameter shells fitting snugly inside protein shells of a larger diameter. The virus-like transport vehicles would be similar in construction to viruses, and such virus-like transport vehicles would carry a payload consisting of ribosomal RNA molecules. The size of the virus-like transport vehicle would depend upon the payload the virus-like transport vehicle would be required to carry. Embedded in the virus-like transport vehicle's outer lipid bilayer surface would be a quantity of probes that are intended to target cell-surface receptors on specific cells. The virus-like transport vehicle would be introduced into a patient's blood stream or tissues so that the virus-like transport vehicle could deliver the therapeutic genetic payload that it carries to Beta cells in the pancreas. When one or more probes on the surface of the virus-like transport vehicle engage one or more cell-surface receptors on a Beta cell located in the pancreas, the virus-like transport vehicle will insert its therapeutic payload of ribosomal RNA into the Beta cell to enhance the Beta cell's biologic function of producing insulin and/or insulin receptors.

[0038] The action of altering the type of probe or probes present on the surface of the modified virus, the modified Hepatitis C virus, or the virus-like transport vehicle would change the target the modified virus or virus-like transport vehicle would seek out. By changing the probe on the surface of the modified virus, the modified Hepatitis C virus, or the virus-like transport vehicle the payload carried by the modified virus, the modified Hepatitis C virus, or the virus-like transport vehicle could be delivered to any cell that carried on its surface a cell-surface receptor that would engage the probes the modified virus, the modified Hepatitis C virus, or the virus-like transport vehicle was carrying on its surface. In this fashion, specific payloads could be delivered to specific cells throughout the body.

[0039] The utilization of ribosomal RNA molecules or messenger RNA molecules does not alter the cell's DNA. Ribosomal RNAs and messenger RNAs degrade due to the presence of RNAases and become unusable after a period of time. Use of RNA as a therapeutic modality offers a therapeutic opportunity that could have a reversible or an attenuable effect when required. Using ribosomal RNA and messenger RNA to produce proteins bypasses the action of decoding the DNA and errors or deficiencies that might occur during the process of transcription. By employing a medically therapeutic virus to carry ribosomal RNA along with messenger RNAs to cells, deficiencies of any of the approximately 30,000 proteins that comprise the tissues that exist in the body and on the surface of the body can be successfully treated or averted.

[0040] Messenger RNA molecules are comprised of three regions (or segments). These three regions include (1) a 5' untranslatable region, (2) a coding region and (3) a 3' untranslatable region. The '5' untranslatable region' acts as the initiation point for a ribosome to attach to the mRNA. The 'coding region' acts as the template from which a protein is constructed. An 'untranslatable region' represents a segment of a messenger RNA molecule that does not code for a protein and is not used to yield a protein and therefore 'translation' does not occur in such a region. The 3' untranslatable region is associated with the degradation of the usefulness of the mRNA. Different mRNAs have different service life expectancies. The half-life of the naturally occurring mRNA that acts as the template responsible for the production of the protein 'glucokinase' is two hours. The half-life of the naturally occurring mRNA that acts as the template that produces the protein 'alcohol dehydrogenase' is ten hours. The half-life of the naturally occurring mRNA that acts as the template to produce the protein 'glucuronidase' is thirty hours. By modifying the nucleotides that comprise the 3' untranslatable unit of an mRNA the service half-life of the mRNA may be altered to be lengthened or shortened depending upon the need for the quantity of protein and timeframe over which the mRNA is required to produce the protein coded in the protein template of the mRNA's coding region.

[0041] Research has demonstrated that natural proteins can be altered to produce medically beneficial effects. The parathyroid hormone (PTH) is one example. Intact PTH is produced by cells in the parathyroid glands. There are four parathyroid glands present in the neck, generally in the vicinity of the thyroid gland. The term 'para-' means 'next to', so early anatomists identified the four glands 'parathyroid glands' because they were generally found 'next to' the thyroid gland in the neck.

Parathyroid hormone is released in response to the cells of the parathyroid gland sensing a decline in the level of serum calcium. Parathyroid hormone, in its natural state, acts to stimulate osteoclast cells present in bone to release calcium from bone, thereby returning the serum calcium level to the normal range. On the other hand, it has been quite well demonstrated that if (1) the amino acid chain of the parathyroid hormone is shortened and (2) the shorter parathyroid hormone molecule is pulsed, by injecting it into the body once a day, the action of this modified parathyroid hormone molecule is opposite of the intact parathyroid hormone. One such form of a shorter length parathyroid hormone molecule is termed 'teriparatide'. Teriparatide (1-34) has the identical sequence from 1 to the 34th N-terminal amino acid of the 84-amino acid endogenous human parathyroid hormone. The skeletal effects of the modified protein molecule act on bone cells to preferentially cause osteoblastic activity over osteoclastic activity, which results in storage of calcium into bone, rather than a release of calcium from bone if the teriparatide is administered once a day. Teriparatide has been a recognized and widely used treatment of osteoporosis since at least as far back as the year 2000.

[0042] Modifying the 'coding region' of a messenger RNA will modify the protein the messenger RNA will produce when the ribosomes decode such a modified messenger RNA. As demonstrated by the case of modifying the naturally occurring parathyroid hormone by administering a molecule that is comprised of fewer amino acids than the original PTH molecule, modifying proteins the messenger RNAs produce may provide health care providers with an entirely new and widely spanning armamentarium of medically beneficial therapies.

[0043] The 5' untranslatable region of a messenger RNA molecule is used to identify the messenger RNA and utilized as a point of attachment by ribosomes to the messenger RNA molecule. Modifying the 5' untranslatable region by altering the nucleotide sequence in the 5' untranslatable region may make it easier to identify a modified messenger ribonucleic acid molecules in a fashion that the modified ribonucleic acid molecules can be engaged by ribosomes. Altering the nucleotide sequence of the 5' untranslatable region of a modified messenger ribonucleic acid molecule to create a unique identifier would facilitate ribosomes to preferentially engage the modified messenger ribonucleic acid molecule to preferentially produce the protein for which the modified messenger ribonucleic acid molecule is acting as a template. Supplying cells with exogenous rRNA molecules and exogenous mRNA molecules that are both coded with a similar unique identifier such that the rRNA molecules will engage the mRNA molecules, facilitates the production of a desired protein.

[0044] A protein is a macromolecule consisting of long series of amino acids in a peptide linkage. A protease is any enzyme that catalyzes the hydrolysis of a protein in its initial stages of degradation to a simpler substance. Proteases either split proteins by removing amino acids from the ends of the protein or by splitting a protein into subunits. Proteases are divided into endopeptidases and exopeptidases. Exopeptidases catalyze the hydrolysis of the terminal amino acid of a protein chain. Exopeptidases include enzymes such as carboxypeptidase, aminopeptidases, dipeptidases. Endopeptidases catalyze the hydrolysis of a peptide chain well within the chain. Endopeptidases include enzymes such as pepsin, trypsin, cathepsins, papain.

[0045] A 'messenger RNA' carried by a modified form of virus, a modified Hepatitis C virus, or a virus-like transport vehicle may code or act as a template for 'multiple proteins'. A messenger RNA may act as a template for multiple copies of the same protein. A messenger RNA may act as a template that will produce various different types of proteins. Viral genomes often code for multiple proteins on a single strand of genetic material. Viruses sometimes carry proteases, which are used to act on proteins generated by the viral genome, once the viral genome has been inserted inside a host cell. Utilizing naturally occurring proteases or exogenous proteases delivered with the messenger RNA or exogenous proteases delivered by a separate transport vehicle, the original protein produced by an exogenous messenger RNA molecule may be split into subunits, with each subunit representing a copy of the same protein or each subunit representing a different protein. By fitting multiple templates for a particular protein into a single exogenous messenger RNA and utilizing proteases to split the proteins generated by the exogenous messenger RNA at specific sites along the proteins, multiple copies of the same smaller protein subunit could be generated. By fitting multiple templates for different proteins into a single exogenous messenger RNA and utilizing proteases to split the proteins generated by this exogenous messenger RNA at specific sites along the proteins, one or more copies of different smaller protein subunits could be generated. The utilization of proteases may significantly increase the efficiency by which medically therapeutic proteins are generated inside a cell.

[0046] A messenger RNA carried by a modified form of virus, a modified Hepatitis C virus, or a virus-like transport vehicle may be comprised of multiple messenger RNA subunits. RNAs are generally degraded by enzymes known as ribonucleases or RNAases. Ribonucleases act to split RNA molecules, which generally represents a means to inactive the RNA molecules, except when ribonucleases are being used to divide the RNA molecule into smaller active components. Utilizing naturally occurring ribonucleases or exogenous ribonucleases delivered with the messenger RNA or exogenous ribonucleases delivered by a separate transport vehicle, the original exogenous messenger RNA molecule may be split into translatable subunits. The original exogenous messenger RNA molecule may be physically split or degraded into subunits, each subunit representing a separate template, that by the process of translation, will produce copies of the same protein or the original exogenous messenger RNA molecule may be physically split or degraded into subunits, each subunit representing a template, that by the process of translation, will produce copies of different proteins. The utilization of ribonucleases represents another technique that could significantly increase the efficiency by which medically therapeutic proteins are generated inside a cell.

BRIEF SUMMARY OF THE INVENTION

[0047] A modified virus is used as a transport medium to carry a payload of one or more ribosomal ribonucleic acid molecules along with one or more messenger ribonucleic acid molecules. The modified virus is intended to make contact with a target Beta cell located in the Islets of Langerhans in the pancreas by means of the modified virus's exterior probes including one or more probes meant to engage GPR40 exterior cell-surface receptors on a Beta cell. Once the virus's exterior probes engage a target Beta cell's receptors, the modified virus inserts into the target cell one or more exogenous ribosomal ribonucleic acid molecules along with one or more exogenous messenger ribonucleic acid molecules it is carrying. A virus-like transport vehicle may be used in the place of a modified virus. Ribosomal RNA molecules connect to ribosome proteins and the resultant complex, referred to as a ribosome, surrounds the beginning segment of a mRNA molecule. Utilizing its own inherent coding, rRNA directs the ribosome pieces to build the ribosome complex around a particular strand of mRNA that the rRNA locates by matching the inherent coding the rRNA is carrying to a unique code on the mRNA. Medical disease states such as diabetes mellitus that are the result of a deficiency of one or more proteins can be successfully treated by utilizing viruses to insert the proper ribosomal RNA molecules along with the proper messenger RNA molecules into specific cells to enhance the production of proteins that are identified as being deficient, thus correcting the deficiency. The deficiency of insulin production is a prime example of a medical condition that is capable of being corrected by utilizing a modified virus to transport ribosomal RNA molecules along with messenger RNA molecules to assist ribosomes with producing the pro-insulin molecule, the insulin molecule, the insulin receptor molecule, prohormone convertase one (PC1), prohormone convertase two (PC2), and/or carboxypeptidase E. Delivering such ribosomal RNA molecules along with messenger RNA molecules to Beta cells for the purpose of enhancing the Beta cells' production of the insulin molecule and/or the insulin receptor offers a new and innovative treatment of diabetes and other protein deficient diseases.

DETAILED DESCRIPTION

[0048] Diabetes mellitus is a medical condition often recognized when an individual's fasting blood glucose level is persistently higher than the generally accepted normal range of 60-110 mg/dl. An elevated blood glucose level may occur as the result of a lack of sufficient insulin; a lack of sufficient biologically effective insulin; a deficiency of the number of insulin receptors available to interact with insulin; a deficiency in the number of biologically active insulin receptors available to properly interact with insulin; insufficient release of insulin into the blood stream.

[0049] Insulin, a protein, is generated in Beta cells located in the Islets of Langerhans in the pancreas. Insulin is produced by decoding DNA through a process called transcription. Initially, transcription of the DNA produces a messenger ribonucleic acid (mRNA) molecule coded for the pro-insulin molecule. This mRNA coded for the 'pro-insulin' molecule, is then decoded by one or more ribosomes through a process called translation to produce a chain of amino acids that is referred to as the 'pro-insulin' molecule. The 'pro-insulin' molecule is modified by enzymes to produce the biologically active 'insulin' protein. Insulin molecules are stored in vacuoles in the Beta cells of the pancreas. Insulin is released from storage vacuoles in response to a rise in the level of glucose in the blood. Other proteins are manufactured in a similar fashion as pro-insulin and insulin.

[0050] Errors in the DNA or errors that occur in the process that generates the messenger RNA or a deficiency in the number of messenger RNA or a deficiency in the number of biologically active messenger RNA results in a deficiency of, or errors in the 'pro-insulin' molecule. Deficiencies in the biologically active enzymes intended to modify the 'pro-insulin' molecule to produce the biologically active insulin protein may result in deficiencies in adequate insulin production.

[0051] Correcting deficiencies or errors associated with the production of the protein insulin would correct diabetes mellitus, when diabetes mellitus is related to an insufficient quantity of biologically active insulin. Correcting deficiencies or errors associated with the production of insulin receptors would correct diabetes mellitus, when diabetes mellitus is related to an insufficient quantity of biologically active insulin receptors.

[0052] Messenger ribonucleic acids (mRNA) act as templates from which proteins are manufactured inside a cell. Ribosomal ribonucleic acids (rRNA) congregate with ribosomal proteins to produce a complex referred to as ribosome. Ribosomes attach to a mRNA and then in conjunction with charged tRNAs amino acid strings are constructed to form proteins.

[0053] The Hepatitis C virus (HCV) is comprised of an outer lipid bilayer envelope and an internal nucleocapsid. The virus's genetic payload is carried within the nucleocapsid. The HCV's naturally occurring genetic payload consists of a single molecule of linear positive sense, single stranded RNA approximately 9600 nucleotides in length, which includes: the structural proteins of C, E1, E2, the nonstructural proteins NS1, NS2, NS3, NS4A, NS4B, NS5A, NS5B, p7 and ARFP/F protein. Present on the surface of the outer envelope of the Hepatitis C virus are probes that detect receptors present on the surface of liver cells. The glycoproteins E1 and E2 have been identified to be affixed to the surface of HCV. Portions of the Hepatitis C virus genome, when separated into individual pieces, behave like messenger RNA. Naturally occurring HCV is constructed within a liver cell. Naturally occurring HCV is constructed with surface probes fashioned to recognize a receptor on the surface of a liver cell. Once the naturally occurring HCV's surface probe E2 engages a liver cell's CD81 receptor, and cofactors on the surface of HCV's exterior envelope engage the low density lipoprotein receptor (LDLR) or the scavenger receptor class B type I (SR-BI) on the liver cell, HCV then has the opportunity to insert its RNA genetic payload into the engaged target liver cell.

[0054] Replicating viruses and constructing viruses to carry DNA payloads is a form of manufacturing technology that has already been well established and is in use facilitating gene therapy. Replicating viruses and designing these viruses to carry ribosomal ribonucleic acid molecules along with one or more messenger ribonucleic acid molecules as the genetic payload would incorporate similar techniques as already proven useful in current gene therapy technologies.

[0055] To carry out the process to manufacture a modified medically therapeutic Hepatitis C virus, messenger RNA would be inserted into the host that would code for the general physical outer structures of the Hepatitis C virus. Messenger RNA would be inserted into the host that would generate surface probes that would target the surface receptors on Beta cells. Messenger RNA would be inserted into the host that would be used to generate copies of the therapeutic ribosomal RNA and therapeutic messenger RNA that would take the place of the Hepatitis C virus's innate genome. Therapeutic messenger RNA that would act as the modified HCV's genome would encode for proteins that would include the pro-insulin molecule, the insulin molecule, the insulin receptor, the enzyme prohormone convertase one, the enzyme prohormone convertase two, the enzyme carboxypeptidase E. Similar to how copies of a naturally occurring Hepatitis C virus are produced, assembled and released from a host cell, copies of the modified medically therapeutic Hepatitis C virus would be produced, assembled and released from a host cell.

[0056] To treat the various different forms of diabetes mellitus various combinations of messenger RNA would be inserted into the host, and the host would produce copies of modified Hepatitis C virus that target Beta cells and carry a genetic payload consisting of ribosomal RNA along with messenger RNA molecules that would consist of one or more copies of a ribosomal RNA along with a messenger RNA that codes for the insulin molecule, the insulin receptor, the enzyme prohormone convertase one, the enzyme prohormone convertase two, the enzyme carboxypeptidase E. Depending upon the physical size of the ribosomal RNA along with messenger RNAs and the available space inside the modified Hepatitis C virus, more than one type of ribosomal RNA or messenger RNA may be packaged inside a single modified Hepatitis C virus, which may produce more than one therapeutic action in a cell.

[0057] The modified Hepatitis C virus would be incapable of replication on its own due to the fact that the messenger RNA, that a naturally occurring Hepatitis C virus would normally carry, would not be present in the modified form of the Hepatitis C virus.

[0058] To treat diabetes, a quantity of modified Hepatitis C virus would be introduced into a patient's blood stream or tissues so that the modified form of virus could deliver the therapeutic genetic payload that it carries to Beta cells in the pancreas. When the probes on the surface of the modified Hepatitis C virus engage a cell-surface receptor or receptors on a Beta cell, the modified Hepatitis C virus will insert its therapeutic payload of ribosomal RNA molecules and messenger RNA molecules into the Beta cell to enhance the Beta cell's biologic function of producing insulin and/or insulin receptors. One such probe would be a probe located on the surface of the modified Hepatitis C virus that engages the exterior receptor GPR40, which appears to be an exterior receptor specific to Beta cells located in the Islets of Langerhans in the pancreas.

[0059] An alternative means to treat diabetes might include the use of a quantity of virus-like transport vehicles. The virus-like transport vehicles would be comprised of a bilayer lipid envelope and a nucleocapsid inner shell, similar to the construction of a virus, and such virus-like transport vehicles would carry a payload consisting of ribosomal RNA and messenger RNA molecules. Embedded in the virus-like transport vehicle's outer lipid bilayer surface envelope would be a quantity of probes that target cell-surface receptors on specific cells. The outer lipid bilayer acting as a matrix structure for the quantity of probes to be fixed into and extend out from the virus-like transport vehicle. The virus-like transport vehicles would be introduced into a patient's blood stream or tissues so that the virus-like transport vehicle could deliver the therapeutic genetic payload that it carries to Beta cells in the pancreas. When the probes on the surface of the virus-like transport vehicle engage a cell-surface receptor or receptors on a Beta cell located in the pancreas, the virus-like transport vehicle will insert its therapeutic payload of ribosomal RNA and messenger RNA into the Beta cell to enhance the Beta cell's biologic function of producing insulin and/or insulin receptors. One such probe could be a probe on the surface of the virus-like transport vehicle that engages the exterior receptor GPR40, which appears to be an exterior receptor specific to Beta cells located in the Islets of Langerhans in the pancreas. The ribosomal ribonucleic acid molecules carried as a payload in the virus-like transport vehicle would consist of a quantity of 5S ribosomal ribonucleic acid molecules, a quantity of 5.8S ribosomal ribonucleic acid molecules, a quantity of 12S ribosomal ribonucleic acid molecules, a quantity of 16S ribosomal ribonucleic acid molecules, a quantity of 18S ribosomal ribonucleic acid molecules, and/or a quantity of 28S ribosomal ribonucleic acid molecules. The quantity of each variety of ribosomal acid molecule determined by the need to decode messenger RNA molecules.

[0060] RNAs are generally degraded by enzymes known as ribonucleases or RNAases. Ribonucleases act to inactive the RNA molecules. Different RNAs are known to have different half-lives. The nucleotide sequencing of the rRNA molecule could be altered from that of the natural occurring molecule to lengthen or shorten the service half-life of the native rRNA. Depending upon the application, the rate of degradation of rRNA molecules by ribonucleases could be varied. By changing the nucleotide sequence of the rRNA molecule or by altering the folding characteristics of the rRNA molecule or by altering both the nucleotide sequence and the folding characteristics of the rRNA molecule, the rate of degradation of the rRNA molecules by ribonucleases could be caused to vary in length of time from seconds to minutes to hours to days to weeks to months to years. The rate of degradation of the rRNA molecules could be tailored to the treatment objectives of the rRNA molecule. Lengthening the service life of rRNA molecules such that the rRNAs could combine with ribosomal proteins to participate in ribosomes over a longer than the naturally occurring period of time would be especially useful in diabetic patients to facilitate a greater production of insulin molecules in the Beta cells and to increase the interval that would be required between treatments.

[0061] Messenger RNA molecules are comprised of three regions (or segments). These three regions include a (1) 5' untranslatable region, (2) a coding region and (3) a 3' untranslatable region. The '5' untranslatable region' acts as the initiation point for a ribosome to attach to the mRNA. The 'coding region' acts as the template from which a protein is constructed. An 'untranslatable region' represents a segment of a messenger RNA molecule that does not code for a protein and is not used to yield a protein and therefore 'translation' does not occur in such a region. The 3' untranslatable region is associated with the degradation of the usefulness of the mRNA. Different mRNAs have different service life expectancies. The half-life of the naturally occurring mRNA that acts as the template responsible for the production of the protein 'glucokinase' is two hours. The half-life of the naturally occurring mRNA that produces the protein 'alcohol dehydrogenase' is ten hours. The half-life of the naturally occurring mRNA that produces the protein 'glucuronidase' is thirty hours. By modifying the nucleotides that comprise the 3' untranslatable unit of an mRNA the service half-life of the mRNA may be altered to be lengthened or shortened depending upon the need for the quantity of protein and timeframe over which the mRNA is required to produce the protein coded in the mRNA's protein coding region.

[0062] Modifying the 'coding region' of a messenger RNA will modify the protein the messenger RNA will produce when the ribosomes decode such a modified messenger RNA. As demonstrated by the case of modifying the naturally occurring parathyroid hormone by administering a molecule that is comprised of fewer amino acids than the original PTH molecule to produce a beneficial therapeutic effect, modifying proteins the messenger RNAs produce will provide health care providers with an entirely new and widely spanning armamentarium of medically beneficial therapies.

[0063] The 5' untranslatable region of a messenger RNA molecule is used to identify the messenger RNA and utilized as a point of attachment by ribosomes to the messenger RNA molecule. Modifying the 5' untranslatable region by altering the nucleotide sequence in the 5' untranslatable region may make it easier to identify a modified messenger ribonucleic acid molecules in a fashion that the modified ribonucleic acid molecules can be engaged by ribosomes. Altering the nucleotide sequence of the 5' untranslatable region of a modified messenger ribonucleic acid molecule to create a unique identifier would facilitate ribosomes to preferentially engage the modified messenger ribonucleic acid molecule to preferentially produce the protein for which the modified messenger ribonucleic acid molecule is acting as a template. Supplying cells with exogenous rRNA molecules and exogenous mRNA molecules that are both coded with a similar unique identifier such that the rRNA molecules will engage the mRNA molecules, facilitates the production of a desired protein.

[0064] The act of altering the type of probe or probes present on the surface of the modified form of virus, the modified Hepatitis C virus, or the virus-like transport vehicle would change the target the modified form of virus or virus-like transport vehicle would seek. By changing the probes on the surface of the modified virus, the modified Hepatitis C virus, or the virus-like transport vehicle the payload carried by the modified virus, the modified Hepatitis C virus, or the virus-like transport vehicle could be delivered to any cell that carried on its surface a cell-surface receptor that would engage the probes the modified virus, the modified Hepatitis C virus, or the virus-like transport vehicle was carrying on its surface. In this fashion, specific payloads could be delivered to specific cells throughout the body.

[0065] A 'messenger RNA' carried by a modified form of virus, a modified Hepatitis C virus, or a virus-like transport vehicle may code or act as a template for 'multiple proteins'. A messenger RNA may act as a template for multiple copies of the same protein. A messenger RNA may act as a template that will produce various different types of proteins. Utilizing naturally occurring proteases or exogenous proteases delivered with the messenger RNA or exogenous proteases delivered by a separate transport vehicle, the original protein produced by an exogenous messenger RNA molecule may be split into subunits, with each subunit representing a copy of the same protein or each subunit representing a different protein. Proteases carried by a modified form of virus, a modified Hepatitis C virus, or a virus-like transport vehicle are carried inside the outer shell of the respective vehicle, generally inside the nucleocapsid inner shell of the modified form of virus, a modified Hepatitis C virus, or a virus-like transport vehicle. By fitting multiple templates for a particular protein into a single exogenous messenger RNA and utilizing proteases to split the proteins generated by the exogenous messenger RNA at specific sites along the proteins, multiple copies of the same smaller protein subunit could be generated. By fitting multiple templates for different proteins into a single exogenous messenger RNA and utilizing proteases to split the proteins generated by this exogenous messenger RNA at specific sites along the proteins, one or more copies of different smaller protein subunits could be generated. The utilization of proteases will significantly increase the efficiency by which medically therapeutic proteins are generated inside a cell.

[0066] A messenger RNA carried by a modified form of virus, a modified Hepatitis C virus, or a virus-like transport vehicle may be comprised of multiple translatable messenger RNA subunits. Utilizing naturally occurring ribonucleases or exogenous ribonucleases delivered with the messenger RNA or exogenous ribonucleases delivered by a separate transport vehicle, the original exogenous messenger RNA molecule may be split into translatable subunits. The original exogenous messenger RNA molecule may be physically split or degraded into subunits representing templates, that by the process of translation, will produce copies of the same protein or the original exogenous messenger RNA molecule may be physically split or degraded into subunits representing templates, that by the process of translation, will produce copies of different proteins. Ribonucleases carried by a modified form of virus, a modified Hepatitis C virus, or a virus-like transport vehicle are carried inside the outer shell of the respective vehicle, generally inside the nucleocapsid inner shell of the modified form of virus, a modified Hepatitis C virus, or a virus-like transport vehicle. Ribonucleases carried by a modified form of virus, a modified Hepatitis C virus, or a virus-like transport vehicle may be required to be in primitive state or inactive state that does not cause degradation of the messenger RNA while the messenger RNA is being packaged into the vehicle during initial production, or cause degradation of the messenger RNA while the messenger RNA is being transported in a modified form of virus, a modified Hepatitis C virus, or a virus-like transport vehicle on its way to a host cell. The utilization of ribonucleases will significantly increase the efficiency by which medically therapeutic proteins are generated inside a cell.

[0067] By providing Beta cells with the above-mentioned ribosomal RNAs along with messenger RNAs, the capacity of Beta cells to carrying out the biologic processes of producing insulin and recognizing and responding to blood glucose levels is enhanced, which results in an efficient means to control the glucose levels in the blood stream on a constant and persistent basis utilizing innate regulatory mechanisms and thus diabetes mellitus can be effectively treated and the harmful effects of this disease can be averted.

[0068] By providing any target cell with medically therapeutic ribosomal RNAs along with medically therapeutic messenger RNAs, to enhance a cell's capacity to produce one or more proteins, any protein deficiency can be effectively treated and the harmful effects of the protein deficiency can be averted.

CLAIMS: Reserved,

No. 7: CHEMO VECTOR THERAPY TO DELIVER CHEMO-THERAPY MOLECULES TO SPECIFIC CELLS TO MANAGE BREAST CANCER, OTHER CANCERS AND INFLAMMATO-RY DISORDERS

INDIVIDUALS REQUESTING PATENT: Dr. Lane B. Scheiber, ScD and Dr. Lane B. Scheiber II, MD

©2010 Lane B. Scheiber and Lane B. Scheiber II. A portion of the disclosure of this patent document contains material which is subject to copyright protection. The copyright owners have no objection to the facsimile reproduction by anyone of the patent document or the patent disclosure, as it appears in the Patent and Trademark Office patent file or records, but otherwise reserves all copyright rights whatsoever.

ABSTRACT

The innovative treatment strategy described here utilizes configurable microscopic medical payload delivery devices to act as a transport means to deliver chemotherapy molecules to specific cell types in the body. Utilizing probes present on the exterior of the transport device, transport device locates specific target cell types in the body. Once a specific target cell type has been encountered, the configurable microscopic medical payload delivery device inserts its payload of chemotherapy molecules into the target cell type. By delivering chemotherapy molecules into specific cells, the growth of the specific cells can be stifled. Delivering chemotherapy molecules into specific cancer cells inhibits the rate of growth and rate of cell reproduction of the cancer cells. Utilizing configurable microscopic medical payload delivery devices to insert chemotherapy into targeted cancer cells or inflammatory cells effectively manages cancer, inflammatory arthritis and other inflammatory conditions, while preventing unwanted side effects.

BACKGROUND OF THE INVENTION

Field of the Invention

This invention relates to any medical device intended to manage breast cancer, other cancers and inflammatory disorders utilizing a configurable microscopic medical payload delivery device to insert one or more chemotherapy molecules into one or more specific cell types.

Description of Background Art

[0001] Methotrexate has been used for decades to treat various forms of cancer. For over twenty years rheumatologists have treated inflammatory arthritis with methotrexate. Low dose methotrexate is used to suppress the growth and division of synovial cells. The benefits of using methotrexate to treat conditions such as rheumatoid arthritis and psoriatic arthritis was first recognized when patients with rheumatoid arthritis and cancer were treated with high dose methotrexate in an attempt to manage the cancer. In addition to retarding the growth of cancer cells, the methotrexate suppressed the growth of synovial cells that are responsible for the destructive features of rheumatoid arthritis.

[0002] Methotrexate is an antimetabolite of the B vitamin. Methotrexate inhibits dihydrofolate reductase (DHFR). Dihydrofolates must be reduced to tetrahydrofolic acid by the enzyme DHFR in the process of deoxyribonucleic acid synthesis. Methotrexate therefore inhibits synthesis of nucleic acids, which in turn inhibits cellular replication. Actively proliferating cells such as malignant cells, bone marrow, fetal cells, buccal mucosa cells, intestinal mucosa cells, and rheumatoid arthritis activated synovial cells are generally more sensitive to the presence of methotrexate. The rate of cellular proliferation in malignant tissues is generally greater than in normal tissues. Methotrexate generally impairs malignant or inflammatory cell growth without irreversibly damaging normal tissues. In many patients, treatment with oral or injectable methotrexate does result in significant unwanted side effects, which prevents effective use of the drug in these patients. Methotrexate is principally excreted from the body by the kidneys.

[0003] When utilized to manage an inflammatory arthritis such as rheumatoid arthritis, suppressing folate production suppresses synovial tissue proliferation, which suppresses erosive joint changes. Treatment of rheumatoid arthritis utilizing methotrexate is a strategy of long-term suppression of the disease. Patients with rheumatoid arthritis will often take methotrexate indefinitely.

[0004] Methotrexate generally is categorized as a chemotherapy and also an antimetabolite.

[0005] Cancer cells generally exhibit a rate of growth and replication that exceeds that of normal healthy cells. Cancer cells whose rate of cell growth and cell division can be slowed down to match that of normal healthy cells would result in such a cancer does not pose a significant health risk to the body.

[0006] Breast cancer is a devastating diagnosis for women and men. The survival rate for breast cancer patients has risen significantly over the years as treatment strategies have evolved and improved. Still, the diagnosis or even the threat of breast cancer strikes fear in many women and men around the world. If the growth or rate of cell division of breast cancer cells could be reduced to the same rate as normal cells in breast tissue, then the resultant threat that the occurrence of breast cancer causes would be greatly diminished for the patient, family and friends.

[0007] Present medical research is attempting to utilize viruses to deliver genetic information into cells. Research in the field of 'gene therapy' has involved certain naturally occurring viruses.

Some of the common viral vectors that have been investigated include: Adeno-associated virus, Adenovirus, Alphavirus, Epstein-Barr virus, Gammaretrovirus, Herpes simplex virus, Letivirus, Poliovirus, Rhabdovirus, Vaccinia virus. Naturally occurring virus vectors are limited to the naturally occurring external probes that are affixed to the outer wall of the virus. The external probes fixed to the outside wall of a virus virion dictate which type of cell the virus can engage and infect. Therefore, as an example, the function of the adenovirus, a respiratory virus, is strictly limited to engaging and infecting specific lung cells. Used as a medical treatment device, the adenovirus can only deliver gene therapy to specific lung cells, which severely limits this vector's usefulness as a deliver device. The therapeutic function of all naturally occurring viral vectors is limited to delivering a DNA or RNA payload to the cell type the viral vector naturally targets as its host cell.

[0008] Naturally occurring viruses also have the disadvantage of being susceptible to detection and elimination by a body's immune system. Viruses have been infecting humans for hundreds of thousands of years. A human's immune system, comprised of an innate system and an adaptable system, is very complex, and very efficient at detecting the presence of most naturally occurring viruses when such a virus breaches the outer perimeter of the body. The human immune system is quite capable of generating a vigorous response to most intruding viruses, attacking and neutralizing virus virions whenever a virus virion physically exists are outside the exterior wall of the virus's host cell. If gene therapy, in its current state, were to become a clinical therapeutic tool, the naturally occurring viruses selected for gene therapy research will have limited effectiveness. Once a naturally occurring viral vector is introduced into the body, the body's the immune system will most likely detect the intrusion, quickly engage and eliminate the viral vectors, possibly before any one of the vectors is able to deliver its payload to its host cell or target cell.

[0009] Cichutek, K., 2001 (US Patent No. 6,323,031 B1) teaches preparation and use of novel lentiviral SiVagm-derived vectors for gene transfer into selected cell types, specifically into proliferatively active and resting human cells.

[0010] Cichutek teaches that it is indeed plausible to re-configure an existing virus and use it as a transport vehicle, though Cichutek's specification and claims are too limited to describe a method that will work for all cell types, if indeed if it will work for any cell type.

[0011] Cichutek describes vectors for 'gene transfer'; in the claims the language that is used is 'genetic information'. Cichutek's Claim 1 of the cited patent states 'A propagation-incompetent SIVagm vector comprising a viral core and a viral envelope, wherein the viral core comprises a simian immunodeficiency virus (SIVagm) viral core of the African vervet monkey Chlorocebus.' Cichutek's does not describe in his claims any further details of the intended payload other than the stating 'SIVagm viral core' in claim 1; in claims 5 & 6 Cichutek describes only 'genetic information'. Transfer of 'genetic information' dramatically limits the useful application of Cichutek's patent in the treatment of medical diseases.

[0012] Cichutek's approach is dependent upon the probes naturally present on the viral vectors reported in the patent, which will direct the viral vectors to only those cells the viruses naturally use as their host cell. Cichutek's approach is very restrictive, limited to gene transfer to only cells the viruses use as their natural host cell.

[0013] Singular type antibodies or ligands can be used for cell-to-cell communication, but to open an access portal into a cell and insert a payload into the cell requires two different types of antibodies or ligands. As an example human immunodeficiency virus requires the use of both the gp120 and gp41 probes to open a portal into a T-Helper cell and inserts its viral genome into the T-Helper cell. The gp120 probe engages the CD4+ cell-surface receptor on the T-cell. Once the gp120 probe has successfully engaged a CD4+ cell-surface receptor on the target T-Helper cell, then the HIV virion's gp41 probe can engage either a CXCR4 or a CCR5 cell-surface receptor on the T-Helper cell in order to open up an access portal for HIV to insert its viral genome into a T-Helper cell. It is well documented in the medical literature that a genetic defect leading to an abnormality in the CXCR4 cell-surface receptor prevents HIV virions from opening an access portal and inserting its genetic payload into such T-Helper cells. This genetic defect in the CXCR4 cell-surface receptors offers the subset of people carrying the genetic defect resistance to HIV infection. This example demonstrates the need for at least two types of glycoprotein probes to be present on the surface of a viral vector in order for a viral vector to be capable of opening an access portal and delivering the payload the vector carries into its host cell or target cell.

[0014] A delivery system that offered a defined means of targeting specific types of cells would invoke minimal or no response by the innate immune system or the adaptable immune system when present in the body, and a delivery system that would be capable of inserting into cells a wide variety of chemotherapy molecules would significantly improve the current medical treatment options available to clinicians treating patients. Such a strategy would increase the effectiveness of the chemotherapy and would result in a dramatic reduction in unwanted side effects posed by such chemotherapy.

[0015] The solution to arriving at a versatile, workable delivery system that will meet the needs of a number of medical treatments involves three important elements. These elements include:

    (1) configurable external probes whereby more than one type of protein structure probe or more than one type

of glycoprotein probe is to be used to engage and access specific target cell types in order to successfully deliver a payload into a specific cell type,

(2) an exterior envelope comprised of a protein shell or lipid layer or a lipid bilayer expressing the least number of cell-surface markers, such as the use of a stem cell to act as the host cell to manufacture the delivery devices,

(3) configuring the core or center of the vector to enable it to carry and deliver a wide variety of chemotherapy molecules.

[0016] Viruses are obligate parasites. Viruses simply represent a carrier of genetic material and by themselves viruses are unable to replicate or carry out any form of biologic function outside their host cell. A 'virion' refers to the physical structure of a single complete virus as it exists outside of the host cell; an older term for 'viral virion' was 'virus particle'. Viruses are generally comprised of one or more nested shells constructed of one or more layers of protein, some with a lipid outer envelope, a genetic payload that represents the instruction code necessary to replicate the virus, and protein enzymes to help facilitate the genetic payload in the function of replicating copies of the virus once the genetic payload has been delivered to a host cell. Located on the outer shell or envelope of a virus are probes. The function of a virus's external probes is to locate and engage a host cell's receptors. The virus's surface probes are designed to detect, make contact with and functionally engage one or more receptors located on the exterior of a cell type that will offer the virus the proper environment in which to construct copies of itself. A host cell provides the virus the proper biologic machinery for the virus to successfully replicate itself. Once the virus's genome is inside the host cell, the viral genome takes command of the cell's production machinery and causes the host cell to generate copies of the virus. As the viral copies exit the host cell, these virions set off in search of other host cells to infect.

[0017] Naturally occurring viruses exist in a number of differing shapes. The shape of a virus may be rod or filament like, icosahedral, or complex structures combining filament and polygonal shapes. Viruses generally have their outer wall comprised of a protein coat or an envelope comprised of lipids.

[0018] An outer envelope comprised of lipids may be in the form of one or two phospholipid layers. When the outer envelope is comprised of two phospholipid layers this is termed a lipid bilayer. For purposes of this text the term 'lipid' includes 'phospholipid' molecules. A phospholipid is a composite molecule comprised of a polar or hydrophilic region on one end and a nonpolar or hydrophobic region on the opposite end. A lipid bilayer covering a virus, like the membrane of a cell, is constructed with the hydrophilic region of one of the phospholipid layers pointed toward the exterior of the virion and the hydrophilic region of the second phospholipid layer pointed inward toward the center of the virus virion; with the hydrophobic regions of each of the two lipid layers pointed toward each other. The outer envelope of some forms of virus may be comprised of an outer lipid layer or lipid bilayer affixed to a protein matrix for support, the protein matrix being located closer to the center of the virus virion than the lipid layer or lipid bilayer.

[0019] Spherical viruses are generally spherical in shape and may be comprised of an outer envelope and one inner shell or an outer envelope and multiple inner shells. Inner shells are approximately spherical in shape; this is because the proteins comprising the protein matrix shell have an irregular shape to their structure. In the case of a spherical virus with an outer envelope and one inner shell, the inner shell is often referred to as a nucleocapsid shell comprised of numerous capsid proteins attached to each other. In the case of a spherical virus being comprised of an outer envelope and multiple inner shells, the outermost inner viral shells may be referred to as comprised of a quantity of matrix proteins, where the innermost shell is referred to as a nucleocapsid and is comprised of a quantity of capsid proteins. The inner protein shells are nested inside each other. The cavity present created by the innermost shell or nucleocapsid is referred to as the 'core' or the 'center of the virus'. Any payload carried by the virus virion is generally carried in the core or center of the virion.

[0020] Viruses carry genetic material in the form of deoxyribonucleic acid (DNA) or ribonucleic acid (RNA) as their payload. DNA or RNA payloads are carried in the cavity of the nucleocapsid referred to as the core. A virus is therefore generally considered to be a DNA virus if its genome is comprised of DNA or the virus is considered a RNA virus if its genome is comprised of RNA that acts as genetic instructions to generate copies of the virus. Viruses may also carry enzymes as part of their payload. An enzyme such as 'reverse transcriptase' transforms a RNA viral genome into DNA. Protease enzymes modify the viral genome once it has entered a host cell. An integrase enzyme assists a DNA viral genome with insertion into the host cell's nuclear DNA. The entire genetic payload is carried inside cavity created by the virus's nucleocapsid shell.

[0021] The probes attached to the exterior of a virus are constructed to engage specific cell-surface receptors on specific cell types in the body. Only a cell that expresses cell-surface receptors that are capable of being engaged by the probes of a specific virus can act as a host for the virus. Viruses generally use two probes to access a host cell. The first probe makes an initial attachment to the host cell, while the action of the virus's second probe often in conjunction with the action of the first probe cause an access portal to be created in the host cell's exterior plasma membrane. Once an access portal is formed, the virus inserts the contents of its payload into the host cell. Once the virus's genome is inside the cytoplasm of the host cell, any enzymes that accompanied the viral genome into the cell, may begin to modify or assist the virus's genome with infecting and taking control of the host cell's biologic functions.

[0022] Probes are attached to the exterior envelope of a virus virion. Probes may be in the form of a protein structure or may be in the form of a glycoprotein molecule. For viruses constructed with a protein matrix as its outer envelope, the probes tend to be protein structures. A portion of the protein structure probe is fixed or anchored in the protein matrix, while a portion of the protein structure probe extends out and away from the protein matrix. The portion of the protein structure probe extending out away from the virus virion is referred to as the 'exterior domain', the portion anchored in the protein matrix is the 'transcending domain'. Some protein probes have a third segment that extends through the envelope and exists inside the virus virion, which is referred to as the 'interior domain'. The exterior domain of a protein structure probe is intended to engage a specific cell-surface receptor on a biologically active cell the virus is targeting as its host cell.

[0023] Viruses that utilize a lipid layer as the outer envelope, are constructed with probes that tend to be glycoproteins. A glycoprotein is comprised of a protein segment and a carbohydrate segment. The carbohydrate segment of the glycoprotein molecule is fixed or anchored in the lipid layer of the outer envelope, while the protein segment extends outward and away from the outer envelope. The protein portion of a glycoprotein probe that extends outward and away from the outer envelope of a virus virion is intended to engage a cell-surface receptor on a biologically active cell the virus is targeting as its host cell.

[0024] Some forms of viruses that utilize a lipid layer as its envelope use protein structure probes. In this case, the portion of the protein structure probe that extends outward and away from the outer envelope is the 'exterior domain', the portion that is anchored in the lipid layer is the 'transcending domain' and again some protein structure probes have an 'interior domain' that exist inside the virion, which may also help anchor the protein structure probe to the virion. The exterior domain of a protein structure probe that extends outward and away from the outer envelope of a virus virion is intended to engage a cell-surface receptor on a biologically active cell the virus is targeting as its host cell.

[0025] When a virus carries a DNA payload and the viral DNA is inserted into the host cell, the virus's DNA travels to the host cell's nucleus and is known to become inserted into the host cell's own native DNA. In the case where a virus is carrying its genetic payload as RNA, the virus inserts the RNA payload into the host cell and may also insert one or more enzymes to facilitate the RNA being utilized properly to replicate copies of the virus. Once inside the host cell, some species of virus facilitate use of the viral RNA by having the RNA converted to DNA. Once the viral RNA has been converted to DNA, the virus's DNA travels to the host cell's nucleus and is known to become inserted into the host cell's native DNA. Once a virus's genetic material has been inserted into the host cell's native DNA, the virus's genetic material takes command of certain cell functions and redirects the resources of the host cell to generate copies of the virus. Other forms of RNA viruses bypass the need to use the nuclear DNA and simply utilize portions of the viral genome to act as messenger RNA. RNA viruses that bypass the host cell's DNA, cause the cell in general to generate copies of the necessary parts of the virus directly from the virus's RNA genome.

[0026] The human immunodeficiency virus (HIV) is a RNA virus and has an outer envelope comprised of a lipid bilayer. The lipid bilayer covers a protein matrix consisting of p17^{gag} proteins. Inside the p17^{gag} protein is nested a nucleocapsid comprised of p24^{gag} proteins. Inside the nucleocapsid HIV carries its payload. HIV's genetic payload consists of two single strands of RNA and several enzymes. The enzymes that accompany HIV's genome include 'reverse transcriptase', 'integrase' and 'protease' molecules.

[0027] The T-Helper cell acts as HIV's host cell. The HIV virion utilizes two types of glycoprotein probes affixed to its exterior envelope to locate and engage a T-Helper cell. HIV utilizes a glycoprotein probe 120 to locate a CD4 cell-surface receptor on a T-Helper cell. Once an HIV glycoprotein 120 probe has successfully engaged a CD4 cell surface-receptor on a T-Helper cell a conformational change occurs in the glycoprotein 120 probe and a glycoprotein 41 probe is exposed. The glycoprotein 41 probe's intent is to engage a CXCR4 or CCR5 cell-surface receptor on the same T-Helper cell. Once a glycoprotein 41 probe on the HIV virion successfully engages a CXCR4 or CCR5 cell-surface receptor, the HIV virion opens an access portal through the T-Helper cell's outer membrane.

[0028] Once the HIV virion has opened an access portal through the T-Helper cell's outer plasma membrane, the HIV virion inserts two positive strand RNA molecules and the associated enzymes it carries into the T-Helper cell. Each RNA strand is approximately 9500 nucleotides in length. Inserted along with the RNA strands are the enzymes reverse transcriptase, protease and integrase. Once the virus's genome gains access to the interior of the T-Helper cell, in the cytoplasm the pair of RNA molecules are transformed to deoxyribonucleic acid by the reverse transcriptase enzyme. Following modification of the virus's genome to DNA, the virus's genetic information migrates to the host cell's nucleus. In the nucleus, with the assistance of the integrase protein, the HIV's DNA becomes inserted into the T-Helper cell's native nuclear DNA. When the timing is appropriate, the now integrated viral DNA is decoded by the host cell's polymerase molecules and the virus's genetic information commands certain cell functions to carry out the replication process to construct copies of the human immunodeficiency virus.

[0029] The outer layer of the HIV virion is comprised of a portion of the T-Helper cell's outer cell membrane. In the final stage of the replication process, as a copy of the HIV virion, carrying the HIV genome, buds through the host cell's cell membrane the outer capsid acquires as its exterior envelope, a wrapping of lipid bilayer from the host cell's cell membrane. In the case of HIV, since the surface of the pathogen is covered by an envelope comprised of lipid bilayer taken from the host T-Helper cells, this feature allows the HIV virion the capacity to eluded the two immune systems, since the detectors comprising the innate immune system and the adaptable immune system may find it difficult to distinguish between the surface of an infectious HIV virion and the surface characteristics of a noninfected T-Helper cell.

[0030] The Hepatitis C virus (HCV) is a positive sense RNA virus, meaning a type of RNA that is capable of bypassing the need for involving the host cell's nucleus by having its RNA genome function as messenger RNA. Hepatitis C infects liver cells. The Hepatitis C viral genome becomes divided once it gains access to the interior of a liver host cell. Portions of the subdivisions of the Hepatitis C genome directly interact with ribosomes to produce proteins necessary to construct copies of the virus.

[0031] HCV belongs to the Flaviviridae family and is the only member of the Hepacivirus genus. There are considered to be at least 100 different strains of Hepatitis C virus based on genome sequencing variability.

[0032] HCV is comprised of an outer lipoprotein envelope and an internal nucleocapsid. The genetic payload is carried within the nucleocapsid. In its natural state, present on the surface of the outer envelope of the Hepatitis C virus are probes that detect receptors present on the surface of liver cells. The glycoprotein E1 probe and the glycoprotein E2 probe have been identified to be affixed to the surface of HCV. The E2 probe binds with high affinity to the large external loop of a CD81 cell-surface receptor. CD81 is found on the surface of many cell types including liver cells. Once the E2 probe has engaged the CD81 cell-surface receptor, cofactors on the surface of HCV's exterior envelope engage either or both the low density lipoprotein receptor (LDLR) or the scavenger receptor class B type I (SR-BI) present on the liver cell in order to effect the mechanism to facilitate HCV breaching the cell membrane and inserting its RNA genome payload through the plasma cell membrane of the liver cell into the liver cell. Upon successful engagement of the HCV surface probes with a liver cell's cell-surface receptors, HCV inserts the single strand of RNA and other payload elements it carries into the liver cell targeted to be a host cell. The HCV RNA genome then interacts with enzymes and ribosomes inside the liver cell in a translational process to produce the proteins required to construct copies of the protein components of HCV. The HCV genome undergoes a method of transcription to replicate copies of the virus's RNA genome. Inside the host, pieces of the HCV virus are assembled together and ultimately loaded with a copy of the HCV genome. Replicas of the original HCV then escape the host cell and migrate the environment in search of additional host liver cells to infect and continue the replication process.

[0033] The HCV's naturally occurring genetic payload consists of a single molecule of linear positive sense, single stranded RNA approximately 9600 nucleotides in length. By means of a translational process a polyprotein of approximately 3000 amino acids is generated. This polyprotein is cleaved post translation by host and viral proteases into individual viral proteins which include: the structural proteins of C, E1, E2, the nonstructural proteins NS1, NS2, NS3, NS4A, NS4B, NS5A, NS5B, p7 and ARFP/F protein. Hepatitis C virus's proteins direct the host liver cell to construction copies of the Hepatitis C virus. A membrane associated replicase complex consisting of the virus's nonstructural proteins NS3 and NS5B facilitate the replication of the viral genome. The membrane of the endoplasmic reticulum appears to be the site of protein maturation and viral assembly. Once copies of the Hepatitis C Virus are generated, they exit the host cell and each copy of HCV migrates in search of another appropriate liver cell that will act as a host to continue the replication process.

[0034] Hepatitis C virus life-cycle demonstrates that copies of a virus virion can be generated by inserting RNA into a host cell that functions as messenger RNA in the host cell. The Hepatitis C viral RNA genome functions as messenger RNA, acting as the template in conjunction with the biologic machinery of a host cell to produce the components that comprise copies of the Hepatitis C virion and the Hepatitis C viral RNA provides the biologic instructions to assemble the components into complete copies of the Hepatitis C virions. The Hepatitis C virus life-cycle clearly demonstrates that viral virions can be manufactured by a host cell without involving the nucleus of the cell.

[0035] Deciphering the existence, replication and behavior of viruses provides clear examples of several fundamental concepts, which include: (1) Viruses target specific cells in the body by means of identifying and engaging such target cells utilizing the probes projecting outward from the virus's exterior shell to make contact with cell-surface receptors located on the surface of their host cells, and (2) Viruses are capable of carrying a variety of different types of payloads including DNA, RNA and a variety of proteins.

[0036] Current gene therapy approach to attempting to deliver a payload to cells in the body use modified forms of existing viruses to act as transport devices to deliver genetic information. This approach is severely limited by restricting the virus virion to the target only cells the viral vector naturally seeks out and infects. Current gene therapy approach is further limited by using the pre-existing size of naturally occurring viruses, rather than being able to modify the size of the structure to be able to tailor the volumetric carrying capacity of the payload portion of the modified virus. Further gene therapy is restricted to utilizing naturally occurring viruses to deliver only genetic information; it has not previously been appreciated by those skilled in the art that virus-like transport devices might deliver to a variety of specific cell types a wide variety of differing payloads including various chemotherapy drug molecules.

[0037] A dramatic necessity, not previously recognized by those expert in the art, is the need to develop a transport vehicle that can be fashioned to seek out specific types of cells and deliver to these cells chemotherapy molecules to treat cancer and inflammatory disorders by inhibiting the rate cell growth and replication of these specific target cells. The exterior envelope of a transport vehicle should be constructed so as not to alert either component of the immune system of its presence to prevent rejection of these transport vehicles. Transport vehicles should be capable of being configured to target any specific cell type and engage and deliver their chemotherapy payload only to that specific cell type. To this point, no such device or process has been documented in the literature.

BRIEF SUMMARY OF THE INVENTION

[0038] Utilization of configurable microscopic medical payload delivery devices to deliver chemotherapy molecules to specific cell types facilitates a dramatic new approach to managing cancer and inflammatory disorders. By selecting the type of probes that will effectively engage cell-surface receptors on target cells and fixing these probes on the surface of the configurable microscopic medical payload delivery devices, specific types of cells can be targeted. By utilizing configurable microscopic medical payload delivery devices to deliver chemotherapy molecules to specific cell types, the rate of cell growth and rate of cell replication can be inhibited without provoking unwanted side effects in other cells. A wide variety of cancers and inflammatory disorders are treatable by utilizing this new and unique approach.

DETAILED DESCRIPTION

[0039] Future medical treatment includes the aggressive, widespread utilization of configurable microscopic medical payload delivery devices (CMMPDD) to deliver chemotherapy molecules directly to specific targeted cell types in the body.

[0040] The configurable microscopic medical payload delivery device transporting chemotherapy molecules represents a very versatile medical treatment delivery device. CMMPDD is used to deliver chemotherapy molecules to a wide variety of cancer cells and inflammatory cells. Utilizing CMMPDD to deliver chemotherapy molecules to cancer cells represents a new means to manage cancer. Using CMMPDD to deliver chemotherapy molecules to inflammatory arthritis represents a new means to treat inflammatory arthritis. By delivering chemotherapy molecules directly to targeted cells and only to the targeted cells by virus-like transport devices, the configurable microscopic medical payload delivery devices represent a significant advancement over current chemotherapy treatment techniques in that this strategy avoids many of the unwanted side effects that conventional chemotherapy cause.

[0041] For purposes of this text an 'external envelope' refers to the outermost covering of a virus or a virus-like transport device or a configurable microscopic medical payload delivery device. The external envelope may be comprised of a lipid layer, a lipid bilayer, the combination of a lipid layer affixed to a protein matrix or the combination of a lipid bilayer affixed to a protein matrix. A protein matrix is equivalent to a protein shell and may be referred to as a protein matrix shell. The terms protein matrix, protein shell, protein matrix shell are equivalent to the term capsid, where the term capsid is meant to represent 'a protein coat or shell of a virus particle, surrounding the nucleic acid or nucleoprotein core'. The term 'particle' is equivalent to the term 'virion'.

[0042] For purposes of this text an 'internal shell' refers to a protein matrix shell nested inside the external envelope. The innermost protein matrix shell is termed the nucleocapsid. The proteins that comprise the nucleocapsid are termed capsid proteins. In the cavity created by the nucleocapsid, referred to as the center or core of the nucleocapsid, is where the payload of chemotherapy molecules is carried.

[0043] For purposes of this text 'external probes' are molecular structures that are utilized to locate and engage cell-surface receptors on biologically active cells. External probes are generally comprised of a portion which is anchored or fixed in the external envelope and a second portion that extends out and away from the external envelope. The portion of the external probe that extends out and away from the external envelope is intended to make contact and engage a cell-surface receptor located on a biologically active cell. External probes may be comprised solely of a protein structure or an external probe may be a glycoprotein molecule.

[0044] For purposes of this text 'glycoprotein molecule' refers to a molecule comprised of a carbohydrate region and a protein region. Glycoprotein molecules that act as probes are generally anchored or fixed to a lipid layer utilizing the carbohydrate portion of the molecule as an anchor. The protein portion of the glycoprotein molecule which extends outward and away from the exterior envelope the glycoprotein has been affixed such that the protein region may function as a probe to locate and attach to the cell-surface receptor it was created to engage.

[0045] The concept of configurable microscopic medical payload delivery devices is modeled after naturally existing viruses. Configurable microscopic medical payload delivery devices in general are spherical in shape; though other shapes may be used as function might warrant the use of a particular shape. The spherical configurable microscopic medical payload delivery devices are comprised of an exterior envelope and one or more inner nested protein shells. A quantity of exterior protein structure probes and/or glycoprotein probes are anchored in the exterior lipid envelope and a portion extends out and away from the exterior lipid envelope. Nesting of protein shells refers to progressively smaller diameter shells fitting snugly inside protein shells of a larger diameter. Inside the inner most protein shell, referred to as the nucleocapsid, is a cavity referred to as the core of the device. The core of the device is the space where the medically therapeutic payload the device carries is located. The payload of the device is comprised of chemotherapy molecules.

[0046] Configurable microscopic medical payload delivery devices (CMMPDD) target specific types of cells in the body. Configurable microscopic medical payload delivery devices engage specific types of cells by the configuration of probes affixed to the exterior envelope of the CMMPDD. By fixing specific probes to the exterior envelope of the CMMPDD, these probes intended to engage and attach only to specific cell-surface receptors located on certain cell types in the body, the CMMPDD will deliver its payload to only those cell types that express compatible and engagable specific cell-surface receptors. In a similar fashion where the exterior probes of a naturally occurring virus engage specific cell-surface receptors present on the surface of the virus's host cell and only the designated host cell, the CMMPDD's exterior probes are configured to engage cell-surface receptors on a specific type of target cell and only those cells. In this manner, the payload of chemotherapy drug molecules carried by CMMPDD will be delivered only to specific types of cells in the body. The configuration of the exterior probes on the surface of a CMMPDD will vary as needed so as to effect the CMMPDD delivery of chemotherapy drug payloads to the specific cell types as needed to effect a particular predetermined medical treatment.

[0047] The size of configurable microscopic medical payload delivery devices is dependent upon the diameter of the inner protein matrix shells and this is dictated by the volume size of the payload the CMMPDD is required to carry and deliver to a target cell. The diameter of each inner protein matrix shell is governed by the number of protein molecules utilized to construct the protein matrix shell at the time the protein matrix shell is generated. Increasing the number of proteins that comprise a protein matrix shell, increases the diameter of the protein matrix shell. When applicable an external lipid envelope wraps around and covers the outermost protein matrix shell. The larger the volume of the core of the CMMPDD, the greater the physical size payload the CMMPDD is able to carry. The size of the configurable microscopic medical payload delivery device is to be the size of cell (approximately 10^{-4} m in diameter) or less, generally detectable by a light microscope or, as needed, an electron microscope. The size of the CMMPDD is not to be too large such that it would generate a burden to the body by damaging organ tissues through clogging blood vessels or glomeruli in the kidneys. The dimensions of each type of CMMPDD are to be tailored to the mission of the CMMPDD, which takes into account factors such as the type of target cell, the size of the payload that is to be delivered to the target cells and the length of time the CMMPDD may have to engage the target cell.

[0048] Being enveloped in an external lipid layer, configurable microscopic medical payload delivery devices possess the advantage of having their exterior appear similar to the plasma membrane that acts as an outside covering for the cells that comprise the body. By appearing similar to existing plasma membranes, the CMMPDDs appear similar to naturally occurring structures found in the body. CMMPDD's are afforded the capability to avoid detection by a body's immune system because the exterior of the CMMPDD mimics the cells comprising the body and the surveillance elements of the immune system find it difficult to discern between the CMMPDD and naturally occurring cells comprising the body.

[0049] To carry out the process of manufacturing a configurable microscopic medical payload delivery device, a primitive cell such as a stem cell is selected. The reason for utilizing primitive cells such as stems cells as the host cell, is that the CMMPDD acquires its outer envelope from the host cell and the more primitive the host cell, the fewer in number the identifying protein markers are present on the surface of the CMMPDD. The fewer the identifying surface proteins present on the outer envelope of the CMMPDD, the less likely a body's immune system will identify the CMMPDD as an intruder and therefore less likely the body's immune system will react to the presence of the CMMPDD and reject the CMMPDD by attacking and neutralizing the CMMPDD.

[0050] Stem cells used as host cells to manufacture quantities of CMMPDD product are selected per histocompatibility markers present on their surface. Certain histocompatibility markers present on the surface of the final CMMPDD product will be less likely to cause a reaction in a specific patient based on the genetic profile of the patient's histocompatibility markers. A similar histocompatibility match is done when donor organs are selected to be given to recipients to avoid rejection of the donor organ by the recipient's immune system.

[0051] The selected stem cells used to manufacture configurable microscopic medical payload delivery devices goes through several steps of maturation before it is capable of generating therapeutic CMMPDD product. Messenger RNA would be inserted into the host stem cell that would code for the general physical outer structures of the CMMPDD. Messenger RNA would be inserted into the host that would generate surface probes that would target the cell-surface receptors on specific target cell types. Messenger RNA would be inserted into the host that would be used to generate the payload of chemotherapy molecules or the chemotherapy molecules are introduced into the CMMPDD post production of the CMMPDD based on the size and complexity of the chemotherapy molecules. Similar to how copies of a naturally occurring virus, such as the Hepatitis C virus or HIV, are produced, assembled and released from a host cell, copies of the CMMPDD would be produced, assembled and released from a host cell. Once released from the stem cell functioning as a de facto host cell, the copies of the CMMPDD would be collected, then pooled together to produce a therapeutic dose that results in a medically beneficial effect.

[0052] The stem cells used as host cells are suspended in a broth of nutrients and are kept at an optimum temperature to govern the rate of production of the CMMPDD product. Similar to the natural production of the Hepatitis C virus, the configurable microscopic medical payload delivery devices 'production genome' is introduced into the host stem cells. The configurable microscopic medical payload delivery devices production genome carries genetic instructions to cause the host cells to manufacture the configurable microscopic medical payload delivery devices' outer protein wall, the inner protein matrixes, the surface probes the configurable microscopic medical payload delivery device is to have affixed to its outer envelope, the chemotherapy molecules the configurable microscopic medical payload delivery devices are to carry, and the instructions to assemble the various pieces into the final form of the configurable microscopic medical payload delivery devices along with the instructions to activate the budding process. The resultant configurable microscopic medical payload delivery devices are collected from the nutrient broth surrounding the host cells and placed together into doses to be used as a treatment for a medical disease.

[0053] The 'production genome' are an array of messenger RNAs that are directly translated by the host cell's ribosomes. The production genome dictates the characteristics of the final version of the CMMPDD that buds from the host stem cell and is released and is to be utilized as a medical treatment. The production genome is specifically tailored to code for the surface probes that will seek and engage a specific type of target cell. The production genome also carries the instructions to code for the production of the type of chemotherapy molecules to be delivered to the specific type of target cell. The 'production genome' varies depending upon the configuration of the CMMPDD and the type of chemotherapy molecules the CMMPDD will transport to effect a specific medical treatment in a specific type of cell.

[0054] The configurable microscopic medical payload delivery device transporting chemotherapy molecules represents a very versatile medical treatment delivery device. CMMPDD is used to deliver chemotherapy molecules to a wide variety of cancer cells and inflammatory cells. Utilizing CMMPDD to deliver chemotherapy molecules to cancer cells represents a new means to manage cancer. Using CMMPDD to deliver chemotherapy molecules to inflammatory arthritis represents a new means to treat inflammatory arthritis.

[0055] As an example of this method, to treat breast cancer utilizing configurable microscopic medical payload delivery devices to deliver to breast cells chemotherapy such as the antimetabolite methotrexate, the following production process is followed in the lab: (1) human stem cells are selected. (2) Into the selected stem cells is placed the production genome constructed, in this case, specifically as a means to treat breast cancer. The RNA production genome contains genetic instructions to cause the host stem cells to manufacture the configurable microscopic medical payload delivery devices' outer protein wall, the inner protein matrix, surface probes to include glycoprotein probes that engage estrogen cell-surface receptors present on the surface of breast cells, and the payload of chemotherapy molecules; and the biologic instructions to assemble the components into the final form of the configurable microscopic medical payload delivery devices; and the biologic instructions to activate the budding process. (3) Upon insertion of the RNA production genome dedicated to producing a configurable microscopic medical payload delivery devices to transport chemotherapy molecules, into the host stem cells, host stem cells respond by (i) simultaneously translating the different segments of the RNA production genome to produce the proteins that comprise the exterior protein wall, the inner protein matrix shell molecules, the surface probes to seek out and engage breast cells, the chemotherapy molecules, and (ii) decoding the RNA instructions to assemble the components into the configurable microscopic medical payload delivery devices. (4) Upon assembly, the configurable microscopic medical payload delivery devices bud through the cell membrane of the host stem cell. (5) At the time of the budding process, the configurable microscopic medical payload delivery devices acquire an outside envelope wrapped over the outer protein shell, this outer envelope comprised of a portion of the plasma membrane from the host stem cell as the configurable microscopic medical payload delivery devices exit the host cell. (6) In some cases dependent upon the treatment application and how tightly packed the configurable microscopic medical payload delivery devices need to be packed with chemotherapy molecules, such chemotherapy molecules may be present in the nutrient broth and diffuse into the configurable microscopic medical payload delivery devices. (7) The resultant configurable microscopic medical payload delivery devices are collected from the nutrient broth surrounding the host stem cells. (8) The configurable microscopic medical payload delivery devices are washed in sterile solvent to remove contaminants. (9) The configurable microscopic medical payload delivery devices are removed from the sterile solvent and suspended in a hypoallergenic liquid medium. (10) The configurable microscopic medical payload delivery devices are separated into individual quantities to facilitate storage and delivery to physicians and patients. (11) The configurable microscopic medical payload delivery devices transported in the hypoallergenic liquid medium is administered to a patient with a diagnosis of breast cancer per injection in a dose that is tailored to receiving patient's severity of breast cancer. (12) Upon being injected into the body, the configurable microscopic medical payload delivery devices migrate to the breast tissues by means of the patient's blood stream. (13) Upon the configurable microscopic medical payload delivery devices reaching the breast cells, the configurable microscopic medical payload delivery devices engage the cell-surface receptors located on the breast cells and insert the payload they carry into the breast cells. The payload, in this case being the chemotherapy methotrexate. Methotrexate molecules inhibit dihydrofolate reductase and therefore prevents breast cells synthesizing nucleic acids, therefore prevents cell division, which prevents the cancer cells from replicating but does not interfere with normal breast cells.

[0056] In a similar fashion, configurable microscopic medical payload delivery devices can be fashioned to deliver a payload of a specific chemotherapy molecule to any type of cancer cell or inflammatory cell in the body. Different cell types express different cell-surface markers on the exterior of their plasma membrane. The differing configurations of cell-surface markers on differing types of cells distinguish one cell type from another cell type. By configuring the exterior probes that extend from the surface of the configurable microscopic medical payload delivery device to seek out and engage specific cell-surface receptors present on normal cells and cancer cells payloads of chemotherapy can be delivered to specific cells in the body.

[0057] Rheumatoid arthritis is an inflammatory disease affecting millions of people worldwide. The chemotherapy drug methotrexate has been used for over twenty years, and is used quite extensively as a treatment of rheumatoid arthritis. Oral and injectable forms of the methotrexate are used to suppress the growth and cell division of synovial tissues. Oral and injectable methotrexate causes many unwanted side effects. Utilizing configurable microscopic medical payload delivery devices to deliver methotrexate molecules specifically to synovial cells and only to synovial cells, increases the efficacy of methotrexate and reduces or eliminates the unwanted side effects of methotrexate.

Conclusions, Ramification, and Scope

[0058] Accordingly, the reader will see that the configurable microscopic medical payload delivery device to deliver chemotherapy molecules to specific targeted cell types provides advantages over existing art by: (1) being a delivery device that seeks out specific types of cells, (2) by being a delivery device that is versatile enough to deliver a variety of potential chemotherapy molecules to accomplish various medical treatments, (3) by being a device that delivers chemotherapy molecules only to targeted cells, thus avoiding unwanted side effects that current chemotherapy causes, and (4) by being a delivery device constructed with a surface envelope that will avoid detection by the innate immune system and the adaptable immune system so as not to activate either immune system to its presence; for these reasons this represents a new and unique medical delivery device that has never before been recognized nor appreciated by those skilled in the art.

[0059] Although the description above contains specificities, these should not be construed as limiting the scope of the invention but as merely providing illustrations of some of the presently preferred embodiments of the invention.

[0060] Thus the scope of the invention should be determined by the appended claims and their legal equivalents, rather than by the examples given.

CLAIMS: Reserved.

No. 8: QUANTUM UNIT OF INHERITANCE

INDIVIDUALS REQUESTING PATENT: Dr. Lane B. Scheiber, ScD and Dr. Lane B. Scheiber II, MD

©2010 Lane B. Scheiber and Lane B. Scheiber II. A portion of the disclosure of this patent document contains material which is subject to copyright protection. The copyright owners have no objection to the facsimile reproduction by anyone of the patent document or the patent disclosure, as it appears in the Patent and Trademark Office patent file or records, but otherwise reserves all copyright rights whatsoever.

ABSTRACT

Quantum genes have a unique identifier assigned to them. By identifying genetic material with a unique identifier a means of locating specific genetic material is plausible. Delivering such quantum genes, that contain a unique identifier, to specific cell types provides a means of inserting specific genetic information into the cell's nuclear deoxyribonucleic acid that can be readily located by the cell's nuclear transcription complexes. These medically therapeutic quantum genes are intended to provide a wide variety of medical therapeutic options to clinicians.

BACKGROUND OF THE INVENTION

Field of the Invention

This invention relates to any medical device associated with gene therapy where the gene therapy is conducted with genetic information labeled with a unique identifying code.

Description of Background Art

[0001] The central dogma of microbiology dictates that in the nucleus of a biologically active cell, genes are transcribed to produce messenger ribonucleic acid molecules (mRNAs), these mRNAs migrate to the cytoplasm where they are translated to produce proteins. One of the great unknowns that has challenged the study of microbiology is the subject of understanding of how the genes, comprising the genome of a species, are organized such that the nuclear transcription machinery can efficiently locate specific transcribable genetic information and instructions that the cell requires to maintain itself, grow and conduct cell replication. Decoding the means as to how the genetic information contained in the nuclear deoxyribonucleic acid (DNA) of a cell is organized, helps to further the efforts to produce an effective gene therapy treatment strategy. Understanding the basis of genetic instruction code information stored in a cell's DNA and utilizing such knowledge of labeling and cataloging of genetic information, makes inserting biologic instruction into the DNA of cells a practical and effective means of treating a wide scope of medical conditions.

[0002] The human genome is comprised of deoxyribonucleic acid (DNA) separated into 46 chromosomes. The chromosomes are further subdivided into genes. Genes represent units of transcribable DNA. Transcription of the DNA refers to generating one or more of a variety of RNA molecules. Regarding the human genome, currently it is estimated that 5% of the total nuclear DNA is thought to represent genes and 95% is thought to represent redundant non-gene genetic material. The DNA genome in a cell is therefore comprised of transcribable genetic information and nontranscribable genetic information. Transcribable genetic information represent the segments of DNA that when transcribed by transcription machinery yield RNA molecules, usually in a precursor form that require modification before the RNA molecules are capable of being translated. The nontranscribable genetic information represent segments that act as either points of attachment for the transcription machinery or act as commands to direct the transcription machinery or act as spacers between transcribable segments of genetic information or have no known function at this time. A segment of nontranslatable DNA that is coded as a STOP command, under the proper circumstances, will cause the transcription machinery to cease transcribing the DNA at that point. A segment of DNA coded to signal a REPEAT command, will cause the transcription machinery to repeat its transcription of a segment of genetic information. The term 'genetic information' refers to a sequence of nucleotides that comprise transcribable portions of DNA and nontranscribable portions of DNA. In the DNA, four different nucleotides comprise the nucleotide sequences. The four different nucleotides that comprise the DNA include adenine, cytosine, guanine, and thymine.

[0003] Computer programs, commonly utilized in desk top computers, laptop computers, mainframe computers are comprised of a series of software instructions and data. In order for a computer program to run its digital programming in an orderly fashion, each software instruction and each element of data is assigned or associated with a unique identifier such that the software instructions can be carried out in an orderly fashion and each element of data can be efficiently located when there is a need to process the data elements. Similarly, each unit of genetic information, often referred to as a gene, comprising the nuclear DNA of a species genome, must have a unique identifier assigned to it such that the genetic information can be readily located by the transcription machinery and utilized when needed by a cell.

[0004] When a gene is to be transcribed, approximately forty proteins assemble together into what is referred to as a transcription complex, which acts as the transcription machinery. The transcription complex forms along a segment of DNA, upstream from the start of the transcribable genetic information. The transcription complex transcribes the genetic information to produce RNA. It is vital to the cell that the transcription complex is able to locate a specific gene amongst the 3 billion base pairs comprising the human genome in an orderly and efficient fashion to enable it to perform functions the cell requires to operate, survive, grow and replicate.

[0005] For purposes of this text there are several general definitions. A 'ribose' is a five carbon or pentose sugar ($C_5H_{10}O_5$) present in the structural components of ribonucleic acid, riboflavin, and other nucleotides and nucleosides. A 'deoxyribose' is a deoxypentose ($C_5H_{10}O_4$) found in deoxyribonucleic acid. A 'nucleoside' is a compound of a sugar usually ribose or deoxyribose with a nitrogenous base by way of an N-glycosyl link. A 'nucleotide' is a single unit of a nucleic acid, composed of a five carbon sugar (either a ribose or a deoxyribose), a nitrogenous base and a phosphate group. There are two families of 'nitrogenous bases', which include: pyrimidine and purine. A 'pyrimidine' is a six member ring made up of carbon and nitrogen atoms; the members of the pyrimidine family include: cytosine (C), thymine (T) and uracil (U). A 'purine' is a five-member ring fused to a pyrimidine type ring; the members of the purine family include: adenine (A) and guanine (G). A 'nucleic acid' is a polynucleotide which is a biologic molecule such as ribonucleic acid or deoxyribonucleic acid that enable organisms to reproduce. A 'ribonucleic acid' (RNA) is a linear polymer of nucleotides formed by repeated riboses linked by phosphodiester bonds between the 3-hydroxyl group of one and the 5-hydroxyl group of the next; RNAs are single stranded macromolecules comprised of a sequence of nucleotides, these nucleotides are generally referred to by their nitrogenous bases, which include: adenine, cytosine, guanine and uracil. The term macromolecule refers to any very large molecule. RNAs are subset into different types which include messenger RNA (mRNA), transport RNA (tRNA), ribosomal RNA (rRNA) and a variety of small RNAs. Messenger RNAs act as templates to produce proteins. A ribosome is a complex comprised of rRNAs and proteins and is responsible for the correct positioning of mRNA and charged tRNA to facilitate the proper alignment and bonding of amino acids into a strand to produce a protein. A 'charged' tRNA is a tRNA that is carrying an amino acid. Ribosomal RNA (rRNA) represents a subset of RNAs that form part of the physical structure of a ribosome. Small RNAs include snoRNA, U snRNA, and miRNA. The snoRNAs modify precursor rRNA molecules. U snRNAs modify precursor mRNA molecules. The miRNA molecules modify the function of mRNA molecules.

[0006] A 'deoxyribose' is a deoxypentose ($C_5H_{10}O_4$) sugar. Deoxyribonucleic acid (DNA) is comprised of three basic elements: a deoxyribose sugar, a phosphate group and nitrogen containing bases. DNA is a macromolecule made up of two chains of repeating deoxyribose sugars linked by phosphodiester bonds between the 3-hydroxyl group of one and the 5-hydroxyl group of the next; the two chains are held antiparallel to each other by weak hydrogen bonds. DNA strands contain a sequence of nucleotides, which include: adenine, cytosine, guanine and thymine. Adenine is always paired with thymine of the opposite strand, and guanine is always paired with cytosine of the opposite strand; one side or strand of a DNA macromolecule is the mirror image of the opposite strand. Nuclear DNA is regarded as the medium for storing the master plan of hereditary information.

[0007] Genes are considered segments of the DNA that represent units of inheritance.

[0008] A chromosome exists in the nucleus of a cell and consists of a DNA double helix bearing a linear sequence of genes, coiled and recoiled around aggregated proteins, termed histones. The number of chromosomes varies from species to species. Most human cells carries twenty two pairs of chromosomes plus two sex chromosomes; two 'x' chromosomes in women and one 'x' and one 'y' chromosome in men. Chromosomes carry genetic information in the form of units which are referred to as genes. The entire nuclear genome, forty six chromosomes, is comprised of 3 billion base pairs (bp) of nucleotides.

[0009] Mitochondria possess numerous circular DNA. The limited information stored in mitochondrial DNA is thought to assist the mitochondria in producing the enzymes needed to convert glucose to adenosine triphosphate.

[0010] Various standard definitions of a gene exist. Per *Stedman's Medical Dictionary*, 24th edition, copyright 1982: 'The functional unit of heredity. Each gene occupies a specific place or locus on a chromosome, is capable of reproducing itself exactly at cell division, and is capable of directing the formation of an enzyme or other protein. The gene as a functional unit probably consists of a discrete segment of purine (adenine and guanine) and pyrimidine (cytosine and thymine) bases in the correct sequence to code the sequence of amino acids needed to form a specific peptide. Protein synthesis is mediated by molecules of messenger RNA formed on the chromosome with the gene unit of DNA acting as a template, which then pass into the cytoplasm and become oriented on the ribosomes where they in turn act as templates to organize a chain of amino acids to form a peptide. Genes normally occur in pairs in all cells except gametes as a consequence of the fact that all chromosomes are paired except the sex chromosomes (x and y) of the male.'

[0011] Per *Dorland's Pocket Medical Dictionary*, 23rd edition, copyright 1982 the definition of 'gene' is 'the biologic unit of heredity, self-producing, and located at a definite position (locus) on a particular chromosome.'

[0012] Per the text *Understanding Biology*, Second Edition, Peter Raven, George Johnson, Mosby, copyright 1991: 'Gene: The basic unit of heredity. A sequence of DNA nucleotides on a chromosome that encodes a polypeptide or RNA molecule and so determines the nature of an individual's inherited traits.'

[0013] Per *The New Oxford American Dictionary*, Second Edition, copyright 2005: 'Gene: A unit of heredity that is transferred from a parent to offspring and is held to determine some characteristic of the offspring: proteins coded directly by genes. In technical use: a distinct sequence of nucleotides forming part of a chromosome, the order of which determines the order of monomers in a polypeptide or nucleic acid molecule which a cell (or virus) may synthesize.'

[0014] Per MedicineNet.com. (*Current as of the time of this publication*): According to the official Guidelines for Human Gene Nomenclature, a 'gene' is defined as "a DNA segment that contributes to phenotype/function. In the absence of demonstrated function a gene may be characterized by sequence, transcription or homology." DNA: Genes are composed of DNA, a molecule in the memorable shape of a double helix, a spiral ladder. Each rung of the spiral ladder consists of two paired chemicals called bases. There are four types of bases. They are adenine (A), thymine (T), cytosine (C), and guanine (G). As indicated, each base is symbolized by the first letter of its name: A, T, C, and G. Certain bases always pair together (AT and GC). Different sequences of base pairs form coded messages. The gene: A gene is a sequence (a string) of bases. It is made up of combinations of A, T, C, and G. These unique combinations determine the gene's function, much as letters join together to form words. Each person has thousands of genes--billions of base pairs of DNA or bits of information repeated in the nuclei of human cells-- which determine individual characteristics (genetic traits).'

[0015] Per Wikipedia.com, referenced to: Group of the Sequence Ontology consortium, coordinated by K. Eilbeck, cited in H. Pearson. (2006). Genetics: what is a gene? *Nature*, 441, 398-401 (*Current as of the time of this publication*): A modern working definition of a gene is '*a locatable region of genomic sequence, corresponding to a unit of inheritance, which is associated with regulatory regions, transcribed regions, and or other functional sequence regions.*'

[0016] The above definitions of a 'gene' are fairly detailed and at present time generally universally accepted in the science and medical communities as representing the definition of a gene. There is a distinct lack of any previous reference in the medical science literature to a unique identifier associated with genetic material.

[0017] Current gene theory is derived from Gregor Mendel (1822-1884), who discovered the basic principles of heredity by breeding garden peas at the abbey where he resided, while teaching at Brunn Modern School. Gregor Mendel built and documented a model of inheritance, often referred to as Mendelian genetics, that has acted as the foundation of modern genetics. Gregor Mendel documented changes in characteristics of the plants he grew and described the physical traits as being related to 'heritable factors'. Over time Mendel's term 'heritable factor' has been replaced by the terms 'gene' and 'allele'. Much of what the current term of a 'gene' describes remains related to and distinctly linked to the physical traits of the live organisms they describe.

[0018] Per J. K. Pal, S.S. Ghaskabi, *Fundamentals of Molecular Biology*, 2009: 'The central dogma of molecular biology…states that the genes present in the genome (DNA) are transcribed into mRNAs, which are then translated into polypeptides or proteins, which are phenotypes.' 'Genome, thus, contains the complete set of hereditary information for any organism and is functionally divided into small parts referred to as genes. Each gene is a sequence of nucleotides representing a single protein or RNA. Genome of a living organism may contain as few as 500 genes as in case of Mycoplasma, or as many as 30,000 genes as in case of human beings.'

[0019] Current computer technology utilizes the binary numeric language. Every task a computer performs is related to the language of 'ones' and 'zeros'. Transistors that comprise the inside of computer chips are either turned 'on' representing a 'one' or turned 'off' representing a 'zero'. At the core of all computer programs is the machine language of 'ones' and 'zeros'. The most sophisticated central processing unit (CPU) in the world only reads and processes the language of 'ones' and 'zeros'. All text, all pictures, all video, all sound and music is diluted down to the form of 'ones' and 'zeros', and consequently all of the computing and storage power of a computer is performed by the computer language of 'ones' and 'zeros'.

[0020] The nucleus of a biologically active cell arguably possesses the most sophisticated and well organized processing power in the world. To run such a powerful processing unit, a form of biologic computer language would seem to be a necessary foundation by which to transfer stored information from the DNA to the remainder of the biologically active portions of a cell as needed. Given that the DNA comprising the chromosomes and mitochondrial DNA are both comprised of four different nucleotides including adenosine, cytosine, guanine and thymine, and RNA is comprised of four nucleotides including adenosine, cytosine, guanine and uracil (uracil in place of thymine), it appears evident the biologic computer language used by a cell's genome is an information language derived from base-four mathematics. Instead of current computer technology utilizing binary computer code comprised of 'ones' and 'zeros', the DNA and RNA in a biologically active cell utilize an information language comprised of 'zeros', 'one's', two's' and 'threes' to store and transfer information, which in effect represents a base-four language or quaternary language.

[0021] The above definitions of a 'gene' refer to genes residing in a specific place or locus on a chromosome. Identifying that a gene is present in a particular location is obvious to the human observer, but from a functional standpoint for cell biology this does not necessarily help a cell find or use the information stored in the nucleotide sequence of a particular gene. To rely on location alone, as a means of identifying a gene, would put the function of the entire genome at peril of failure if even a single base pair of nucleotides were added or deleted from the genome. To this point, no discussion regarding genes being organized utilizing a coding system of any form within the genome, other than the mention of physical location in a chromosome, has been made in the medical literature.

[0022] The current understanding of the actual biologic structure of a gene is far more elaborate than the standard definition of a gene leads a casual reader to believe; this knowledge has evolved greatly since Gregor Mendel's work in the 19th century. A gene appears to be comprised of a number of segments loosely strung together along a particular section of DNA. In general there are at least three global segments associated with a gene which include: (1) the Upstream 5' flanking region, (2) the transcriptional unit and (3) the Downstream 3' flanking region.

[0023] The Upstream 5' flanking region is comprised of the 'enhancer region', the 'promoter-proximal region', and 'promoter region'.

[0024] The 'transcriptional unit' begins at a location designated 'transcription start site' (TSS), which is located in a site called the 'initiator region' (inR), which may be described in a general form as Py_2CAPy_5. The transcription unit is comprised of the combination of segments of DNA nucleotides to be transcribed into RNA and spacing units known as 'introns' that are not transcribed or if transcribed are later removed post transcription, such that they do not appear in the final RNA molecule. In the case of a gene coding for a mRNA molecule, the transcription unit will contain all three elements of the mRNA, which includes: (1) the 5' noncoding region, (2) the translational region and (3) the 3' noncoding region. Interspersed between these regions are exons, which will not be transcribed and introns that if transcribed, are removed from the precursor form of mRNA prior to the mRNA reaching its final form. Exons and introns appear to be likened to spacers. The exact role exons and introns play in the transcription process is undetermined.

[0025] The Downstream 3' flanking region contains DNA nucleotides that are not transcribed and may contain what has been termed an 'enhancer region'. An enhancer region in the Downstream 3' flanking region may promote the gene previously transcribed to be transcribed again.

[0026] On either side of the DNA sequencing comprising a gene and its flanking regions, may be inactive DNA which act as boundaries which have been termed 'insulator elements'. The term 'upstream' refers to DNA sequencing that occurs prior to the TSS if viewed from the 5' end to the 3' end of the DNA; where the term 'downstream' refers to DNA sequencing located after the TSS.

[0027] The 'enhancer region' may or may not be present in the Upstream 5' flanking region. If present in the Upstream 5' flanking region, the enhancer region helps facilitate the reading of the gene by encouraging formation of the transcription mechanism. An enhancer may be 50 to 1500 base pairs in length occupying a position upstream from the transcription starting site.

[0028] The 'transcription mechanism', also referred to as 'the transcription machinery' or the 'transcription complex' (TC), in humans, is reported to be comprised of over forty separate proteins that assemble together to ultimately function in a concerted effort to transcribe the nucleotide sequence of the DNA into RNA. The transcription mechanism includes elements such as 'general transcription factor Sp1', 'general transcription factor NF1', 'general transcription factor TATA-binding protein', 'TF$_{II}$D', 'basal transcription complex', and a 'RNA polymerase protein' to name only a few of the forty elements that exist. The elements of the transcription mechanism function as (1) a means to recognize the location of the start of a gene, (2) as proteins to bind the transcription mechanism to the DNA such that transcription may occur or (3) as means of transcribing the DNA nucleotide coding to produce a RNA molecule or a precursor RNA molecule.

[0029] There are at least three RNA polymerase proteins which include: RNA polymerase I, RNA polymerase II, and RNA polymerase III. RNA polymerase I tends to be dedicated to transcribing genetic information that will result in the formation of rRNA molecules. RNA polymerase II tends to be dedicated to transcribing genetic information that will result in the formation of mRNA molecules. RNA polymerase III appears to be dedicated to transcribing genetic information that results in the formation of tRNAs, small cellular RNAs and viral RNAs.

[0030] The 'promoter proximal region' is located upstream from the TSS and upstream from the core promoter region. The 'promoter proximal region' includes two sub-regions termed the GC box and the CAAT box. The 'GC box' appears to be a segment rich in guanine-cytosine nucleotide sequences. The GC box binds to the 'general transcription factor Sp1' of the transcription mechanism. The 'CAAT box' is a segment which contains the nucleotide sequence 'GGCCAATCT' located approximately 75 base pairs (bps) upstream from the transcription start site (TSS). The CAAT box binds to the 'general transcription factor NF1' of the transcription mechanism.

[0031] The 'core promoter' region is considered the shortest sequence within which RNA polymerase II can initiate transcription of a gene The core promoter may include the inR and either a TATA box or a 'downstream promoter element' (DPE). The inR is the region designated Py_2CAPy_5 that surrounds the transcription start site (TSS). The TATA box is located 25 base pairs (bps) upstream from the TSS. The TATA box acts as a site of attachment of the $TF_{II}D$, which is a promoter for binding of the RNA polymerase II molecule. The DPE may appear 28 bps to 32 bps downstream from the TSS.

The DPE acts as an alternative site of attachment for the $TF_{II}D$ when the TATA box is not present.

[0032] The transcription mechanism or transcription complex appears to be comprised of different elements depending upon whether rRNA is being transcribed versus mRNA or tRNA or small cellular RNA or viral RNA. The proteins that assemble to assist RNA Polymerase I with transcribing the DNA to produce rRNA appear different from the proteins that assemble to assist RNA polymerase II with transcribing the DNA to produce mRNA and from the proteins that assemble to assist RNA polymerase III with transcribing the DNA to produce tRNA, small cellular RNA or viral RNA. A common protein that appears to be present at the initial binding of all three types of RNA polymerase molecules is TATA-binding protein (TBP). TBP appears to be required to attach to the DNA, which then facilitates RNA polymerase to bind to the promoter along the DNA. TBP assembles with TBP-associated factors (TAFs). Together TBP and 11 TAFs comprise the complex referred to as $TF_{II}D$, which has been previously mentioned in the above text.

[0033] Upstream from the TATA box is the 'initiator element', which may be considered as part of the 'core promoter' region. The initiator element is a segment of the nuclear DNA that binds the basal transcription complex. The basal transcription complex is comprised of a number of proteins that make initial contact with the DNA prior to the RNA polymerase binding to the transcription mechanism. The basal transcription complex is associated with an activator.

[0034] An activator is a protein comprised of three components. The three components of the activator include: (1) DNA binding domain, (2) Connecting domain, and (3) Activating domain. When the activator's DNA binding domain attaches to the DNA at a specific point along the DNA, the activator's activating domain then causes the other elements of the transcription mechanism to assemble at this location. Generally the assembly of the other proteins occurs downstream from where the activator's DNA binding domain attached to the DNA. There is evidence that the activator is associated with the activity of small RNAs.

[0035] The design of the cell is so complex, all of its functions so diverse and intricate that some form of practical order is necessitated. The genes must be ordered in some fashion, especially in a human, where there are at least 30,000 different genes used by the cells. Some estimates put the total number of genes present in the human nuclear DNA genome to be closer to 100,000. If no means of order existed as to how the genes could be identified, then 'random circumstance' would dictate a cell locating a particular portion of genetic information that it requires, at any given time. Randomness tends to favor the occurrence of random events rather than a purposeful order. A 'random circumstance' approach to any living cell would tend to favor failure of the cell rather than survival of the cell.

[0036] To allow a cell to utilize the biologic information stored in a gene a 'unique identifier' needs to be associated with or attached to the gene's specific nucleotide sequence. In the human genome, the cell's transcription mechanism require an organized means to locate and transcribe any given gene's nucleotide sequence amongst the 3 billion nucleotides that reside in the 46 chromosomes that comprise human DNA. Given how the transcription mechanism assembles upstream from the portion of the gene to be transcribed, the nucleotide sequence acting as a unique identifier associated with a specific gene would be positioned upstream from the transcription start site.

[0037] The transcription complex (TC) engages the DNA upstream from the genetic information segment the TC transcribes. The unique identifier may be attached directly to the RNA coding segment of genetic material, or there may exist one or more base pairs physically separating the unique identifier and the RNA coding portion of genetic material. Regarding some genes, there may be numerous base pairs separating the unique identifier from the transcribable region of the gene.

[0038] For any form of 'gene therapy' to work efficiently, medically therapeutic genetic material inserted into the native DNA of a cell needs to be associated with a unique identifier. Attaching a unique identifier to medically therapeutic genetic material is essential in making it possible for the components of a transcription complex to, in a timely organized fashion, locate the exogenous medically therapeutic genetic material, assemble around this exogenous genetic material, and decode the information contained therein. If no such unique identifier is used, then utilization of such exogenous transcribable genetic information occurs based on the occurrence of random events rather than dictated by therapeutic design.

[0039] Naturally occurring unique identifiers in the nuclear genome may occur in numerous forms. Since humans share 47% of their DNA with bananas and 95% of their DNA with monkeys, a portion of the unique identifiers associated with genes in the nuclear DNA may not be specific to a human. Unique identifiers may have a global utility, with a portion of the genome of any organism being shared amongst numerous species. The rational would be that once Nature developed an adequate fundamental design for a particular facet of biologic organisms, this information may be shared amongst numerous species that would benefit from the design. An example might be the basic design of a eukaryote cell; this information would be shared amongst all life that utilized the eukaryote cell design rather than each successive multi-celled species having to repeatedly re-invent the design of a eukaryote cell.

[0040] In order for the knowledge base of cellular genetics to progress forward, the definition of a gene must be expanded to include the presence of a 'unique identifier' associated with each gene present within the DNA. The basis for the presence of this unique identifier (UI) associated with each active gene is so that the cell can locate the biologic information stored in the DNA nucleotide sequencing of the gene. An active gene refers to those genes present in the genome that are utilized by a particular species to support conception, development and maintenance of a species.

[0041] Upon adding a unique identifier to a gene, the current term 'gene' is thus expanded to the term 'quantum gene'. The term 'quantal' in biology generally refers to an 'all or nothing' state or response. The term 'quantal' is a derivative of the word quantum. The term 'quantum' means a quantity or amount, and a discrete quantity of energy or a discrete bundle of energy or a discrete quantity of electromagnetic radiation.

[0042] A 'quantum gene' is comprised of a sequence of nucleotides that represents a 'unique identifier' physically linked to a sequence of nucleotides that represent a discrete quantity of genetic information; these sequences of nucleotides being comprised of some combination of the nucleotides being referred to by their nitrogenous base as adenine (A), thymine (T), cytosine (C), and guanine (G). The genetic information associated with the above-mentioned unique identifier may be comprised of a portion of transcribable genetic information and a portion of nontranscribable genetic information which together define a specific gene, otherwise referred to as a discrete quantity of genetic information.

[0043] Similar to how a gene is described, with regards to a quantum gene, the term 'upstream' refers to DNA sequencing that occurs prior to the transcription start site (TSS) if viewed from the 5' end to the 3' end of the DNA; where the term 'downstream' refers to DNA sequencing located after the TSS.

[0044] Similar to the previously described organization of a standard gene found in nuclear DNA, a quantum gene is structured with at least three global segments which include: (1) the Upstream 5' flanking region, (2) the transcriptional unit and possibly instructional units and (3) the Downstream 3' flanking region. The 'unique identifier' is located in the Upstream 5' flanking region. The current standard definition of a gene strictly encompasses the concept that a gene is comprised of a segment of nuclear DNA that when transcribed produces RNA. Therefore, the differences between the current standard definition of a 'gene' and the definition of a 'quantum gene' is that a quantum gene includes both a unique identifier and a segment of nuclear DNA that when transcribed produces RNA. The segment of nuclear DNA that when transcribed produces RNA is comprised of one or more segments of transcribable genetic information that may be accompanied by one or more segments of nontranscribable genetic information. Nontranscribable segments of genetic information include segments that are removed or ignored during the transcription process or segments that act as commands which includes a START code, STOP code or a REPEAT code. When present, a START code signals initiation of the transcription process. When present, a STOP code signals the discontinuation of the transcription process. When present, a REPEAT code signals that the transcription process should repeat the transcription of the segment of DNA that was just transcribed.

[0045] Similar to the standard description of a 'gene', a quantum gene's Upstream 5' flanking region is comprised of the 'enhancer region', the 'promoter-proximal region', and 'promoter region'.

[0046] Similar to the standard description of a 'gene', a quantum gene's 'transcriptional unit' begins at a location designated 'transcription start site' (TSS), which is located in a site called the 'initiator region' (inR), which may be described in a general form as Py_2CAPy_5. The transcription unit is comprised of the combination of segments of DNA nucleotides to be transcribed into RNA and spacing units known as 'exons' AND 'introns', whereby exons represent segments that are not transcribed and introns represent segments that are transcribed but later removed post transcription, such that they do not appear in the final RNA molecule. In the case of a gene coding for a mRNA molecule, the transcription unit will contain all three elements of the mRNA, which includes: (1) the 5' noncoding region, (2) the translational region and (3) the 3' noncoding region. Interspersed between these regions are exons, which will not be transcribed and introns that if transcribed, are removed from the precursor form of mRNA prior to the mRNA reaching its final form. Exons and introns present in nuclear DNA appear to be likened to spacers interspersed in the nuclear DNA. The exact role exons and introns play in the transcription process is undetermined.

[0047] Similar to the standard description of a gene, with regards to the quantum gene the Downstream 3' flanking region contains DNA nucleotides that are not transcribed and may contain what has been termed an 'enhancer region'. An enhancer region in the Downstream 3' flanking region may promote the gene previously transcribed to be transcribed again.

[0048] On either side of the DNA sequencing comprising a gene and a quantum gene are flanking regions which represent inactive DNA, which act as boundaries which have been termed 'insulator elements'. Insulator elements are areas that are not transcribed to produce RNA. The function of insulator elements, other than acting as boundary markers between differing genes, is unknown.

[0049] In nuclear DNA, quantum genes are comprised of a segment of deoxyribonucleic acid where the portion that represents a unique identifier may be separated from the portion that represents transcribable genetic information by a quantity of base pairs of nucleotides that do not represent a unique identifier and do not represent transcribable genetic information. The purpose of the separation of the portion of the unique identifier from the portion of the genetic information by a quantity of base pairs of nucleotides that do not represent a unique identifier and does not represent genetic information may be to act to facilitate a transcription complex attaching to the quantum gene upstream from the portion of the quantum gene that represents genetic information so that transcription of the biologic information associated with the quantum gene may occur at the designated starting point.

[0050] The unique identification or identifier of a quantum gene could be in the form of nucleotide sequence that represents a name assigned to the quantum gene, or a number assigned to a quantum gene or the combination of a name and number assigned to a quantum gene. Irrespective of whether the unique identifier incorporated in a quantum gene is considered a 'name', or a 'number' or a combination of a name or number, the unique identifier is comprised of a sequence of nucleotides linked to the transcribable genetic information for which it acts as a unique identifier; these sequences of nucleotides being comprised of some combination of the nucleotides being referred to by their nitrogenous base as adenine (A), thymine (T), cytosine (C), and guanine (G). It has been estimated that there are as many as 100,000 separate genes stored in the DNA of the 46 chromosomes comprising the human genome. In a base four language, a string of nine nucleotides is needed to code for 256,144 individual genes. If there were over a million quantum genes, then a string of ten nucleotides could be used since ten nucleotides could represent 1,024,576 unique numbers in a base-four number system.

[0051] Utilizing a base four number system a string of twenty-five nucleotides would represent the number 1,125,899,906,842,624, which could account for 200,000 different quantum genes in 5 billion different species. Therefore 200,000 different quantum genes could be dedicated to producing a biped form of life. In the human genome 5% of the 3 billion base pairs are considered to represent genes by the current definition of a gene. If 5% of the human genome represents the 100,000 quantum genes in the nuclear DNA, then on average 1500 nucleotides can be dedicated to each gene. If 25 nucleotides are dedicated to a unique address or unique identifier, then there remain 1475 nucleotides, on average, to be utilized for coding the biologic information associated with each of the 100,000 quantum genes estimated to exist in the human genome.

[0052] A unique identifier (UI) incorporated in quantum genes could be comprised of a unique number or a unique name or the unique combination of a number and a name. A name might be represented as a single letter or a series of letters. The current convention utilized in science is to apply the four letter alphabet A, C, G, T to represent the four different bases of the nucleotides comprising the DNA, which include adenosine, cytosine, guanine, and thymine respectfully. With regards to RNA, the four letter alphabet A, C, G, U is utilized to represent the bases of the nucleotides which include adenosine, cytosine, guanine, and uracil. Regarding utilizing a unique identifier for DNA, a name could be comprised of a series of letters derived from the four letters A, C, G, and T. Regarding utilizing a unique identifier for purposes of use within an RNA molecule, a unique identifier could be comprised of a series of letters derived from the four letters A, C, G, and U. The current scientific convention does not recognize a mathematical base-four nomenclature regarding DNA or RNA. The unique identifier could be represented as a number. Names can be translated into numbers and vice versa.

[0053] In the nuclear DNA, there are several places in the upstream segment of a quantum gene where a segment of twenty-five or more base pairs could exist that acts as the unique identifying code that uniquely identifies the segment of transcribable genetic information. The transcription start site (TSS) is present upstream from a segment of transcribable genetic information. There exists a segment of 25 bps upstream from the TSS that occupies the space along the DNA between the TSS and the TATA box. There exists the downstream promoter element (DPE) 28 bps to 32 bps downstream from the TSS. The DPE acts as an alternative site of attachment for the TF$_{II}$D when the TATA box is not present. Within the 28 bps to 32 bps of DNA separating the DPE from the TSS may also be a convenient location for a unique identifying code to reside and be associated with the genetic information located just downstream. The cell exists with numerous variability. There exists variation in the arrangement of the elements upstream from the transcribable genetic information, therefore various sites upstream from the transcribable genetic information may function as the unique identifying code for some quantum genes. The unique identifying code may be represented as subsegments of DNA, where subsegments are physically separated from each other, but in combination, the subsegments act in unison to identify a segment of transcribable genetic information.

[0054] By delivering quantum genes containing the genetic information required to produce insulin directly to the cells responsible for the production of insulin, the medical treatment of diabetes mellitus is significantly improved. Diabetes mellitus represents a state of hyperglycemia, a serum blood sugar that is higher than what is considered the normal range for humans. Glucose, a six-carbon molecule, is a form of sugar. Glucose is absorbed by the cells of the body and converted to energy by the processes of glycolysis, the Krebs cycle and phosporylation. Insulin, a protein, facilitates the transfer of glucose from the blood into cells. Normal range for blood glucose in humans is generally defined as a fasting blood plasma glucose level of between 70 to 110 mg/dl. For descriptive purposes, the term 'plasma' refers to the fluid portion of blood.

[0055] Diabetes mellitus is classified as Type One and Type Two. Type One diabetes mellitus is insulin dependent, which refers to the condition where there is a lack of sufficient insulin circulating in the blood stream and insulin must be provided to the body in order to properly regulate the blood glucose level. When insulin is required to regulate the blood glucose level in the body, this condition is often referred to as insulin dependent diabetes mellitus (IDDM). Type Two diabetes mellitus is noninsulin dependent, often referred to as noninsulin dependent diabetes mellitus (NIDDM), meaning the blood glucose level can be managed without insulin, and instead by means of diet, exercise or intervention with oral medications. Type Two diabetes mellitus is considered a progressive disease, the underlying pathogenic mechanisms including pancreatic Beta cell (also often designated as β-Cell) dysfunction and insulin resistance.

[0056] The pancreas serves as an endocrine gland and an exocrine gland. Functioning as an endocrine gland the pancreas produces and secretes hormones including insulin and glucagon. Insulin acts to reduce levels of glucose circulating in the blood. Beta cells secrete insulin into the blood when a higher than normal level of glucose is detected in the serum. For purposes of this description the terms 'blood', 'blood stream' and 'serum' refer to the same substance. Glucagon acts to stimulate an increase in glucose circulating in the blood. Beta cells in the pancreas secrete glucagon when a low level of glucose is detected in the serum.

[0057] Glucose enters the body and then the blood stream as a result of the digestion of food. The Beta cells of the Islets of Langerhans continuously sense the level of glucose in the blood and respond to elevated levels of blood glucose by secreting insulin into the blood. Beta cells produce the protein 'insulin' in their endoplasmic reticulum and store the insulin in vacuoles until it is needed. When Beta cells detect an increase in the glucose level in the blood, Beta cells release insulin into the blood from the described storage vacuoles.

[0058] Insulin is a protein. An insulin protein consists of two chains of amino acids, an alpha chain and a beta chain, linked by two disulfide (S-S) bridges. One chain, the alpha chain consists of 21 amino acids. The second chain the beta chain consists of 30 amino acids.

[0059] Insulin interacts with the cells of the body by means of a cell-surface receptor termed the 'insulin receptor' located on the exterior of a cell's 'outer membrane', otherwise known as the 'plasma membrane'. Insulin interacts with muscle and liver cells by means of the insulin receptor to rapidly remove excess blood sugar when the glucose level in the blood is higher than the upper limit of the normal physiologic range. Recognized functions of insulin include stimulating cells to take up glucose from the blood and convert it to glycogen to facilitate the cells in the body to utilize glucose to generate biochemically usable energy, and to stimulate fat cells to take up glucose and synthesize fat.

[0060] Diabetes Mellitus may be the result of one or more factors. Causes of diabetes mellitus may include: (1) mutation of the insulin gene itself causing miscoding, which results in the production of ineffective insulin molecules; (2) mutations to genes that code for the 'transcription factors' needed for transcription of the insulin gene in the deoxyribonucleic acid (DNA) to create messenger ribonucleic acid (mRNA) molecules, which facilitate the manufacture of the insulin molecule; (3) mutations of the gene encoding for the insulin receptor, which produces inactive or an insufficient number of insulin receptors; (4) mutation to the gene encoding for glucokinase, the enzyme that phosphorylates glucose in the first step of glycolysis; (5) mutations to the genes encoding portions of the potassium channels in the plasma membrane of the Beta cells, preventing proper closure of the channel, thus blocking insulin release; (6) mutations to mitochondrial genes that as a result, decreases the energy available to be used facilitate the release of insulin, therefore reducing insulin secretion; (7) failure of glucose transporters to properly permit the facilitated diffusion of glucose from plasma into the cells of the body.

[0061] A 'eukaryote' refers to a nucleated cell. Eukaryotes comprise nearly all animal and plant cells. A human eukaryote or nucleated cell is comprised of an exterior lipid bilayer plasma membrane, cytoplasm, a nucleus, and organelles. The exterior plasma membrane defines the perimeter of the cell, regulates the flow of nutrients, water and regulating molecules in and out of the cell, and has embedded into its structure receptors that the cell uses to detect properties of the environment surrounding the cell membrane. The cytoplasm acts as a filling medium inside the boundaries of the plasma cell membrane and is comprised mainly of water and nutrients such as amino acids, oxygen, and glucose. The nucleus, organelles, and ribosomes are suspended in the cytoplasm. The nucleus contains the majority of the cell's genetic information in the form of double stranded deoxyribonucleic acid (DNA). Organelles generally carry out specialized functions for the cell and include such structures as the mitochondria, the endoplasmic reticulum, storage vacuoles, lysosomes and Golgi complex (sometimes referred to as a Golgi apparatus). Floating in the cytoplasm, but also located in the endoplasmic reticulum and mitochondria are ribosomes. Ribosomes are complex macromolecule structures comprised of ribosomal ribonucleic acid (rRNA) molecules and ribosomal proteins that combine and couple to a messenger ribonucleic acid (mRNA) molecule. The rRNAs and the ribosomal proteins congregate to form a macromolecule structure that surrounds a mRNA molecule. Ribosomes decode genetic information in a mRNA molecule and manufacture proteins to the specifications of the instruction code physically present in the mRNA molecule. More than one ribosome may be attached to a single mRNA at a time.

[0062] Proteins are comprised of a series of amino acids bonded together in a linear strand, sometimes referred to as a chain; a protein may be further modified to be a structure comprised of one or more similar or differing strands of amino acids bonded together. Insulin is a protein structure comprised of two strands of amino acids; one strand comprised of 21 amino acids long and the second strand comprised of 30 amino acids, the two strands attached by two disulfide bridges. There are an estimated 30,000 different proteins the cells of the human body may manufacture. The human body is comprised of a wide variety of cells, many with specialized functions requiring unique combinations of proteins and protein structures such as glycoproteins (a protein combined with a carbohydrate) to accomplish the required task or tasks a specialized cell is designed to perform. Forms of glycoproteins are known to be utilized as cell-surface receptors. Messenger RNAs (mRNA) are created by transcription of DNA, they generally migrate to other locations inside the cell and are utilized by ribosomes as protein manufacturing templates. A ribosome is a protein complex that manufactures proteins by deciphering the instruction code located in a mRNA molecule. When a specific protein is needed, pieces of the ribosome complex, which include rRNA molecules and ribosomal proteins, bind around the strand of a mRNA that carries the specific instruction code that will generate the required protein. The ribosome traverses the mRNA strand and deciphers the genetic information coded into the sequence of nucleotides that comprise the mRNA molecule to produce a protein molecule and this process is referred to as translation.

[0063] The insulin molecule is a protein produced by Beta cells located in the pancreas. The 'insulin messenger RNA' is created in a Beta cell by a polymerase complex transcribing the insulin gene from nuclear DNA in the nucleus of the cell. The native messenger RNA (mRNA) for insulin then travels to the endoplasmic reticulum where numerous ribosomes, comprised of rRNA and ribosomal proteins, engage these mRNA molecules. Many ribosomes may be attached to a single strand of mRNA simultaneously, each generating an identical copy of the protein as dictated by the information encoded in the mRNA. Insulin is produced by ribosomes translating the information in a mRNA molecule coded for the insulin protein, which produce strands of amino acids that are coded for an immature form of the biologically active insulin molecule referred to as 'pro-insulin'. Once the pro-insulin molecule is generated it then undergoes modification by several enzymes including prohormone convertase one (PC1), prohormone convertase two (PC2) and carboxypeptidase E, which results in the production of a biologically active insulin molecule. Once the biologically active insulin protein is generated it is stored in a vacuole in the Beta cell to await being released into the blood stream.

[0064] Insulin receptors, which appear on the surface of cells, offer binding sites for insulin circulating in the blood. When insulin binds to an insulin receptor, the biologic response inside the cell causes glucose to enter the cell and undergo processing in the cytoplasm. Processed glucose molecules then enter the mitochondria. The mitochondria further process the modified glucose molecules to produce usable energy in the form of adenosine triphosphate molecules (ATP). Thirty-eight ATP molecules may be generated from one molecule of glucose during the process of aerobic respiration. ATP molecules are utilized as an energy source by biologic processes throughout the cell.

[0065] The current medical therapeutic approach for the management of diabetes mellitus has produced limited results. Patients with diabetes generally struggle with an inadequate production of insulin, or an ineffective release of biologically active insulin molecules, or a release of an insufficient number of biologically active insulin molecules, or an insufficient production of cell-surface receptors, or a production of ineffective cell-surface receptors, or a production of ineffective insulin molecules that are unable to interact properly with insulin receptors to produce the required biologic effect. Type One diabetes requires administration of exogenous insulin. The traditional approach to Type Two diabetes has generally first been to adjust the diet to limit the caloric intake the individual consumes. Exercise is used as an initial approach to both Type One and Type Two diabetes as a means of up-regulating the utilization of fats and sugar so as to reduce the amount of circulating plasma glucose. When diet and exercise are inadequate in properly managing Type Two diabetes, oral medications are often introduced. The action of sulfonylureas, a commonly prescribed class of oral medication, is to stimulate the Beta cells to produce additional insulin receptors and enhance the insulin receptors' response to insulin. Biguanides, another form of oral treatment, inhibit gluconeogenesis, the production of glucose in the liver, thereby attempting to reduce plasma glucose levels. Thiazolidinediones (TZDs) lower blood sugar levels by activating peroxisome proliferator-activated receptor gamma (PPAR-γ), a transcription factor, which when activated regulates the activity of various target genes, particularly ones involved in glucose and lipid metabolism. If diet, exercise and oral medications do not produce a satisfactory control of the level of blood glucose in a diabetic patient, exogenous insulin is injected into the body in an effort to normalize the amount of glucose present in the serum. Insulin, a protein, has not successfully been made available as an oral medication to date due to the fact that proteins in general become degraded when they encounter the acid environment present in the stomach.

[0066] Despite strict monitoring of blood glucose and potentially multiple doses of insulin injected throughout the day, many patients with diabetes mellitus still experience devastating adverse effects from elevated blood glucose levels. Microvascular damage and elevated tissue sugar levels contribute to such complications as renal failure, retinopathy involving the eyes, neuropathy, and accelerated heart disease despite aggressive efforts to maintain the blood sugar within the physiologic normal range using exogenous insulin by itself or a combination of exogenous insulin and one or more oral medications. Diabetes remains the number one cause of renal failure in the United States. Especially in diabetic patients that are dependent upon administering exogenous insulin into their body, though dosing of the insulin may be four or more times a day and even though this may produce adequate control of the blood glucose level to prevent the clinical symptoms of hyperglycemia; this does not unerringly supplement the body's natural capacity to monitor the blood sugar level minute to minute, twenty-four hours a day, and deliver an immediate response to a rise in blood glucose by the release of insulin from Beta cells as required. The deleterious effects of diabetes may still evolve despite strict and persistent control of the glucose level in the blood stream.

[0067] The current treatment of diabetes may be augmented by the unique approach to utilizing modified viruses as vehicles to transport quantum genes into cells in order to increase the production of biologically active insulin. By utilizing modified viruses to transport quantum genes to facilitate and enhance the production of mRNAs, which would then facilitate the assembly of proteins would offer a new treatment option for patients with diabetes.

[0068] Present medical care is attempting to utilize viruses to deliver genetic information into cells. Research in the field of gene therapy has involved certain naturally occurring viruses. Some of the common viral vectors that have been investigated include: Adeno-associated virus, Adenovirus, Alphavirus, Epstein-Barr virus, Gammaretrovirus, Herpes simplex virus, Letivirus, Poliovirus, Rhabdovirus, Vaccinia virus. Naturally occurring virus vectors are limited to the naturally occurring external probes that are affixed to the outer wall of the virus. The external probes fixed to the outside wall of a virus virion dictate which type of cell the virus can engage and infect. Therefore, as an example, the function of the adenovirus, a respiratory virus, is strictly limited to engaging and infecting specific lung cells. Used as a medical treatment device, the adenovirus can only deliver gene therapy to specific lung cells, which severely limits this vector's usefulness as a deliver device. The therapeutic function of all naturally occurring viral vectors is limited to delivering a DNA or RNA payload to the cell type the viral vector naturally targets as its host cell.

[0069] Cichutek, K., 2001 (US Patent No. 6,323,031 B1) teaches preparation and use of novel lentiviral SiVagm-derived vectors for gene transfer into selected cell types, specifically into proliferatively active and resting human cells.

[0070] Cichutek teaches that it is indeed plausible to re-configure an existing virus and use it as a transport vehicle, though Cichutek's specification and claims are too limited to describe a method that will work for all cell types, if indeed if it will work for any cell type.

[0071] Cichutek describes vectors for 'gene transfer'; in the claims the language that is used is 'genetic information'. Cichutek's Claim 1 of the cited patent states 'A propagation-incompetent SIVagm vector comprising a viral core and a viral envelope, wherein the viral core comprises a simian immunodeficiency virus (SIVagm) viral core of the African vervet monkey Chlorocebus.' Cichutek's does not describe in his claims any further details of the intended payload other than the stating 'SIVagm viral core' in claim 1; in claims 5 & 6 Cichutek describes only 'genetic information'. Transfer of 'genetic information' dramatically limits the useful application of Cichutek's patent in the treatment of medical diseases.

[0072] The necessity for labeling genetic material with a unique identifier has not yet been recognized by those skilled in the art.

[0073] For purposes of this text, the term 'exogenous' refers to an item which originates outside the boundaries of a particular cell or cell type and is caused to become a part of a particular cell or cell type. The term 'endogenous' refers to an item which originates as a part of a particular cell or cell type and remains a part of that particular cell or cell type.

BRIEF SUMMARY OF THE INVENTION

[0074] Quantum genes are comprised of a unique identifier linked to a segment of genetic information, at least a portion of this genetic information coding for the production of one or more ribonucleic acids. By delivering one or more quantum genes to a specific cell type or an array of cell types for installation into the DNA of the cells, the exogenous easily identifiable genetic instructions made available to the cells can be located and transcribed in an efficient manner and thus utilized in one or more specific cell types in a timely fashion. A wide variety of medical conditions are manageable by utilizing this new and unique approach.

DETAILED DESCRIPTION

[0075] The future of medical treatment will be the widespread utilization of quantum genes delivered directly to targeted cell types in the body in order to manage protein deficient states.

[0076] For the purposes of this text a 'quantum gene' is comprised of a sequence of nucleotides that represents a 'unique identifier' physically linked to a sequence of nucleotides that represent a discrete quantity of genetic information; these sequences of nucleotides being comprised of some combination of the nucleotides being referred to by their nitrogenous base as adenine (A), thymine (T), cytosine (C), and guanine (G). The genetic information associated with the above-mentioned unique identifier may be comprised of a portion of transcribable genetic information and a portion of nontranscribable genetic information which together define a specific gene, otherwise referred to as a discrete quantity of genetic information. The nontranscribable segments of a quantum gene may represent segments that act as instructions such as a START code,

STOP code and REPEAT code or may help facilitated the attachment of a transcription complex or be simply ignored during the transcription process. Quantum gene molecules can be comprised of a segment of nucleotides where the portion that represents a unique identifier is separated from the portion that represents genetic information by a quantity of base pairs of nucleotides that do not represent a unique identifier and do not represent genetic information. The purpose of the separation of the portion of the unique identifier from the portion of the genetic information by a quantity of base pairs of nucleotides that do not represent a unique identifier and does not represent genetic information is to facilitate a transcription complex attaching to the quantum gene upstream from the portion of the quantum gene that represents genetic information so that transcription of the biologic information associated with the quantum gene may occur.

[0077] The genetic information in a quantum gene codes for some combination of protein coding RNA (pcRNA), non-coding RNAs (ncRNA) and spacers. Spacers represent segments of nucleotides that do not code for a RNA molecule. The genetic information in a quantum gene, when transcribed, produces protein coding RNA and non-coding RNA. Protein coding RNAs, usually referred to as messenger RNAs, undergo the process of translation in the cytoplasm of the cell and produce proteins. Non-coding RNAs are highly abundant and functionally important for the cell's operation. Non-coding RNAs have also been referred to by such terms as non-protein-coding RNAs (npcRNA) or non-messenger RNA (nmRNA) or small non-messenger RNA (snmRNA) or functional RNAs (fRNA). The non-coding RNAs include: transfer RNAs (tRNA), ribosomal RNAs (rRNA), small nuclear RNAs (snRNA), small nucleolar RNAs (snoRNA), signal recognition particle RNA (SRP RNA), antisense RNA (aRNA), micro RNA (miRNA), small interfering RNA (siRNA), and Y RNA, telomerase RNA.

[0078] Transfer RNAs (tRNA), are RNAs that carries amino acids and deliver them to a ribosome. Ribosomal RNAs (rRNA), are RNAs that couple with ribosomal proteins and participate in translation of mRNA to produce protein molecules. Small nuclear RNAs (snRNA) are RNAs involved in splicing and other nuclear functions. Small nucleolar RNAs (snoRNA) are RNAs involved in nucleotide modification. Signal recognition particle RNA (SRP RNA) are RNAs involved in membrane integration. Antisense RNA (aRNA) are RNAs involved in transcription attenuation, mRNA degradation, mRNA stabilization, and translation blockage. Micro RNA (miRNA) are RNAs involved in gene regulation and have been implicated in a wide range of cell functions including cell growth, apoptosis, neuronal plasticity, and insulin secretion. Small interfering RNA (siRNA) are RNAs involved in gene regulation, often interfering with the expression of a single gene. Y RNA are RNAs involved in RNA processing and DNA replication. Telomerase RNA are RNAs involved in telomere synthesis.

[0079] In addition to a unique identifier, a quantum gene is comprised of the biologic instruction code, which when transcribed produce one or more of the same RNA molecules or different RNA molecules. A quantum gene must be comprised of a unique identifier and the genetic material to code for at least one RNA molecule. The definition of a 'quantum gene' differs from all previous definitions of a 'gene' due to the requirement that the quantum gene must have a unique identifier that accompanies a segment of genetic information. From a medical treatment perspective, the quantum gene's unique identifier allows the genetic information present in the quantum gene to be located by a cell's transcription machinery, once the quantum gene is inserted into a cell's nuclear DNA.

[0080] Ribonucleic acid molecules directly transcribed from the DNA or quantum gene, may be precursor ribonucleic acid molecules that require modification by nuclear enzymes prior to being translatable or may be ribonucleic acid molecules which are directly translatable without further modification.

[0081] In the DNA there are a number of nucleotides physically existing along the deoxyribonucleic acid between the unique identifier and the transcribable genetic information; or in other terms a number of nucleotides that are not a part of the identification code and are not transcribable, exist downstream from the unique identifier and upstream from the transcribable genetic information.

[0082] It is well recognized that within the transcribable genetic information there exist subsegments of nucleotides that are not transcribable and there are subsegments of nucleotides that are transcribed but are not found in the final version of the RNA molecule. Subsegments of transcribable genetic information that are not transcribed are subsegments such as 'STOP' codes, which indicate to the transcription complex a potential point at which to cease transcribing the genetic information. Certain factors may influence whether a transcription complex actually ceases transcription at that point or whether the transcription complex continues transcribing when the transcription complex reaches a 'STOP' code. Subsegments of nucleotides that are transcribed and appear in the final active form of a RNA are referred to as exons. Subsegments of nucleotides that are transcribed, but do not appear in the final active form of a RNA are referred to as introns. Precursor RNA molecules include both exons and introns. Introns are removed by modification of the initial RNA segment directly transcribed from the transcribable genetic information.

[0083] Utilization of the sigma summation symbol to show summation over a series of indexed variables or expression can be represented as:

$$\sum_{j=1}^{n} [K]_j = [K]_1 + [K]_2 + \ldots + [K]_n$$

[0084] An equation to represent a quantum gene would be:

Quantum gene = [unique identifier] $+\sum_{a=0}^{n}$[nontranscribable connector nucleotide]$_a$ + $\sum_{b=1}^{n}$[nucleotide segment transcribable for RNA]$_b$ + $\sum_{c=0}^{n}$[nontranscribable spacer nucleotide]$_c$ + $\sum_{d=0}^{n}$[nontranscribable nucleotide commands]$_d$

Where 'unique identifier' represents a number, a name or the combination of a number and a name that the transcription complex utilizes to locate a specific quantum gene amongst the DNA material present in a biologically active cell.

Where 'nontranscribable connector nucleotide' represents one or more nucleotides that physically exists between the 'unique identifier' and the segment of 'transcribable genetic information'.

Where a 'nontranscribable spacer nucleotide' represents one or more nucleotides comprising the transcribable genetic information that is not transcribed when the transcription complex transcribes the genetic information of the quantum gene.

Where a 'nontranscribable nucleotide command' represents one or more nucleotides comprising the transcribable genetic information that is not transcribed when the transcription complex transcribes the genetic information of the quantum gene, but acts as an instruction to the transcription complex to cause the transcription complex to function in a certain manner; examples include a STOP code that causes the transcription complex to cease transcription and a REPEAT code that causes the transcription complex to repeat its transcription of a segment of genetic material.

Where 'a' represents the range of 'zero to any positive whole number.

Where 'b' represents the range of 'one to any positive whole number'.

Where 'c' represents the range of 'zero to any positive whole number'.

Where 'd' represents the range of 'zero to any positive whole number'.

Where the DNA segment that is transcribable for RNA may transcribe RNAs that may exist in a precursor form; such a precursor form may include elements such as introns that are removed following transcription by modifying proteins.

[0085] As an example of this method, to treat diabetes mellitus utilizing configurable microscopic medical payload delivery devices to deliver to Beta cells quantum genes that code for messenger RNA that when translated produce insulin molecules, the following production process is followed in the lab: (1) human stem cells are selected. (2) Into the selected stem cells is placed the production genome constructed, in this case, specifically as a means to treat diabetes mellitus. The RNA production genome contains genetic instructions to cause the host stem cells to manufacture the quantum genes to activate the production of the insulin molecules in Beta cells; the biologic instructions to assemble the components into the final form of the configurable microscopic medical payload delivery devices; and the biologic instructions to activate the budding process. (3) Upon insertion of the RNA production genome dedicated to producing a quantum genes configured to activate the genes to generate messenger RNA that will result in the production of insulin, into the host stem cells, host stem cells respond by simultaneously translating the different segments of the RNA production genome to produce the proteins that comprise the exterior protein wall, the inner protein matrix molecules, and the quantum gene to produce insulin. Upon production the gene molecules are packaged into vacuoles and expressed from the host cell. (4) The quantum gene molecules are collected from the nutrient broth surrounding the host stem cells. (5) The quantum stem cells are separated from the nutrient. (6) The configurable quantum gene molecules are suspended in a hypoallergenic liquid medium. (7) The quantum gene molecules are divided into individual quantities to facilitate storage and delivery to physicians and patients. (8) Modified virus vectors or configurable microscopic medical payload delivery devices containing the quantum gene molecules suspended in a hypoallergenic liquid medium are administered to a diabetic patient per injection in a dose that is tailored to receiving patient's requirement to produce sufficient amount of insulin to control the blood sugar. (9) Upon being injected into the body, the modified viruses or the configurable microscopic medical payload delivery devices migrate to the Beta cells located in the Islets of Langerhans by means of the patient's blood stream. (10) Upon the modified virus or the configurable microscopic medical payload delivery devices reaching the Beta cells, the configurable microscopic medical payload delivery devices engage the cell-surface receptors located on the Beta cells and insert the payload of quantum genes they carry into the Beta cells. The payload of quantum genes migrate to the nucleus of the Beta cells. The quantum gene becomes inserted into the nuclear DNA of the Beta cell. Transcription machinery present in the nucleus transcribes the quantum gene. Messenger RNAs generated by transcribing the exogenous quantum genes enhances the Beta cells' production of insulin molecules. The increase in insulin production by Beta cells successfully manages diabetes mellitus.

[0086] The transcribable genetic information linked to the unique identifier may occur in the form of naturally found transcribable genetic information or may occur as artificially created transcribable genetic information, referred to as 'artificial transcribable genetic information'. Naturally found transcribable genetic information would be a segment of transcribable genetic information that would be found in a cell's genome otherwise referred to as a gene. Artificial transcribable genetic information would be transcribable genetic information that would represent either (i) a modified form of a naturally occurring gene or (ii) a segment of nucleotides that represents transcribable genetic information that is artificially created to produce a medically beneficial result.

[0087] A quantum gene, as it exists as a functional part of the deoxyribonucleic acid of a cell, is a segment of deoxyribonucleic acid, comprised of both a unique identifier and a segment of transcribable biologic information, that is capable of being inserted into a cell's nuclear DNA. DNA is comprised of two parallel strands of nucleotides. Each strand of DNA is a mirror image of each other since adenine must combine with thymine and cytosine must combine with guanine. Therefore since each strand of DNA is a mirror image of each other, one strand of DNA possesses the nucleotide sequence that codes for both strands; one strand represents the DNA code, while the second strand represents the mirror image of the first strand. In this manner, a quantum gene can be defined in its most elemental form as a sequence of nucleotides comprising a single strand of nucleotides.

[0088] A quantum gene could thus be represented as a single strand of nucleotides comprised of the nucleotides adenine, cytosine, guanine and thymine. The double stranded form of a quantum gene would be the single strand of nucleotides attached in parallel to a second strand of nucleotides that represents the mirror image of the single strand of nucleotides. Double stranded deoxyribonucleic acid segments is the form quantum genes take when a quantum gene is inserted into a cell's nuclear genome.

Conclusions, Ramification, and Scope

[0089] A 'quantum gene' is comprised of a sequence of nucleotides that represents a 'unique identifier' physically linked to a sequence of nucleotides that represent a discrete quantity of genetic information; these sequences of nucleotides being comprised of some combination of the nucleotides being referred to by their nitrogenous base as adenine (A), thymine (T), cytosine (C), and guanine (G). The genetic information associated with the above-mentioned unique identifier may be comprised of a portion of transcribable genetic information and a portion of nontranscribable genetic information which together define a specific gene, otherwise referred to as a discrete quantity of genetic information.

[0090] Accordingly, the reader will see that the concept and utilization of the quantum gene has never before been recognized nor appreciated by those skilled in the art.

[0091] Although the description above contains specificities, these should not be construed as limiting the scope of the invention but as merely providing illustrations of some of the presently preferred embodiments of the invention.

[0092] Thus the scope of the invention should be determined by the appended claims and their legal equivalents, rather than by the examples given.

CLAIMS: Reserved.